Pediatric PRIMARY CARE

Practice Guidelines for Nurses

SECOND EDITION

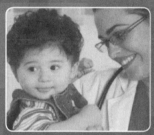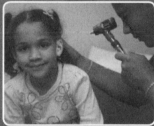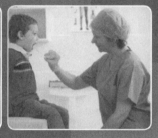

Edited by

Beth Richardson, PhD, RN, CPNP, FAANP

Professor Emeritus
School of Nursing
Indiana University
Pediatric Nurse Practitioner
HealthNet, Inc.
Indianapolis, Indiana

JONES & BARTLETT
LEARNING

D1543798

World Headquarters
Jones & Bartlett Learning
5 Wall Street
Burlington, MA 01803
978-443-5000
info@jblearning.com
www.jblearning.com

Jones & Bartlett Learning books and products are available through most bookstores and online booksellers. To contact Jones & Bartlett Learning directly, call 800-832-0034, fax 978-443-8000, or visit our website, www.jblearning.com.

Substantial discounts on bulk quantities of Jones & Bartlett Learning publications are available to corporations, professional associations, and other qualified organizations. For details and specific discount information, contact the special sales department at Jones & Bartlett Learning via the above contact information or send an email to specialsales@jblearning.com.

The authors, editor, and publisher have made every effort to provide accurate information. However, they are not responsible for errors, omissions, or for any outcomes related to the use of the contents of this book and take no responsibility for the use of the products and procedures described. Treatments and side effects described in this book may not be applicable to all people; likewise, some people may require a dose or experience a side effect that is not described herein. Drugs and medical devices are discussed that may have limited availability controlled by the Food and Drug Administration (FDA) for use only in a research study or clinical trial. Research, clinical practice, and government regulations often change the accepted standard in this field. When consideration is being given to use of any drug in the clinical setting, the health care provider or reader is responsible for determining FDA status of the drug, reading the package insert, and reviewing prescribing information for the most up-to-date recommendations on dose, precautions, and contraindications, and determining the appropriate usage for the product. This is especially important in the case of drugs that are new or seldom used.

Production Credits
Publisher: Kevin Sullivan
Acquisitions Editor: Amanda Harvey
Editorial Assistant: Sara Bempkins
Production Editor: Amanda Clerkin
Associate Marketing Manager: Katie Hennessy
Associate Photo Researcher: Lauren Miller
V.P., Manufacturing and Inventory Control: Therese Connell
Composition: Laserwords
Cover Design: Kristin E. Parker
Cover Images: © Rmarmion/Dreamstime.com, © Morgan Lane Photography/ShutterStock, Inc., © michaeljung/ShutterStock, Inc., © Sergii Teplov/Dreamstime.com
Printing and Binding: Malloy, Inc.
Cover Printing: Malloy, Inc.

Library of Congress Cataloging-in-Publication Data
Pediatric primary care: practice guidelines for nurses / [edited by] Beth Richardson.—2nd ed.
  p. ; cm.
  Rev. ed. of: Practice guidelines for pediatric nurse practitioners / [edited by] Beth Richardson.
  Includes bibliographical references and index.
  ISBN-13: 978-1-4496-0043-3
  ISBN-10: 1-4496-0043-3
  1. Pediatric nursing. I. Richardson, Beth, CPNP. II. Practice guidelines for pediatric nurse practitioners.
  [DNLM: 1. Pediatric Nursing—methods. 2. Primary Care Nursing. 3. Child. 4. Infant. 5. Nurse Practitioners. WY 159]
  RJ245.P73 2012
  618.92′00231—dc23
                                                                                                2011023318

6048
Printed in the United States of America
15 14 13 12 11   10 9 8 7 6 5 4 3 2 1

Contents

CHAPTER 31
Neurologic Disorders: Altered States of Consciousness   477
Kristin Miller

Preface

Pediatric Primary Care: Practice Guidelines for Nurses can be used as a resource for a variety of information including treatment strategies. It is divided into three sections. The first section includes taking a medical history with a family seen for the first time, taking an interval history, newborn rounding, and breastfeeding. Well-child visits are included along with information about nutrition, elimination, sleep patterns, growth and development, and injury prevention. The second section is organized by body system and is written in outline format, making it easy to read and find information quickly. Common medical conditions are presented with information about etiology, occurrence, clinical manifestations, physical findings, diagnostic tests, differential diagnosis, treatment, follow up, complications, and patient/family education. The third section (the Appendices) includes common medications used in pediatrics, and information is provided about common uses, availability, adverse effects, and nursing implications.

The Appendices provide several charts, including growth charts, BMI, asthma guidelines, and fluoride dosing. The charts are to be used to locate needed information quickly.

—BETH RICHARDSON

Acknowledgments

I would like to thank my children, Jason and Sarah; my grandchildren, Caroline and Darren; my friends; and all the students I've had the privilege of meeting. Thank you for teaching me.

To students, friends, and colleagues—thank you for all you do in caring for children.

Contributors

Mary J. Alvarado, MSN, RN, CPNP
Pediatric Nurse Practitioner
HealthNet, Inc.
Indianapolis, Indiana

Patricia Clinton, PhD, ARNP, PNP, FAANP
Clinical Professor & Assistant Dean for Graduate Programs
University of Iowa College of Nursing
Iowa City, Iowa

Karen M. Corlett, RN, CPNP-AC/PC
Pediatric Nurse Practitioner
Cardiac Intensive Care Unit
Children's Medical Hospital
Dallas, Texas

Mary Jo Eoff, MSN, RN, CPNP
Clinical Associate Professor
School of Nursing
Indiana University
Indianapolis, Indiana

Amy L. Feldman, MSN, RN, CPNP, IBCLC, CIMI
Nurse Consultant
Early Intervention
Shapiro Center for Infant Development
East Orange, New Jersey

Jane A. Fox, EdD, PNP-BC
Professor
School of Nursing
University of North Carolina Wilmington
Wilmington, North Carolina

Linda S. Gilman, EdD, RN, CPNP
Associate Professor Emeritus
School of Nursing
Indiana University
Pediatric Nurse Practitioner
HealthNet, Inc.
Indianapolis, Indiana

Donna Hallas, PhD, PNP-BC, CPNP, FAANP
Clinical Associate Professor
Director of PNP Program
College of Nursing
New York University
New York, New York

Betsy Atkinson Joyce, EdD, MSN, CPNP
Pediatric Nurse Practitioner
Northpoint Pediatrics
Associate Professor Emeritus
School of Nursing
Indiana University
Indianapolis, Indiana

Susan J. Kersey, PMHCNS-BC
Child/Adolescent/Mental Health Clinical Nurse Specialist
Wabash Valley Alliance
Lafayette, Indiana
Lecturer Purdue University School of Nursing
West Lafayette, Indiana

Shelly J. King, MSN, RN, CPNP
Pediatric Nurse Practitioner
Director of Children's Continence Center and Pediatric Urology
Riley Hospital for Children
Indianapolis, Indiana

Julie LaMothe, RN, MSN, CPNP, PNP
Riley POWER Clinic
Riley Hospital for Children
Indianapolis, Indiana

Marti Michel, MSN, CPNP, CNS, RN, AE-C
Pediatric Nurse Practitioner
Indiana University Health
Indianapolis, Indiana

Kristin Miller, MSN, RN, CPNP
Pediatric Nurse Practitioner
Pediatric Neurology
Peyton Manning Children's Hospital at St. Vincent Hospital
Indianapolis, Indiana

Meg Moorman, RNC, MSN, WHNP
Assistant Clinical Professor
School of Nursing
Indiana University
Indianapolis, Indiana

Pamela Meador Nickell, MSN, RN, CPNP
Pediatric RN Case Manager
IU Health Hospice
Indianapolis, Indiana

Miki M. Patterson, PhD, PNP, ONP
Director of Clinical Solutions
Stryker Performance Solutions
Assistant Professor Nursing
University of Massachusetts, Lowell
Lowell, Massachusetts

Frances K. Porcher, EdD, RN, CPNP
Pediatric Nurse Practitioner
Pediatric Emergency Department
Medical University of South Carolina
Charleston, South Carolina

Susan G. Rains, BSN, MA, CPNP
Pediatric Nurse Practitioner
HealthNet, Inc.
Indianapolis, Indiana

Beth Richardson, PhD, RN, CPNP, FAANP
Pediatric Nurse Practitioner
HealthNet, Inc.
Associate Professor Emeritus
Indiana University School of Nursing
Indianapolis, Indiana

Mary Lou C. Rosenblatt, MS, RN, CPNP
Senior Pediatric Nurse Practitioner
Harriet Lane Primary Care Center for Children and Adolescents
Johns Hopkins Hospital
Baltimore, Maryland

Robin Shannon, MS, RN, CPNP
Pediatric Nurse Practitioner
Pediatric Gastroenterology, Hepatology, and Nutrition
University of Minnesota Amplatz Children's Hospital
Minneapolis, Minnesota

Elizabeth Godfrey Terry, MSN, RN, CPNP
Health Editor
Children's Better Health Institute/US Kids Magazines
Indianapolis, Indiana

Peggy Vernon, RN, MA, CPNP
Dermatology Nurse Practitioner
Alta Vista Dermatology
Highlands Ranch, Colorado

Kim Walton, MSN, CNS
Director Youth Services
Community Health Network
Indianapolis, Indiana

Candace F. Zickler, MSN, RN, CPNP
Nurse Supervisor
MSD of Perry Township
Indianapolis, Indiana

SECTION ONE

Child Health Care

CHAPTER 1

Obtaining an Initial History

Beth Richardson

I. INTRODUCTION

    A. The complete health history taken at the first visit is an opportunity for the practitioner to establish a relationship with the child and family, gain insight into family relationships, and obtain pertinent health information.

II. INITIAL INFORMATION

    A. Parent(s).
        1. Name(s).
        2. Age(s).
        3. Health status.
    B. Sibling(s).
        1. Age(s).
        2. Health status.

III. REASON FOR CURRENT VISIT

    A. Current problem or illness.
        1. Background information.
            a. When did it start?
            b. What are the symptoms?
            c. Are others in family ill with similar symptoms?
            d. What has been done to treat symptoms?

IV. PAST HISTORY

A. Prenatal history and care if child younger than 5 years.
1. Was pregnancy planned?
2. Did the mother smoke? Drink alcohol? Take any medications or drugs?
3. Any problems such as:
   a. Vaginal infection?
   b. Kidney infection?
   c. High blood pressure?
   d. Diabetes?
   e. Edema?
   f. Bleeding?
   g. Any accidents during pregnancy?
B. Natal history and care.
1. Labor and delivery.
   a. Where was infant born?
   b. Type of delivery?
   c. Length of labor?
   d. Anesthesia used during labor?
   e. Any problems with mother or infant after birth?
   f. Infant's birth weight? Length? Head circumference? Gestational age?
   g. Did infant go home with the mother?
2. Feeding.
   a. Baby fed by bottle or breast?
   b. Type of formula used?
   c. Frequency of feedings?
   d. Pattern of weight gain?
3. Childhood illness.
   a. Rheumatic fever, chickenpox, number of ear infections, strep throat, respiratory syncytial virus (RSV), whooping cough, mononucleosis, sexually transmitted infections (STIs).
4. Hospitalizations.
   a. Dates, names of hospitals, diagnoses.
5. Surgeries.
   a. Dates, names of hospitals, diagnoses, complications.
6. Immunizations (see Appendix A).
   a. Dates, reactions.
7. Screening tests.
   a. Vision, hearing, speech, hemoglobin, urine, tuberculosis skin test, X-rays, other laboratory tests.

  8. Allergies.
    a. Medications, environment, foods.
  9. Transfusions.
    a. Dates, number of units transfused, reactions.
 10. Medications.
    a. Prescription; over the counter; herbal; current/recent medications including dosage, length of time taking medication, adverse reactions/ side effects.

V. REVIEW OF SYSTEMS

A. History.
  1. Head, eyes, ears, nose, throat.
    a. Head: Headaches or head injuries?
    b. Eyes: Tearing, strabismus? Has child had vision test? Does child wear glasses/contacts?
    c. Ears: Ear infections? Drainage? Has child had a hearing test?
    d. Nose: Allergies? Frequency of colds? Does child snore, have nose-bleeds, or postnasal drip?
    e. Throat: Sore throat, dental hygiene, lymph glands, hoarseness?
  2. Cardiovascular.
    a. Heart murmur.
    b. Congenital heart disease.
    c. Cyanosis.
    d. Edema.
    e. Activity tolerance, shortness of breath, syncope.
  3. Respiratory.
    a. Pneumonia, bronchitis.
    b. Asthma.
    c. Cystic fibrosis.
    d. Croup, cough.
  4. Gastrointestinal.
    a. Diarrhea, constipation.
    b. Vomiting, reflux, upset stomach, abdominal pain.
    c. Bloody stools, rectal bleeding.
    d. Fissures, ulcer.
    e. Jaundice.
  5. Genitourinary.
    a. When did child achieve night dryness?

      b. Frequency of urination, urinary tract infections, dysuria, polyuria.

      c. Hematuria.

      d. Menstrual history (pain, flow), vaginal drainage.

      e. Penis or testes abnormalities, STIs, sexual activity.

6. Musculoskeletal.

      a. Painful joints, swelling, strains, sprains, fractures.

      b. Deformities.

      c. Activity tolerance.

7. Neurologic.

      a. Headaches.

      b. Seizures, epilepsy.

      c. Fainting, dizziness, tremors.

      d. Clumsy, uncoordinated.

      e. ADD/ADHD, learning disability, developmental delay.

8. Endocrine.

      a. Sexual maturation.

      b. Diabetes.

      c. Thyroid or adrenal diseases.

9. Skin.

      a. Rashes, birth marks.

VI. FAMILY HISTORY

A. History of any of following in family members:

    1. High blood pressure.

    2. Heart disease, stroke.

    3. Diabetes.

    4. Cataracts, glaucoma.

    5. Anemia.

    6. High cholesterol levels.

    7. Asthma, allergies.

    8. Kidney infections.

    9. Colitis, ulcers.

   10. Cancer.

   11. Thyroid problems.

   12. Epilepsy.

   13. Dysplasia of hip.

14. Mental retardation.
15. Alcoholism or substance abuse.

VII. DISEASE HISTORY

A. Disease/problem.
   1. When was patient diagnosed?
   2. How was patient treated? Response to treatment?
   3. How have symptoms changed? How is patient doing now?
   4. Is patient taking medications to treat problem?

VIII. SOCIAL HISTORY

A. Parents'/guardians' employment site(s) and hours worked.
B. Child care.
   1. Daycare or sitter?
   2. Preschool or after-school programs?
C. Family relationships: How do family members get along?
D. Home life.
   1. Does home have a yard where child can play?
   2. Stairs in house?
   3. City, well, or bottled water?
   4. Is home in safe neighborhood?
E. School life.
   1. How is child's progress?
      a. What are child's grades?
      b. What are child's strengths and weaknesses in learning? Does child need extra help in learning?
      c. What type of classroom (advanced, regular, learning disability)?
   2. Behavior.
      a. Does this child bully others or is child a victim of bullying?
      b. What is child's behavior in learning situations?
      c. History of absenteeism or truancy?
   3. Classmates/friends.
      a. How does child relate to and play with those in classroom, daycare, or preschool?
      b. Does child have a best friend?
      c. What does child like to play?

IX. DEVELOPMENT

    A. For child younger than 2 years ask when first:
        1. Smiled.
        2. Rolled.
        3. Sat without assistance.
        4. Crawled.
        5. Walked without assistance.
        6. Said 2 words.
        7. Fed self.
        8. Said 10 words.
    B. Behavior.
        1. Temper tantrums, whining.
        2. Thumb sucking.
        3. Sleep patterns.
        4. Temperament.

BIBLIOGRAPHY

Bickley L. *Bates' Physical Examination and History Taking*. 10th ed. Philadelphia, Lippincott; 2008.
Duderstadt K. *Pediatric Physical Examination*. Philadelphia, Elsevier; 2006.

CHAPTER 2

Obtaining an Interval History

Donna Hallas

I. THE INTERVAL HISTORY

A. Definition.
 1. Interval history: data collection that occurs at subsequent visits to one in which comprehensive history and physical examination were completed.
 2. Amount of information reviewed and collected for interval history depends on child's age and length of time since either comprehensive history was obtained and/or prior appointments in which interval history was updated.
 3. General guideline for obtaining interval history: review and update data every 6 months for infants, toddlers, preschool-age children and every year for school-age children, adolescents.
B. Significance of interval history.
 1. Although comprehensive history is used to establish initial health promotion plan, analysis of data collected during interval history is often used in one of four ways:
  a. To continue established health promotion plan.
  b. To identify new healthcare problems.
  c. To make changes to health promotion plan based on new data.
  d. To establish new health promotion plan.
C. Preparation for obtaining interval history.
 1. Prior to beginning data collection for interval history, review comprehensive history and any prior interval histories available on medical record.
  a. Helps nurse practitioner focus questions that will elicit data needed to complete interval history.
  b. Sample data contained in comprehensive history that may need further exploration during interval history are listed in **Table 2-1**.

Table 2-1 Focusing the Interval History from Details in the Comprehensive History

Comprehensive history	Interval history
Past medical history	Any data in past medical history that is significant and requires further clarification.
	Consider previous acute illnesses including hospitalizations, injuries, accidents, surgeries, chronic illnesses.
	Review problem list.
	If all prior problems are listed as resolved, then no further data should be elicited at this visit.
	If problems still exist, then ask questions specific to identified problem.
Allergies	Always obtain update on allergies to foods, medications, environmental pollutants.
Developmental history	Review results of prior DDST or the Ages and Stages Questionnaires.
	Note achievement of developmental milestones at each interval visit.
	If delays are noted, question status of intervention services (early intervention for children 5 years old, OT, PT, speech, special education services for all children).
Social history	Exercise and activity.
	Wellness behaviors.
	Behavior issues at home or at school.
Family history	Review family structure and family support systems.
	If data contained in comprehensive history suggest dysfunctional family, ask about present family structure and function.
	Review genogram.
	Review significant family history prior to interview.
	Pay particular attention to strong family history of conditions in which family lifestyle modifications can have significant impact (e.g., cardiovascular conditions, hypertension, diabetes, obesity).

Table 2-1 (Continued)

Comprehensive history	Interval history
	Implementing lifestyle modifications in early childhood years may significantly affect health throughout lifetime.
Medication history	Prescription.
	Over the counter.
	Homeopathic remedies.
Nutritional history	Timing and frequency of meals.
	Ethnic and cultural considerations in food choices.
Immunization history	Immunization records should be reviewed at each visit.
Mental health	Assess mental health status for school age and adolescence at each interval visit.
	Anxiety and depression frequently occur in these populations.

D. Elements of an interval history.
   1. Elements included in interval history should be related to the age of the child.
   2. Major focus for interval history for each age child and adolescent should include questions concerning eating, sleeping, bladder and bowel patterns, and any unusual behaviors or changes in behaviors. Additional questions are then age related.
   3. Infant, toddler, and preschool-age children.
      a. Ask questions related to achievement of developmental milestones.
      b. Denver Developmental Screening Test (DDST) may be used as a guide for questioning patterns concerning achievement of developmental milestones.
      c. Toddlers and preschoolers: Assess information regarding speech and language development and development of social skills.
      d. Use the Surveillance and Screening Algorithm: Autistic Spectrum Disorders for toddlers at the 18, 21, and/or 24 month old episodic visit if it had not been completed at a maintenance health visit.

Table 2-2 Review of System (ROS) in an Interval History

System	ROS—gathering the interval history*
On a regular basis, do you have problems with:	
Head and neck	Headaches
	Blurred vision or any vision problems
	Earaches
	Nosebleeds
	Sore throats
	Difficulty swallowing
	Any lumps in head or neck area
Chest and lungs	Chest pain
	Heart beating fast in chest (palpitations)
	Shortness of breath
	Fainting
	Frequent cough
Abdomen	Nausea
	Vomiting
	Diarrhea
	Urinating or bowels
	Menstruation
	Testicular pain
Musculoskeletal	Leg pain or cramps
	Stiffness, swelling, bone deformities
Skin, hair, and nails	Rashes
	Moles
	Darkened or discolored areas
	Abnormal hair growth
	Clubbing of nails
	Bruising easily
Sexual history	History of sexually transmitted infections

*This information is gathered in addition to the details related to eating, sleeping, bladder, and bowel patterns.

4. School-age children.
   a. Should also include questions related to sociobehavioral development with peers and progress in school.
   b. If female school-age child has secondary sex characteristics, then ask about menstrual cycle: Age of onset, frequency, length of cycle, any discomfort prior to or during menstruations.
   c. Children older than 10 years of age should be asked: Have they or their friends tried alcohol or drugs? Use a brief alcohol/drug screening tool at each episodic visit.
      • What is their diet?
      • Happy with appearance/weight?
      • Thought about harming themselves or others?
      • Sexually active?
5. Adolescents.
   a. Use the HEADSSS assessment (home, education/employment, activity, drugs/alcohol, sexuality, suicide/depression, safety and exposure to violence).
   b. Adolescent female: Ask questions related to menstrual cycle.
   c. Ask about high-risk social behaviors (smoking; alcohol/drug use; sexual activity, including diagnosis and treatment of sexually transmitted infections [STIs]; driving motor vehicle in reckless manner; use of guns; etc.).
E. Review of systems (ROS).
1. Age-appropriate ROS: Conduct in head-to-toe manner as identified in comprehensive physical examination (**Table 2-2**).

II. INTERVAL HISTORY FOR ATHLETIC CHILD OR ADOLESCENT

A. Pre-participation sports history and physical have well-established guidelines; follow explicitly.
B. Interval history is integral part of assessment.
1. Question parent and child about significant family history changes (e.g., sudden death of relative who was 50 years old from cardiovascular condition). Include questions that elicit information about significant episodes (red flags) of chest pain, dyspnea, syncope, palpitations, loss of consciousness, history of concussions (**Table 2-3**).

Table 2-3 Red Flags: The Interval History for the Athletic Child or Adolescent

Interval history questions that may elicit red flag data	System	Red flag data
Any relatives < 50 years of age die as result of sudden unexpected cardiac death?	Cardiovascular	Change in family history
		Sudden death of relative < 50 years of age
Child report chest pain or palpitations, syncope during or after exercise?		Chief complaint from child:
		Chest pain
		Palpitations
		Syncope
Child report any breathing problems during or after exercise?	Respiratory	Chief complaint from child:
		Dyspnea
		Wheezing
Child had any episodes of dizziness, syncope, fainting, concussion?	Neurologic	Chief complaint from child:
		Syncope
		Loss of consciousness

III. FOCUSED HISTORY

    A. Focused history: Used to collect data about a specific problem, usually chief complaint identified by parent/child (**Tables 2-4** and **2-5**).

    B. Focus all questions on eliciting data about chief complaint.

    C. Focused history usually limited to one or two systems.

IV. APPLYING DATA OBTAINED IN INTERVAL HISTORY TO CLINICAL PRACTICE

    A. After completing interval history and physical examination, compare findings in comprehensive history to data obtained in interval history.

        1. If no significant changes found in interval history, advise parent, infant/child to continue to follow established health promotion plan.

Table 2-4 Sample Focused History: Medical

Subjective data	Questions to focus the history
"My child has a chronic cough."	What do you mean by a chronic cough?
"My child begins coughing each night. I cannot remember the last time he didn't cough at night."	Does child cough during day or just at night?
	What time of night does child begin coughing?
	Describe the cough.
	Is cough productive or nonproductive?
	Does cough affect child's sleeping pattern?
	Any products currently being used in household that weren't being used before child began having this "chronic" cough?
	Pets in your household?
	Did you change pillow your child uses?
	Use any over-the-counter or prescription medications to treat this cough?
	Has child been evaluated for asthma or allergies?
	Anything make cough better or worse?

Table 2-5 Sample Focused History: Mental Health

Subjective	Questions to focus the history
"My child's behavior has become so difficult at home."	Describe what you mean by "difficult behavior."
	Does anything trigger these behaviors?
	What do you do when this behavior becomes "so difficult?"
	What is your child's response?
	Does this behavior pattern occur at school or outside the home, such as at a friend's house or relative's home?
	Has there been a change in your family lifestyle—such as parents arguing at home, parental separation, new family member living in the home?
	Has there been any change in your child's physical abilities—such as change in cognitive or psychomotor skills?
	Does your child complain of headaches?

2. If significant changes are found in interval history, revise health promotion plan.
    a. Example: If interval family history reveals family members have diabetes mellitus, evaluate and modify family/child exercise and dietary patterns.
3. If significant changes are found in interval history in relation to child's health, establish new health promotion plan with parent and child/adolescent active participation.
    a. Example: If interval history reveals significant change in frequency of coughing and upper respiratory symptoms, complete a detailed focused history and establish a new health promotion plan.

BIBLIOGRAPHY

Bickley LS, Hoekelman RA. *Bates' Guide to Physical Assessment*. 10th ed. Philadelphia, PA: Lippincott; 2008.

Burns CE, Dunn AM, Brady MA, et al. *Pediatric Primary Care*. 4th ed. St. Louis, MO: Saunders; 2009.

Duderstadt KG. *Pediatric Physical Examination: An Illustrated Handbook*. St. Louis, MO: Mosby; 2006.

Johnson CP, Myers SA, and the Council on Children with Disabilities. Identification and evaluation of children with autistic spectrum disorders. *Pediatrics*. 2007;120:1183-1215. American Academy of Pediatrics website: http://www.aap.org/pressroom/AutismID.pdf. Accessed June 1, 2011.

CHAPTER 3

Performing a Physical Examination

Mary Jo Eoff

I. INTRODUCTION

A. Pediatric physical assessment is a continual process that includes interviews, inspection, observation of children.

B. Physical growth, motor skills, cognitive, and social development change as the child matures.

C. The assessment of the pediatric patient must include what is considered to be normal within the child's age limits.

D. Children will differ among themselves at various stages of development.

E. The following is an outline that can be used as a guide in doing a comprehensive physical assessment.

II. PEDIATRIC PHYSICAL EXAMINATION

A. Growth measurements.
   1. Length/height.
      a. Recumbent (2 years).
      b. Standing height.
   2. Weight.
   3. Head circumference (occipital frontal circumference [OFC]).
   4. Chest circumference (up to 1 year).
   5. Skinfold thickness.
B. Vital signs.
   1. Temperature, heart rate, respirations, blood pressure.
C. General appearance.
   1. Cleanliness, posture, hygiene.
   2. Nutrition.

       3. Behavior, ability to cooperate.

       4. Development.

       5. Alertness.

D. Skin.

       1. Color: pallor, cyanosis, erythema, ecchymosis, petechiae, jaundice.

       2. Texture.

       3. Temperature.

       4. Turgor.

       5. Describe size, shape, and location of rashes, eruptions, and lesions.

       6. Sweating.

E. Hair: color, texture, quantity, distribution, infestations (nits).

F. Nails.

       1. Inspect color, texture, quality, distribution, hygiene.

       2. Observe for nail biting.

G. Hands and feet.

       1. Observe flexion crease on palm.

       2. Assess for foot and ankle deformities.

H. Lymph nodes.

       1. Palpate for nodes in following areas:

          a. Submaxillary.

          b. Cervical.

          c. Axillary.

          d. Inguinal.

       2. Note size, mobility, or tenderness of any enlarged node.

I. Head.

       1. Assess shape and symmetry.

       2. Assess head control; should be well established by 6 months of age.

       3. Palpate skull.

          a. Fontanels (2 years of age).

          b. Suture ridges and grooves (up to 6 months of age).

          c. Nodes.

          d. Any swelling.

       4. Examine scalp for hygiene, lesions, signs of trauma, loss of hair, or discoloration.

       5. Percuss frontal sinuses (children 7 years of age).

J. Neck.

       1. Palpate trachea for deviation.

       2. Palpate thyroid, noting size, shape, symmetry, tenderness, or nodules.

       3. Palpate carotid arteries.

       4. Palpate neck structure.

       a. Pain or tenderness.

       b. Enlargement of parotid gland.

       c. Web like tissue.

K. Eyes.
1. Check peripheral vision.
2. Check visual acuity.
   a. Snellen E chart.
   b. Allen test.
3. Note whether eyelashes curl away from eye.
4. Note whether eyebrows are above eye and do not meet at midline.
5. Test for any strabismus.
   a. Hirschberg test.
   b. Cover–uncover test.
6. Observe for nystagmus or ptosis.
7. Inspect conjunctiva for drainage, redness, swelling, pain.
8. Inspect sclera, cornea, iris.
9. Check: pupils equal, round, react to light.
10. Examine with ophthalmoscope.
    a. Optic disk, macula, arteriole/vein, fovea centralis, red reflex.
11. Inspect lachrymal ducts: tears, drainage.
12. Inspect placement, alignment of outer eye: palpebral slant, epicanthus, lids.

L. Ears.
1. Inspect placement and alignment of pinna.
2. Inspect auditory canal: color, cerumen, patency.
3. Observe for skin tags and hygiene.
4. Examine middle ear with otoscope.
   a. Color of tympanic membrane, light reflex, bony landmarks.
5. Check hearing.
   a. Rinne test.
   b. Weber test.

M. Nose.
1. Observe mucosal lining for color, discharge, patency.
2. Observe color of the turbinates and meatus.
3. Note if septum is midline.

N. Mouth and throat.
1. Observe internal structures.
   a. Hard and soft palate, palatoglossal arch, palatine tonsil, tongue, oro-pharynx, palatopharyngeal arch, uvula.
2. Palpate ethmoid, frontal, and maxillary sinuses.
3. Observe lip edges.

    4. Observe eruption of teeth.
       a. Number appropriate for age.
       b. Color and hygiene.
       c. Occlusion of upper and lower jaw.
    5. Check salivation.
    6. Check drooling.
    7. Check swallowing reflex.
    8. Note color, texture, or any lesions of the lips.
    9. Observe gingiva and mucous membranes for color, texture, moistness.
O. Tongue.
    1. Observe for smoothness, fissuring, coating, or redness.
    2. Tongue able to extend forward to lips?
    3. Tongue interfere with speech?
P. Chest.
    1. Observe shape of thorax.
    2. Check costal angles; should be between 45 and 50°.
    3. Check that points of attachments between ribs and costal cartilage are smooth.
    4. Check movement.
       a. Inspiration: chest expands, costal angle increases, diaphragm descends.
       b. Expiration: reverse occurs.
Q. Lungs.
    1. Evaluate respiratory movement: rate, rhythm, depth, quality, character.
    2. Auscultate breath sounds.
       a. Vesicular breath sounds.
       b. Bronchovesicular breath sounds.
       c. Bronchial breath sounds.
    3. Note adventitious breath sounds.
       a. Crackles, wheezes, stridor, pleural friction rub.
    4. Check for cough.
       a. Productive/nonproductive.
       b. Color of secretions.
    5. Check retractions.
    6. Check abdominal breathing.
    7. Check thoracic expansion.
    8. Palpate tactile fremitus.
R. Heart.
    1. Auscultate heart sounds.
       a. Aortic area, pulmonic area, Erb's point, tricuspid area, mitral or apical area.

    2. Check S1–S2.

    3. Palpate for thrill.

    4. Record murmurs.

        a. Area best heard.

        b. Timing within S1–S2 cycle.

        c. Change with position.

        d. Loudness and quality.

        e. Grade intensity of murmur.

S. Vascular.

    1. Assess capillary refill; should occur in 1–2 seconds.

    2. Assess circulation.

        a. Color and texture of skin.

        b. Nail and hair distribution.

    3. Assess perfusion.

        a. Edema.

        b. Pulses (4–0).

    4. Assess collateral circulation.

T. Abdomen.

    1. Inspect contour and size of abdomen.

    2. Note condition of skin.

    3. Inspect umbilicus for hernias, fistula, discharge.

    4. Auscultate bowel sounds.

    5. Auscultate for any aortic pulsations.

    6. Percuss abdomen.

    7. Palpate outer edge of liver.

    8. Palpate spleen.

    9. Elicit abdominal reflux.

   10. Palpate femoral pulses.

U. Neurologic.

    1. Observe behavior, mood, affect, interaction with environment, level of activity, positioning, level of consciousness, orientation to surroundings.

    2. Check reflexes of the infant.

        a. Rooting (present birth to 6 months of age).

        b. Sucking (present birth to 10 months of age).

        c. Palmer grasp (present birth to 4 months of age).

        d. Tonic neck (present at 6–8 weeks of age and lasts until 6 months).

        e. Stepping (present birth to 3 months of age).

        f. Plantar grasp (present birth to 8 months of age).

        g. Moro (present birth to 4–6 months of age).

      h. Babinski (child 15–18 months of age normally fans toes outward and dorsiflexes greater toe).

      i. Galant (present birth to 1–2 months of age).

      j. Placing (lack of response is abnormal).

      k. Landau (present 3 months to 2 years of age).

   3. Test cranial nerves.

      a. I: Olfactory.

      b. II: Optic.

      c. III: Oculomotor.

      d. IV: Trochlear.

      e. V: Trigeminal.

      f. VI: Abducens.

      g. VII: Facial.

      h. VIII: Acoustic.

      i. IX: Glossopharyngeal.

      j. X: Vagus.

      k. XI: Spinal accessory.

      l. XII: Hypoglossal.

   4. Test cerebellar functioning: finger-to-nose test, heel-to-shin test, Romberg.

   5. Test deep tendon reflexes (grading 4–0): biceps, triceps, brachioradialis, patellar, Achilles.

   6. Check sensory functioning: pain, temperature, touch.

V. Musculoskeletal.

   1. Inspect curvature and symmetry of spine.

   2. Test for scoliosis.

   3. Inspect all joints for size, temperature, color, tenderness, mobility.

   4. Test for developmental dysplasia of the hips (DDH).

      a. Ortolani maneuver (evaluate up to 12 months of age).

      b. Barlow's maneuver.

      c. Trendelenburg's test (used after child is walking).

   5. Examine tibiofemoral bones: knock knee, bow legs.

   6. Inspect gait: waddling gait (DDH), scissor (cerebral palsy [CP]), toeing-in.

   7. Note flexibility and range of motion of joints.

   8. Elicit planter reflex.

   9. Test motor strength of arms, legs, hands, feet (grading 4–0).

W. Breast.

   1. Pigmentation.

  2. Location.

  3. Tanner stages (sexual maturity rating).

X. Genitalia.

  1. Male.

    a. Inspect size of penis.

    b. Inspect glands and shaft for swelling, skin lesions, inflammation.

    c. Inspect uncircumcised male: prepuce.

    d. Inspect location of urethral meatus, note any discharge.

    e. Inspect scrotum for size, location, skin, and hair distribution.

    f. Palpate each scrotal sac for testes.

    g. Tanner stages (sexual maturing rating).

  2. Female.

    a. Palpate genitalia for any masses, cysts.

    b. Observe for any venereal warts.

    c. Inspect for location of urethral meatus, Skene glands, mons pubis, Bartholin gland, clitoris, labia majora, labia minora.

    d. Note any discharge: color and odor.

    e. Tanner stages (sexual maturity rating).

Y. Anus.

  1. Inspect anal area for firmness and condition of skin.

  2. Elicit anal reflex.

BIBLIOGRAPHY

Bickley L. *Bates' Physical Examination and History Taking.* 10th ed. Philadelphia, PA: Lippincott; 2008.
Duderstadt K. *Pediatric Physical Examination.* Philadelphia, PA: Elsevier; 2006.

CHAPTER 4

Making Newborn Rounds

Candace F. Zickler

Asthma, 493.9	Jaundice, 774.6
Breathing difficulties, 786.09	Meconium stools, 777.1
Café au lait spots, 709.09	Nares patent (choanal atresia), 748
Coarctation of aorta, 747.1	Neck short/masses (cystic hygroma),
Cyanosis, 770.83	228.1
Cytomegalovirus (CMV), 078.5	No urine in 12 hours, 788.2
Decreased bowel movements, 564	Pallor, 782.61
Epispadius, 752.62	Petechiae, 772.6
Gestational diabetes (GD), 648.8	Poor feeding, 779.3
Gonorrhea, 098	Port wine stain, 757.32
Group B streptococcus, 041.02	Pregnancy-induced hypertension
Heart rate with murmur, 785.2	(PIH), 642.9
Hemangioma, 228.01	Rash or pustules, 782.1
Hematoma/caput succedaneum, 767.19	Rubella, 056.9
Herpes simplex virus (HSV), 054.9	Seizures, 779
Human immunodeficiency virus (HIV),	Sickle cell disease, 282.6
042	Spontaneous abortions, 634.9
Hypoglossia/macroglossia, 529.8	Stillbirths/perinatal deaths, 779.9
Hypospadias, 752.6	Supernumerary nipples, 757.6
Infant galactosemia, 271.1	Toxoplasmosis, 130.9
Infertility, 628.9	Umbilicus with hernia, 553.1
Irritability, 799.2	Vomiting, 787.03

I. MAKING NEWBORN ROUNDS

    A. Determine number of newborns delivered in last 24 hours.
    B. Prioritize assessments by birth time and concerns of nurses.
    C. Evaluate each infant within 12–24 hours of age and daily until discharge.

II. REVIEW OF THE INDIVIDUAL RECORDS

    A. Mother.
        1. Past obstetric history: infertility, spontaneous abortions, stillbirths/perinatal deaths, parity, gravity, length of pregnancy, congenital anomalies in other infants, assistive reproductive technology (ART) used, isoimmune disease (Rh, ABO), pregnancy-induced hypertension (PIH), Cesarean births, vaginal birth after Cesarean, gestational diabetes. Current pregnancy history: maternal age, overall health (asthma, sickle cell disease), estimated date of confinement (EDC), prenatal care, number of previous pregnancies, multiple or single fetus, presentation/position of fetus, amount of amniotic fluid, fetal growth/size (small, appropriate, or large for gestational age), nationality, public assistance.
        2. Results of prenatal lab work: blood type; rubella IgG level; hepatitis B immunization status; serologic tests; HIV status (elective); gonorrhea and chlamydia cultures; maternal alpha fetal protein; urinalysis (bacteria, blood, protein); glucose screen; exposure to drugs, alcohol, tobacco, or teratogenic medications (valproate, tetracycline); exposure to viruses (TORCH: toxoplasmosis, rubella, cytomegalovirus, herpes simplex virus); sexually transmitted infections; Group B streptococcus status.
    B. Newborn.
        1. Prenatal history: vaginal or Cesarean delivery; length of labor and delivery; tocolytics used during labor; narcotics, anesthesia, or analgesics mother received; presentation; placental abnormalities (three-vessel cord); amniotic fluid color/volume; Apgar scores (heart rate, respirations, muscle tone, reflex irritability, color) with 5-minute Apgar > 7.
        2. Since birth: delivery weight/length/occipital frontal circumference (OFC), temperature, blood pressure, pulse, respirations, feeding/nursing with breast or bottle, voiding spontaneously, passage of meconium, infant contact with mother/parents.

III. PHYSICAL ASSESSMENT OF THE NEWBORN

A. General appearance.
1. Current weight, length, OFC, color, heart rate, respirations, temperature, blood glucose at birth, response to stimuli, posture, determination of gestational age from the New Ballard Score (physical maturity and neuromuscular maturity).
B. Full-term infant > 37 weeks but < 42 weeks, premature infant < 37 weeks, late preterm infant > 34 weeks to 36 weeks and 6 days, post-term infant > 42 weeks.
C. Late preterm infants at greater risk for airway instability when upright, respiratory distress, apnea/bradycardia, excessive sleepiness, excessive weight loss, poor feeding, hyperbilirubinemia, hypoglycemia, hypothermia, sepsis, weak suck, and rehospitalization.

IV. ABNORMAL PHYSICAL FINDINGS (CONSULT WITH STAFF PHYSICIAN AND/OR REFER FOR EVALUATION, AS INDICATED)

A. Dysmorphic facies hyper- or hypotelorism, epicanthal folds, symmetrical facies and extremities.
1. Skin and scalp with plethora, pallor, jaundice, cyanosis, bruising, abrasions, petechiae, hemangioma, port wine stain, café au lait spots.
2. Shape of skull.
3. Bruising, hematoma/caput succedaneum.
4. Size and tone of anterior and posterior fontanels.
B. Pupils without red reflex and unequal pupillary sizes, nares patent (choanal atresia), mouth with teeth, hypoglossia/macroglossia, palate high arched or missing. External ears with tags or pinhole openings. Neck short/masses (cystic hygroma) or webbing.
C. More/less than five fingers/toes on each hand/foot.
D. Check clavicles for fractures. Chest shape with pectus excavatum/carinatum, and supernumerary nipples. Breath sounds that are moist and grunting/retractions after 4 hours of age, apnea/respirations < 30 or > 60 per minute.
E. Heart rate with murmur (soft III/IV systolic murmur normal for first 12–24 hours since patent ductus may not be closed), or an irregular rate/rhythm < 100 or > 180 bpm, a cuff blood pressure < 65 or > 95 mm Hg of systolic

pressure, and diastolic < 30 or > 60 mm Hg. Absent or decreased femoral pulses (coarctation of aorta), slow capillary refill is indicative of poor perfusion.

F. Temperature instability < 97.7°F (36.5°C) after 4 hours of age.

G. Abdominal skin thin or missing, asymmetrical, distended, umbilicus with hernia, discharge, redness, odor. Missing or overactive bowel sounds. Lower liver edge 3 cm below costal margin (heart disease), infection, hemolysis, palpable spleen (infection or hemopoiesis), enlarged bladder (1–4 cm above symphysis).

H. Female.

   1. Masses in labia (hernia, enlarged Bartholin gland), vesicles.

I. Male.

   1. Meatal opening on penis placed abnormally (hypospadias or epispadius), absence of testes in either inguinal canals or scrotal sac, hydrocele, bifid scrotum, discoloration, or bruising.

J. Anus absent or not patent.

K. Absent or missing extremities, bands, masses, inequality from side to side. Abnormal Ortolani or Barlow sign. Bowing of extremities, abnormal foot positions, flaccid upper extremity. Lesions or dimpling of lower spine.

L. Abnormal posturing, floppy or very jittery, abnormal cry. Exaggerated tonic neck, Moro reflex, poor sucking, or poor rooting.

V. LABORATORY ASSESSMENT OF NEWBORN

A. Glucose screening (normal 40–90 mg/dL), venous hematocrit (normal 45–65%), cord blood (ABO, Rh). If baby is Rh–, maternal RhoGAM status should be Rh+.

B. Bilirubin: Determine etiology of any jaundice, i.e., physiologic or pathologic. Obtain baseline total serum bilirubin, plus a direct and indirect level.

Sixty percent of all term newborns and 80% of preterm infants will have some jaundice in the first week of life.

Any jaundice within the first 24 hours after birth is considered pathologic. If the total serum bilirubin (TSB) rises more than 5 mg/dL/day or is higher than 12 mg/dL in full-term infants or 10–14 mg/dL for preterm, further evaluation and treatment is indicated. If the infant has signs of sepsis, irritability, or lethargy, this needs further evaluation. In infants 25–48 hours old, a TSB level above 15 mg/dL is indicative of rapid rise and infant needs further evaluation. In infants 49–72 hours old a TSB above 18 mg/dL or any infants more than 72 hours old with a TcB of 20 mg/dL needs further evaluation and treatment.[7]

When obtaining serial bilirubins, utilize noninvasive transcutaneous (TcB) bilirubinometer and nomogram.
C. Newborn hearing screening. To be done no later than 1 month of age. Most hospitals offer this screening for newborns prior to discharge. Risk factors for infants include family history of sensorineural hearing loss, in utero infections (TORCH), craniofacial anomalies, hyperbilirubinemia, post natal bacterial meningitis, findings indicative of a syndrome with hearing loss, neurodegenerative disorders, sensory motor neuropathies, parental concerns for hearing, head trauma, and recurrent/persistent otitis media. If infant fails the hearing screening, an audiologic evaluation needs to be done as follow up by 3 months of age.

VI. MEETING WITH THE PARENT

A. Introduce self, sit by bedside. Describe your role. Answer parent's questions, describe the general process of how you will be working with them over the next day or so.
B. Praise parents, compliment baby.
C. Call baby by name.
D. Determine mother's health/wellness/contact with infant so far.
E. Review your findings, briefly.
F. If male, determine if baby is to be circumcised. Discuss pros and cons.
G. Ask about method of feeding, car seat, help when home, concerns.

VII. NUTRITION

A. Breastfeeding is encouraged for all newborns (see Chapter 5). Late preterm infants may not be as vigorous an eater as expected and may need close monitoring of weight. Obtain a breastfeeding consult and encourage nursing every 2 hours around the clock until infant is nursing at least 20 minutes during feedings.
   1. No breastfeeding if HIV infected, active herpes of breast, untreated tuberculosis, maternal debilitating disease (cancer), illicit drug use by mother, infant galactosemia.
B. If bottle-feeding, reassure that baby will grow and thrive on formula.
   1. Only commercially prepared, iron-fortified formulas should be used: powder, concentrate, ready-to-feed. Do not dilute ready-to-feed; do not reuse if > 4 hours since opened.
   2. Mix formulas with bottled water for first month, continue if on well or unsure of water quality. Store in refrigerator if open no longer than 24 hours.

      3. Specialized formulas have similar preparation directions. Goat's milk, whole cow's milk, rice milk have inadequate amounts of vitamins and minerals.

      4. Serve formula at room temperature. Do not microwave to heat. Do not let formula sit out at room temperature to warm for more than 15–20 minutes.

C. Clean technique is sufficient for mixing formulas. Clean off cans with soap and water before opening. Use hot soapy water and bottlebrush to clean nipples and bottles or clean in dishwasher.

D. Hold during feedings; burp every 1–2 oz.

E. Hold in upright, semi-reclined position for feedings. No bottle propping.

F. Newborn will suckle 0.5–1 oz of formula/feeding every 2–3 hours for first 24 hours (60–100 mL/kg/day). Volume increases to 12–24 oz/day and interval between feedings > 3–4 hours in first month. May be days when baby takes more or less, depending on sleep pattern. Baby should take in 90% of feeding in first 20 minutes.

VIII. ELIMINATION

A. Meconium stools in first 48 hours, transition stools green-brown, change to yellow pasty after 2–3 days of oral feeding.

B. Infant should have 1–6 yellow pasty stools for 24 hours.

C. Breastfed baby may have upper range of frequency, bottle-fed may have less.

D. Void every 1–3 hours or with each feeding and diaper change.

IX. SLEEP

A. Awake for feedings; feed every 2–4 hours. Should be alert, nurse vigorously for 15–20 minutes, then fall back to sleep. Respirations may be slightly irregular.

B. Babies should sleep on back in their crib. No pillows/toys in the crib that baby could get face against and be smothered.

C. Babies should sleep in own cribs, not with parents, to minimize potential for rollovers, suffocation, and falls.

X. GROWTH AND DEVELOPMENT

A. Newborn can lose up to 10% of body weight in first 10 days of life. Should regain birth weight by 2 weeks of age.

B. Infant grows 1 in., on average, per month for first 6 months.
C. Head circumference increases 9 cm in first year.
D. Has minimal head control.
E. Looks at person during feeding.
F. Tracks 45°.

XI. SOCIAL DEVELOPMENT

A. Babies have different cries, will fuss/cry 1 to 2 hours/day.
  1. Similar time/pattern daily.
  2. Provide for infant's needs and crying should cease.
  3. Cry gradually decreases by 3 months of age.
B. Refer all high-risk infants/mothers to social worker before release. High-risk situations include:
  1. Adolescent pregnancy.
  2. No prenatal care.
  3. Consideration about giving up the baby for adoption.
  4. Unwanted pregnancy.
  5. Insufficient support from those at home.
  6. Physical limitations of parent.
  7. Inadequate housing/finances.
  8. Domestic violence.
  9. Positive toxicology.
  10. Incarcerated parent.
  11. Emotional disorders.
  12. Parent with mental retardation.
  13. Multiple small children in home.

XII. IMMUNIZATIONS (SEE APPENDIX A)

A. Only monovalent hepatitis B can be used for birth dose. If mother is hepatitis B surface antigen (HBsAg) positive, administer hepatitis B vaccine and 0.5 mL of hepatitis B immune globulin (HBIG) within 12 hours of birth. If mother's HBsAg status is unknown, administer hepatitis B vaccine within 12 hours of birth and determine mother's HBsAg status as soon as possible. If she is then positive, the newborn should receive HBIG within 1 week of life. Monovalent hepatitis B should be given if second dose is given less than 6 weeks of age. Monovalent or combination vaccine can be used to complete series.

XIII. SAFETY/ANTICIPATORY GUIDANCE

A. Sleep position "back to sleep."
B. Not safe for baby to sleep in adult bed; must discuss with parents.
C. Use federal motor vehicle safety standards (FMVSS) tested and approved car seat; install properly in backseat, facing backward in automobile. Contact local hospital, fire department, or March of Dimes chapter for car seat rental program. Infants should ride in the rear-facing position in either an infant seat or a convertible car seat until they are at least 1 year of age and 20 lbs.
D. No smoking around infant.
E. One-piece pacifiers only.
F. No corn syrup (Karo) for constipation, but may give 1 oz of sterile water/ 24 hours.
G. No solids, only breastmilk or formula fed to infant.
H. When to call healthcare provider.
　　1. Breathing difficulties—too fast or too slow or color changes; seizures; irritability; poor feeding; vomiting; no urine in 12 hours; black or decreased bowel movements; reddened, draining umbilical site; jaundice; rash or pustules not present on discharge; concerns.
I. Give office phone number, explain how to use system.

XIV. DISCHARGE TO HOME

A. Review all records/progress.
B. Repeat complete physical examination.
C. Identify abnormal findings that require ongoing monitoring.
D. Review hearing screening results and if not done, schedule before discharge.
E. Collect newborn blood screen.
F. Administer hepatitis B immunization.
G. Complete all consults.
H. Staff nurses will have covered discharge instructions of bathing, cord care, bulb syringe, diapering, dressing, fingernail care, holding, feeding.
I. If concerns, infants should be scheduled for office visit within two days, otherwise parents need a two-week follow-up appointment assigned before discharge. Make them comfortable knowing they can call with any concerns.

BIBLIOGRAPHY

Ballard JL, Khoury JC, Wedeg K, et al. New Ballard Score expanded to Include extremely premature infants. *Pediatrics.* 1991;119:417-423.

Fouzas S, Mantagou L, Skylogianni SM, et al. (2009). Transcutaneous bilirubin levels for the first 120 postnatal hours in healthy neonates. *Pediatrics.* 2009;125(1):e52-e57. Retrieved from American Academy of Pediatrics website: http://www.pediatrics.org/cgi/content/full/125/1/e52. Accessed June 2, 2011.

Car Safety Seats: A Guide For Families 2010. American Academy of Pediatrics Healthy Children website: http://www.healthychildren.org/English/safety-prevention/on-the-go/pages/Car-Safety-Seats-Information-for-Famiies-2010.aspx. Accessed June 2, 2011.

DeMichele AM, Ruth RA. Newborn Hearing Screening. Medscape Reference; 2010: http://emedicine.medscape.com/article/836646. Accessed June 2, 2011.

Hagan JF, Shaw JS, Duncan P, eds. *Bright Futures Guidelines for Health Supervision of Infants, Children, and Adolescents.* 3rd ed. American Academy of Pediatrics; 2008: http://brightfutures.aap.org/3rd_Edition_Guidelines_and_Pocket_Guide.html. Accessed June 2, 2011.

Porter ML, Dennis BL. Hyperbilirubinemia in the term newborn. *Am Family Physician.* 2002;65(4):599-607. American Academy of Family Physicians website: http://www.aafp.org/afp/2002/0215/p599.html. Accessed June 2, 2011.

Recommended Immunization Schedule for Persons Aged 0 through 6 Years—United States 2010. Centers for Disease Control and Prevention website: http://www.cdc.gov/vaccines/recs/acip. Accessed June 2, 2011.

Thureen PJ, Hall D, Deacon J, et al. Obstetric considerations in the management of the well newborn. In: *Assessment and Care of the Well Newborn.* 2nd ed. Philadelphia: W.B. Saunders; 2005:3-20.

Wolf A, Hubbard E, Stellwagen LM. The late preterm infant: A little baby with big needs. *Contemporary Pediatrics.* 2007;24(11):51-59.

CHAPTER 5

Guidelines for Breastfeeding

Amy L. Feldman

Candida albicans, 112.9	Pathologic jaundice, 774.6
Engorgement, 611.79	*Staphylococcus aureus,* 041.11
Galactosemia, 271.1	Thrush, 771.7
Jaundice, 782.4	Weight gain, 783.1
Mastitis, 611	

I. INTRODUCTION

A. Breastfeeding provides optimal nutrition for newborns and infants, protecting against many diseases and infections and improving maternal and infant health. Exclusive breastfeeding is recommended for the first 6 months of life, with continued breastfeeding throughout the first year and beyond with the addition of appropriate complementary foods.

II. PHYSIOLOGY OF LACTATION

A. Mammary glands are complex organs that function independently in response to an intricate combination of hormones and stimulation to produce milk. After expulsion of the placenta following delivery, a significant drop in progesterone readies the body for milk production (**Figure 5-1**).

B. Oxytocin and prolactin are two of many important hormones in controlling lactation.

C. Optimal milk production depends on several factors including release of lactation hormones, frequent, effective milk removal, and adequate breast stimulation.

D. Full lactation can be produced by breasts from 16 weeks of pregnancy forward.

Figure 5-1 Physiology of lactation.

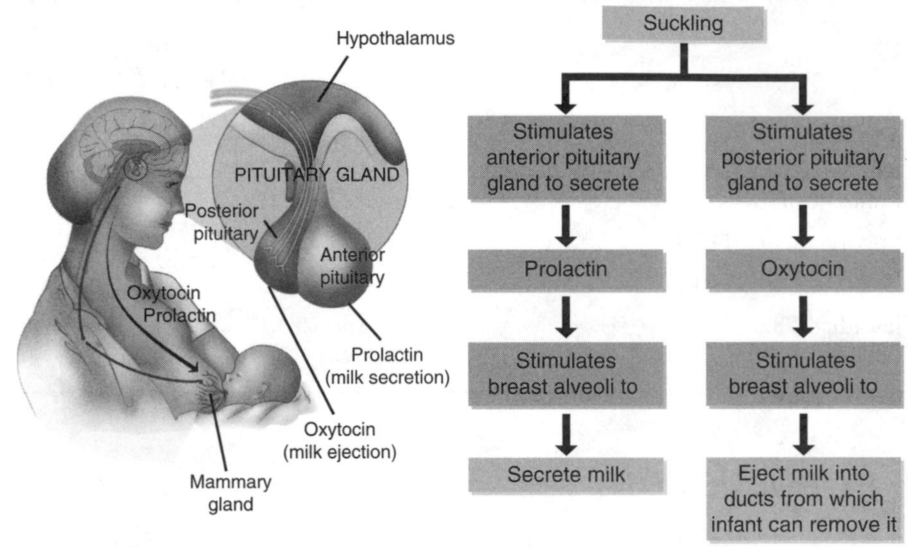

Source: Thibodeau GA, Patton KT. *Anatomy and Physiology.* 5th ed. St Louis: Mosby; 2003.

E. Important to understand balance of supply and demand to optimize lactation.
F. Lactation begins as a result of hormonal control (endocrine) but changes to autocrine (frequent emptying of breasts) over time.

III. HUMAN MILK

A. Human milk is exceptional in its ability to sustain appropriate growth and development for infants.
B. "Liquid gold," as human milk is often referred to, is living tissue, which encompasses fats, proteins, carbohydrates, antibodies, and hundreds of components.
C. Composition of human milk changes to provide optimal nutrition as infant grows.
    1. Colostrum, the first milk, is produced during pregnancy and is considered the infant's first immunization, providing protection to the newborn from viruses and bacteria.
    2. Transitional milk is produced after colostrum, then mature milk as lactogenesis stage II (production of large quantities of milk) begins.

IV. CONTRAINDICATIONS FOR BREASTFEEDING

A. Occasionally there are circumstances that preclude mothers from breastfeeding.
   1. Maternal contraindications include:
      a. HIV positive mother (in the United States).
      b. Maternal drug abuse.
      c. Maternal chemotherapy.
      d. Herpetic lesions on mother's nipple, areola.
      e. Untreated, active tuberculosis.
      f. Certain radioactive compounds and other medications may require temporary cessation of breastfeeding.
      g. Positive HTLV-I and HTLV-II (human T-cell lymphotropic virus).
   2. Infant contraindications include:
      a. Galactosemia.

V. MATERNAL ASSESSMENT

A. Breastfeeding goals and family support.
B. Previous breastfeeding experience.
C. General health and nutritional status.
D. Breast, nipple, or thoracic surgery.
E. Medications, prescriptions, supplements, and OTC.
F. Pregnancy, labor, birth history.
G. Inverted or flat nipples.

VI. INFANT ASSESSMENT

A. General health, including gestational age.
B. Congenital circumstances.
C. Birth history.
D. Medications received and procedures experienced.
E. Initial feeding attempts.
F. Oral facial assessment.

VII. BREASTFEEDING IN THE EARLY DAYS

A. Initial feedings.
   1. Facilitate skin-to-skin contact immediately after birth and as often as possible.

2. Encourage breastfeeding within first hour after birth during quiet alert phase. Do not restrict length or frequency of feedings.
3. Promote rooming in 24 hours a day.
4. Encourage exclusive breastfeeding; this helps to establish and maintain a sufficient milk supply.
5. Instruct parents in correct latch-on techniques.
6. Educate parents regarding initial feedings of colostrum: quantity is very small, but sufficient nutrition as baby is learning to breastfeed.
7. Discourage use of any supplements unless medically indicated.
8. Avoid use of bottles and pacifiers until breastfeeding is well established.
9. Teach parents to breastfeed in response to infant feeding cues (rooting, increased alertness, fists in mouth), at least 8–12 times/day. Crying is a late sign of hunger.
10. Baby should finish feeding on one breast, then be offered second if he/she will take more. Fat content of milk is higher at end of feeding than at beginning. Forcing baby to switch breasts too soon may decrease amount of higher calorie milk consumed.
11. Babies who sleep for long periods of time without eating or feed only for few minutes should be encouraged to nurse (i.e., unwrap, rub feet).

B. Positioning and latch.
1. Mother and infant should be comfortable with infant on his/her side at nipple height supported by pillows or blankets.
2. Support infant's head so he/she can easily reach areola without turning neck.
3. Infant's ear, shoulder, hips should be in alignment.
4. Mother can align her nipple with infant's nose, quickly bringing infant to breast only when his mouth opens widely getting more of the areola on the bottom than top into his mouth, creating an asymmetrical latch (see **Figure 5-2**).
5. Infant's lips should be flanged outward with chin touching breast. When latched properly, the tongue is drawn back to the junction of the hard and soft palate (see **Figure 5-3**).
6. Infant's tongue will protrude over gum ridge and "cup" breast.
7. If baby latches incorrectly, the mother can insert her finger to break the suction, and repeat latch-on attempts until baby is latched correctly.
8. Common breastfeeding positions are cradle position (see **Figure 5-4**), cross cradle and football holds, (see **Figure 5-5**) and side-lying position (see **Figure 5-6**).
9. Trained practitioners should regularly observe latch-on, milk transfer, and feeding during hospitalization.

Figure 5-2 Positioning the baby nipple to nose (3 photos).

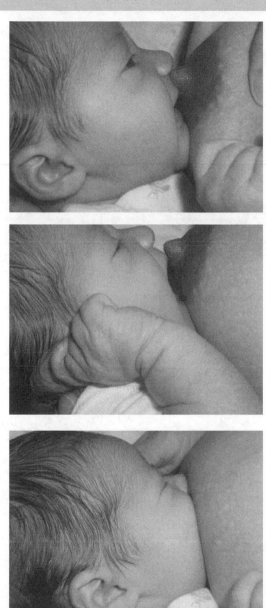

Source: Lauwers J, Swisher A. *Counseling the Nursing Mother: A Lactation Consultant's Guide.* 5th ed. Sudbury, MA: Jones & Bartlett Learning; 2011.

Figure 5-3 Sucking action (breast and bottle).

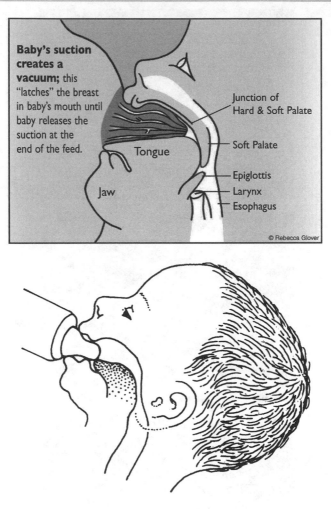

Source: Lauwers J, Swisher A. *Counseling the Nursing Mother: A Lactation Consultant's Guide.* 5th ed. Sudbury, MA: Jones & Bartlett Learning; 2011.

Figure 5-4 Madonna (cradle) position: A) front view, B) side view.

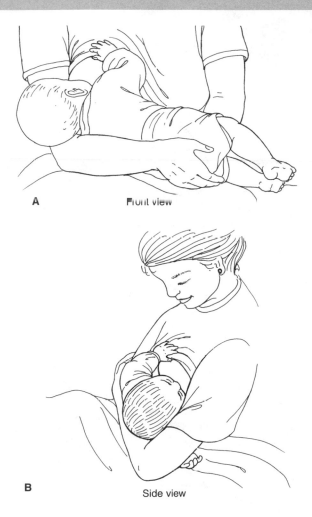

A   Front view

B   Side view

Source: Riordan J, Wambach K. *Breastfeeding and Human Lactation.* 4th ed. Sudbury, MA: Jones & Bartlett Learning; 2010.

Figure 5-5 A) Cross-cradle hold, B) football hold.

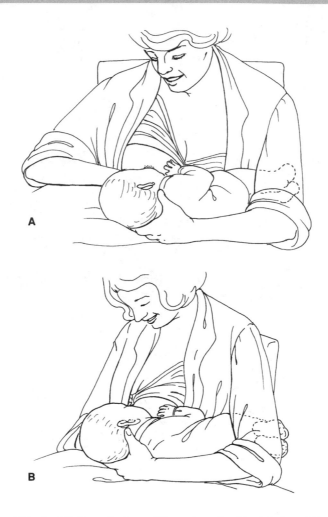

A

B

Source: Riordan J, Wambach K. *Breastfeeding and Human Lactation.* 4th ed. Sudbury, MA: Jones & Bartlett Learning; 2010.

     10.   The mother's nipple should not be pinched, bruised, or creased at the end of a feeding (see **Figure 5-7**).

  C. Signs of milk transfer in infant.

      1.   Observe sustained, rhythmic suck/swallow pattern with intermittent pauses.

Figure 5-6 Side-lying position.

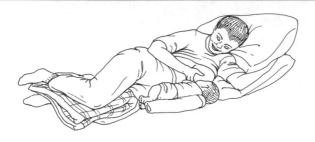

Source: Riordan J, Wambach K. *Breastfeeding and Human Lactation.* 4th ed. Sudbury, MA: Jones & Bartlett Learning; 2010.

   2.   Listen for audible swallowing.
   3.   Baby's arms and hands should be relaxed at the end of the feeding.
   4.   Baby's oral mucous membranes should be moist after feedings.
   5.   Baby should appear satisfied after feedings.
D.   Signs of milk transfer in mother.
   1.   Mother feels strong tugging sensation when baby is sucking that is not painful.
   2.   Mother feels uterine contractions and increased lochia flow during initial days postpartum.
   3.   Milk may leak from opposite breast during feedings.
   4.   Mother may feel relaxed or drowsy during feedings.
   5.   Breast softens after feeding (after milk supply is established).
   6.   Nipples are elongated, but not pinched or bruised after release of latch.
E.   Assessing infant weight gain.
   1.   Parents should be aware of baby's birth and discharge weight.
   2.   Encourage parents to keep daily journal of first week to track feedings, output.
   3.   Healthy, breastfeeding infants may lose 3–7% of birth weight in initial days.
   4.   After Mom's milk is in, infant should gain 0.5–1 oz/day (4–7 oz/week).
   5.   Babies often regain birth weight by 10–14 days of age, double it by 6 months, triple it by 1 year.
   6.   Exclusively breastfed infants tend to be leaner than bottle-fed infants in second 6 months of life.

Figure 5-7 Normal nipple postfeed and creased nipple postfeed.

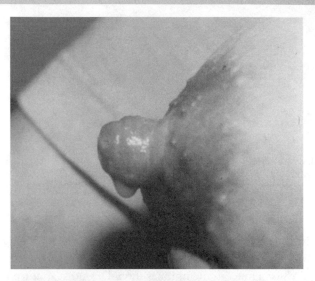

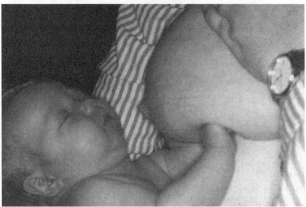

Source: Riordan J, Wambach K. *Breastfeeding and Human Lactation.* 4th ed. Sudbury, MA: Jones & Bartlett Learning; 2010.

    F.   Assessing infant output.
        1.   Colostrum acts as laxative, encouraging expulsion of meconium in first days.
        2.   Effective and regular breastfeeding helps to prevent jaundice in early days.
        3.   Infants showing signs of jaundice should be assessed carefully for ineffective breastfeeding.

4. Bowel movements become lighter in color, then turn to a mustard color, seedy consistency by day 4 or 5.
5. Babies who are breastfeeding well should have 2–3 large mustard color, seedy stools/day.
6. Inadequate stools are a red flag for ineffective breastfeeding.
7. Stool output may decrease to one stool every few days after first few weeks.
8. Urine output is less helpful than stool output in assessing adequate milk intake.
9. Exclusively breastfed baby should produce one wet diaper on day 1, two on day 2, three on day 3, and so on, for first week.
10. By end of first week, baby should have six soaking wet, pale yellow diapers/day.

VIII. SEPARATION OF MOTHER AND INFANT

A. Pumping.
1. All mothers should be taught how to hand express their milk after birth.
2. If small number of feedings must be missed, Mom can hand express or use a battery-operated pump to express milk from both breasts every few hours.
3. Lengthy separation warrants use of hospital-grade, piston-style pump with double hookup system to efficiently remove breastmilk 6–8 times/ 24 hours for approximately 15 minutes each session.
4. Even the smallest quantity of expressed colostrum or milk can be fed to infant via eyedropper, syringe, or cup.
B. Milk collection and storage.
1. Recommendations for collection and storage of mother's milk for hospitalized infant differ from that of the following instructions for the well child at home.
2. Mothers should wash hands thoroughly prior to pumping.
3. Follow manufacturer's instructions for cleaning of pump parts.
4. Glass containers with lids are a good choice for storing milk. Hard plastic (polypropylene) can also be used. Avoid bottles made with bisphenol A.
5. Mother can encourage milk let down by looking at picture of baby, smelling piece of baby's clothing.
6. Warm, wet washcloths on breast combined with breast massage may be helpful in starting milk flow.
7. Breastfeeding on one breast while pumping from other breast is an option.

8. All pumps are different. Encourage mother to find one that creates comfortable seal, which provides appropriate suction. Pumping should not be painful.

9. For specific information on storing milk for home use for full-term infants see the Academy of Breastfeeding Medicine Revised Protocol #8 March 2010.

IX. SUPPORTING BREASTFEEDING PAST THE EARLY DAYS

A. Follow up.
   1. Breastfeeding infants should be evaluated by an appropriate healthcare professional at 3–5 days of age and again at 2–3 weeks for successful feeding and appropriate weight gain. Infants should always be evaluated in between scheduled visits for any concerns.
   2. Breastfeeding mothers should be referred to a breastfeeding support group following hospital discharge.

B. Maternal diet.
   1. Encourage mother to eat a wide variety of healthy foods, eating when hungry, drinking to quench her thirst.
      a. Forcing large quantities of fluids will not increase her milk production.
      b. No specific foods must be avoided by breastfeeding mothers.
      c. Most foods do not bother most babies.
      d. If particular food seems to bother baby, decrease/eliminate for a week to 10 days.
   2. It is recommended that all breastfed babies be supplemented with vitamin D 400 IU starting soon after birth.
   3. Families with significant allergies should receive knowledgeable dietary counseling regarding possible need to eliminate certain foods while breastfeeding.

C. Growth spurts.
   1. Regardless of culture, women frequently worry about ability to provide enough milk for baby.
   2. Teach parents that growth spurts (periods when babies want to nurse more frequently to meet rapid growth) usually occur around 2–3 weeks, 6 weeks, 3 months.
   3. Feed as often as baby wants to nurse to increase, then maintain adequate milk supply.
   4. Reinforce concept of supply and demand.

5. Supplementing with formula is strongly discouraged; mother's milk supply will not increase without adequate stimulation to meet baby's growing demand for more milk.

D. Medications and breastfeeding.

1. It is imperative that healthcare providers give information to mothers who breastfeed on the safety of medications based on appropriate, current research, citing the source. Each infant's individual situation must be assessed prior to determining the appropriate use of any medication during breastfeeding. An excellent reference guide such as Hale (2010) should be available in every clinical setting that deals with breastfeeding mothers. Drugs listed are assigned a lactation risk category from L1 (safest) to L5 (contraindicated).

2. Many of the medications likely to be prescribed to breastfeeding mothers should not affect maternal milk supply or infant's safety. Ibuprofen is a commonly used analgesic postpartum and is considered compatible with breastfeeding. Penicillins and cephalosporins, along with several of the selective serotonin reuptake inhibitors (SSRIs) often used for depression, are also generally considered compatible.

3. Dose of medication transferred through breastmilk is almost always too low to be clinically significant or it is poorly bioavailable to infant.

4. It is preferable for mothers to avoid using medication whenever possible.

5. Extensive benefits of breastfeeding far outweigh any potential risks in majority of cases.
   a. Medications should be safe for infants to consume.
   b. Choose drugs with breastfeeding information whenever possible.
   c. Choose shortest acting form of medication.
   d. Encourage feeding when maternal drug level is lowest.
   e. Educate parents as to potential side effects to observe in infant, and affect on milk supply.
   f. Be extra cautious with preterm, low birth-weight or sick infants.
   g. Certain herbal substances may be harmful to infants.
   h. Drugs of abuse are contraindicated in breastfeeding and temporary cessation of breastfeeding is necessary with certain radioactive compounds, and a few medications. Consult appropriate resources for detailed information.

E. Maternal employment.

1. Women who return to work must be well supported in effort to continue providing breastmilk for infant.

2. Women need a private, clean place to pump every few hours while separated from infant.

3. Expressed milk can be kept at room temperature for short periods, in insulated bag with cooler pack, or, if available, in refrigerator. Encourage mothers to rent or purchase pump that is comfortable and is efficient for their particular needs.

4. Provide information on how to introduce bottle to the infant, as well as suggestions for caregiver that will promote extended breastfeeding (i.e., not bottle feeding immediately before mother will pick up infant, proper handling, storage of breastmilk).

5. Returning to workplace while continuing to provide breastmilk for baby may initially seem overwhelming to some mothers. Strong encouragement, praise, support can make difference between mother being successful and giving up.

6. Some employers are now required to provide break time for nursing mothers under the Patient Protection and Affordable Care Act, signed in to law on March 23, 2010.

X. COMMON PROBLEMS

A. Mothers can complain about pain even when damage is not visible on the breast or nipple. Determine that baby is positioned properly at breast height with adequate support and is latching on correctly. Mothers often describe sensation of baby feeding as strong tugging sensation. Breastfeeding should not be painful. Nipples do not "toughen up" as breastfeeding proceeds. Assess for other causes of sore nipples such as trauma, improper latch and release, thrush, milk plugs on nipple, incorrect use of breastfeeding devices or tight frenulum (see **Figure 5-8**). Paget's disease, an uncommon type of breast cancer, must also be ruled out. Breastfeeding issues that do not resolve quickly should promptly be referred to pediatric or maternal experts for further management.

B. Sore nipples management includes:
1. Correct positioning and latch-on.
2. Teach mothers to express colostrum/hindmilk to apply to nipples after each feeding.
3. Allow nipples to dry before putting bra back on.
4. Offer use of breast shells to prevent fabric from rubbing against sore nipples.
5. Breastfeed from least sore side first.
6. Change positions at each feeding to decrease pressure on sore area.

Figure 5-8 Tight frenulum.

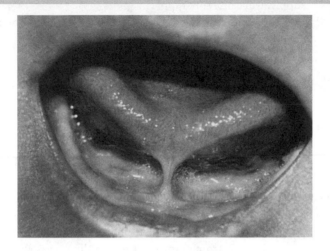

Source: Riordan J, Wambach K. *Breastfeeding and Human Lactation.* 4th ed. Sudbury, MA: Jones & Bartlett Learning; 2010.

7. Suggest moist wound healing methods (i.e., modified lanolin or hydrogel dressings).
8. Analgesics as needed.
C. Flat or inverted nipples.
1. Can initially make breastfeeding more of a challenge, may be difficult for baby to latch on, suck well. Provide adequate support to ensure successful feedings.
2. "Pinch test": determines if nipple is flat or inverted upon compression. With thumb behind nipple and first two fingers underneath, grasp about 1 in. back from base of nipple and compress skin.
   a. Normal nipple will evert.
   b. Flat nipple remains flat with compression.
   c. Inverted nipple looks sunken in.
   d. Nipples can look flat or inverted, but evert on compression.
3. Flat or inverted management includes:
   a. Encouraging deepest possible latch onto breast.
   b. Making sure infant is at breast height and well supported to prevent sliding to base of nipple.

      c. Release latch and repeat attempts until proper latch is obtained. Allowing baby to suck at base of nipple prevents stimulating milk supply, will cause sore nipples.

      d. Encourage offering flat/inverted breast first when baby is hungriest and sucking is strongest.

      e. Teach mother to evert nipple with gentle pulling/rolling immediately prior to latch.

      f. Hand express few drops of colostrum to entice baby to latch on.

      g. Use hand/electric pump for few minutes immediately prior to latch.

      h. If supplement is medically indicated, use expressed milk first using an eyedropper, syringe, cup, or feeding tube at the breast.

      i. Avoid pacifiers and bottle nipples until breastfeeding is well established.

D. Severe engorgement.

   1. Milk stasis caused by inefficient, infrequent removal of milk, results in extremely full, swollen, lumpy, painful breasts.

   2. Result is different from transient breast fullness associated with milk "coming in" 2–4 days after birth.

   3. Breastfeeding emergency: milk stasis can cause damage to tissue, decrease milk supply, and make it difficult to impossible for infant to compress areola and remove milk.

   4. Severe engorgement management includes:

      a. Analgesics as necessary.

      b. Warm, wet compresses to breast prior to feedings to help increase milk flow.

      c. Soften areola using hand expression so baby can latch properly.

      d. Use breast compression during feedings to improve milk flow. Using her thumb on top of breast and her fingers underneath, the mother brings her fingers together, which compresses breast.

      e. Use of cold compresses may help to decrease engorgement after feeding. Some mothers like to use this prior to feeding as well.

      f. Use of chilled green cabbage leaves left on breast for short period several times/day can be helpful to some mothers. Stop using this as soon as engorgement decreases.

      g. Express milk after feeding as needed for comfort. Any expressed milk can be fed to baby using alternative feeding methods.

E. Mastitis.

   1. Infection of breast, usually caused by *Staphylococcus aureus*.

   2. Frequently occurs in upper outer quadrant of breast, often by 2–3 weeks postpartum.

3. Symptoms commonly include hard, swollen, reddened area on breast accompanied by flu-like symptoms.
4. Difficult to differentiate between engorgement, plugged duct, mastitis (**Table 5-1**).
5. Mastitis management includes:
   a. Rest (decrease stress and fatigue by enlisting support from friends, family).
   b. Antibiotics; encourage completing full course as prescribed.
   c. Increase maternal fluid intake.
   d. Frequent, effective emptying of breasts (important to continue breast-feeding, milk is not infected, fine for baby).
   e. Abrupt weaning can predispose to an abscess.
   f. Analgesics as needed.
   g. Correct latch to prevent further nipple trauma (cracked, bleeding nipples allow bacteria to enter milk ducts).
   h. Mother's preference of warm or cool packs for comfort.

Table 5-1 Comparison of Findings of Engorgement, Plugged Duct, and Mastitis

Characteristics	Engorgement, 611.79	Plugged duct	Mastitis, 611
Onset	Gradual, immediately postpartum	Gradual, after feedings	Sudden, after 10 days
Site	Bilateral	Unilateral	Usually unilateral
Swelling and heat	Generalized	May shift a little or no heat	Localized, red, hot, and swollen
Pain	Generalized	Mild but localized	Intense but localized
Body temperature	38.4°C	38.4°C	38.4°C
Systemic symptoms	Feels well	Feels well	Flu-like symptoms

Source: Lawrence RA, Lawrence RM. *Breastfeeding: A Guide for the Medical Profession.* 6th ed. St Louis: Mosby; 2005.

F. Jaundice.
1. Rarely requires cessation of breastfeeding.
2. Pathologic jaundice, with onset in first 24 hours of life, warrants medical evaluation in addition to lactation support.
3 Encourage early initiation of breastfeeding, then frequent, effective, unrestricted feedings to minimize jaundice.
4. Colostrum acts as laxative, eliminating bilirubin through meconium expulsion.
5. Physiologic jaundice, which begins 48–72 hours after birth and peaks on day 3–5, is seen in thriving infants with normal weight gain and output.
6. Observe for effective breastfeeding and continue assessment for normal weight gain and output. Onset and peak of breastfeeding associated with jaundice is similar to physiologic jaundice, but infant is fussy/sleepy with poor feeding and inadequate weight gain, output.
7. Assist with frequent, unrestricted, effective breastfeeding.
8. Teach parents to watch for signs of milk transfer during feedings. If necessary, express milk in addition to feedings, use alternate feeding methods to give baby milk.

G. Thrush.
1. Often described as burning, itching, stinging lasting throughout feeding and beyond, radiating from nipple and breast to shoulder and back.
2. Nipple or areolar skin is often red and shiny.
3. May have period of pain-free nursing, then have sudden onset of pain.
4. Pain from poor latch is often described as feeling like a knife or being stabbed, dissipates as feeding progresses, frequently limited to nipple and areola.
5. Regardless of nipple pain, poor latch must be corrected immediately.
6. Broken skin is perfect environment for organisms to invade.
7. Signs in infant may range from nothing to white patches on buccal mucosa, tongue, and palate, which may bleed when scraped with tongue blade. Fiery red diaper rash with shiny red patches and pustules may also be present.
8. Both mother and baby should be treated simultaneously with appropriate antifungal medications to prevent reinfection from one to the other.
9. All objects (pumping supplies, pacifiers, bottles) coming in contact with baby's mouth should be boiled daily.
10. Mothers should be encouraged to continue breastfeeding while treating infection.

11. *Candida albicans* thrives in warm, moist, dark areas. Nipples can be rinsed with clear water or vinegar solution of 1 tablespoon vinegar in 1 cup of water after each feeding, exposing to air after each feeding.
12. Bed linens, sheets, bras can be rinsed in vinegar solution after hot wash cycle. Breast pads should be disposable and changed as soon as wet.
13. Sexual contact between mother and partner can spread infection. Partner should be treated appropriately.

H. Weight gain concerns.
   1. Breastfed infants gaining less than appropriate amount for age should be carefully evaluated. Often, correcting latch and positioning is enough to facilitate efficient breastfeeding and improve weight gain.
   2. Do not recommend formula supplementation without evaluating breast-feeding. If extra calories are needed, have mother hand express or pump in addition to breastfeeding and use alternative feeding methods to give baby milk.
   3. Allowing baby to finish feeding on one breast before feeding on second allows sufficient amounts of higher calorie breastmilk.
   4. Review with parents appropriate signs of infant hunger, encourage frequent (8–12 or more/24 hours) unrestricted feedings.
   5. Keeping written log of feedings and output is also helpful. Imperative that infant have adequate caloric intake.
   6. If after evaluation and management with skilled breastfeeding consultant, breastfeeding is not going well, formula supplementation is appropriate. Plan for maintaining/increasing mother's milk supply must be implemented.
   7. Return office visit within 24–48 hours to monitor situation should be scheduled. Frequent phone follow up, support are necessary.
   8. Global growth charts released by the World Health Organization (WHO) in 2006 reflect standards on how children should grow based on breast-feeding as the norm.

XI. HELPFUL BREASTFEEDING RESOURCES

A. Locating a board-certified lactation consultant:
   International Lactation Consultant Association
   919-861-5577
   www.ilca.org

International Board of Lactation Consultant Examiners
703-560-7330
www.iblce.org
Breastfeeding National Network (BNN)
1-800-TELL-YOU
www.medela.com

B.   Books.
Biancuzzo M, *Breastfeeding the Newborn: Clinical Strategies for Nurses*. 2nd ed. St. Louis, MO: Mosby; 2003.
Hale TW. *Medications and Mother's Milk*. 14th ed. Amarillo, TX: Hale Publishing, L.P.; 2010.
Lauwers J, Swisher A. *Counseling the Nursing Mother: A Lactation Consultant's Guide*. 5th ed. Sudbury, MA: Jones & Bartlett Learning; 2011.
Newman J, Pitman T. *The Ultimate Breastfeeding Book of Answers*. NY: Three Rivers Press; 2006.
Riordan J, Wambach K. *Breastfeeding and Human Lactation*. 14th ed. Sudbury, MA: Jones & Bartlett Learning; 2010.
Wilson-Clay B, Hoover K. *The Breastfeeding Atlas*. 4th ed. Manchaca, TX: LactNews Press; 2008.

C.   Online resources.
American Academy of Breastfeeding Medicine: www.bfmed.org
American Academy of Pediatrics: www.aap.org
Breastfeeding Pharmacology (Dr. Thomas Hale): http://neonatal.ttuhsc.edu/lact/
Human Milk Banking Association of North America: www.hmbana.com
La Leche League International: www.lalecheleague.org
UNICEF's 10 Steps to Successful Breastfeeding: www.unicef.org/newsline/tenstps.htm
U.S. Breastfeeding Committee: www.usbreastfeeding.org
World Alliance for Breastfeeding Advocacy: http://waba.org/my/

BIBLIOGRAPHY

Academy of Breastfeeding Medicine. ABM Clinical Protocol #8: Human Milk Storage Information for Home Use for Full-Term Infants (original Protocol March 2004 Revision #1 March 2010). Academy of Breastfeeding website: http://www.bfmed.org/Resources/Protocols.aspx. Accessed September 2, 2010.

American Academy of Breastfeeding Section on Breastfeeding. Breastfeeding and the use of human milk. *Pediatrics*. 2005;115(2):496–506.

American Academy of Family Physicians. Position Paper on Breastfeeding. American Academy of Family Physicians website: http://www.aafp.org/online/en/home/policy/policies/b/breastfeedingpositionpaper.html. Accessed September 2, 2010.

American Academy of Pediatrics Committee on Drugs. The transfer of drugs and other chemicals into human milk. *Pediatrics.* 2001;108(3):776–789.

American Academy of Pediatrics. Wagner CL, Greer FR, and the Section on Breastfeeding and Committeee on Nutrition. Clinical report—Prevention of rickets and vitamin D deficiency in infants, children, and adolescents. *Pediatrics.* 2008;122(5):1142–1152. doi:10.1542/peds.2008-1862.

Riordan J, Wambach K. *Breastfeeding and Human Lactation.* 4th ed. Sudbury, MA: Jones & Bartlett Learning; 2010.

Hale TW. *Medications and Mother's Milk.* 14th ed. Amarillo, Texas: Hale Publishing, L.P.; 2010.

International Lactation Consultant Association. *Clinical Guidelines for the Establishment of Exclusive Breastfeeding.* 2nd ed. 2005: http://www.ilca.org/files/education_and_research/independent_study_modules/ILCA%20documents/Doc%20ClinicalGuidelines2005.pdf. Accessed September 2, 2010.

Lu MC, et al. Provider encouragement of breast-feeding: Evidence from a national survey. *Obstet Gynecol.* 2001;97(2):290–295.

Marks JM, Spatz DL. Medications and lactation: What PNPs need to know. *J Pediatr Health Care* 2003;17(6):311–319.

NAPNAP Position statement on breastfeeding. *J Pediatr Health Care.* 2007;21:39A–40A.

Newman J, Pitman T. *The Ultimate Breastfeeding Book of Answers.* New York: Three Rivers Press; 2006.

U.S. Breastfeeding Committee. *Breastfeeding in the United States: A National Agenda.* Rockville, MD: U.S. Department of Health and Human Services, Health Resources and Services Administration, Maternal and Child Health Bureau; 2001.

U.S. Department of Health and Human Services. *HHS Blueprint for Action on Breastfeeding.* Washington, DC: U.S. Department of Health and Human Services, Office on Women's Health; 2000.

U.S. Dept of Labor-Wage and Hour Division (WHD). Fact Sheet #73: Break Time for Nursing Mothers under the FLSA. http://www.dol.gov/whd/regs/compliance/whdfs73.htm. Accessed September 1, 2010.

World Health Organization. The launch of the WHO Child Growth Standards. http://www.who.int/childgrowth/launch/en/index.html. Accessed September 3, 2010.

CHAPTER 6

Two-Week Visit

Candace F. Zickler

Breathing difficulties, 786.09	Poor feeding, 783.3
Decreased bowel movements, 564	Rash, 782.1
Irritability, 799.2	Reddened, draining umbilical site, 789.9
Jaundice, 782.4	Seizures, 780.39
Jaundice, newborn, 774.6	Vomiting, 787.03
No urine in 12 hours, 788.2	

I. GENERAL IMPRESSION

   A. Parents are settling in with 2-week old; each getting acquainted with other. If infant was still losing weight at discharge, the bilirubin was above 10 mg/dL, or the infant had a heart murmur, he/she needs to be seen in the office within 2 days.

   B. Infant should have a naked weight, length on length board, and head circumference performed. Compare the birth weight and the discharge weight with the weight obtained today. Determine daily weight gain since discharge.

   C. A brief exam noting muscle tone, symmetry, and heart sounds, murmurs should be done. Check for hip clicks by doing the Orolani and Barlow tests.

   D. At 2 weeks of age, the infant's cord should have fallen off or be dry and looking like it will likely fall off soon.

   E. Jaundice should be resolved except in some breastfed infants. If unresolved, do a transcutaneous bilirubin.

   F. Newborn screen results should be reviewed and be negative. Share report with parents.

   G. Review the newborn hearing screen. If hearing is within normal limits, share with the parents. If abnormal, schedule baby for an auditory brainstem response (ABR) or an otoacoustic emissions test (OAE) before leaving the office.

   H. Reflexes present should be rooting, Galant's (trunk incurvation), placing and stepping, Landau (infant lifts head when suspended in prone position), asymmetric tonic neck.

II. NUTRITION

A. Breastfeeding is encouraged for all newborns. If mother is breastfeeding, ask specific questions:
  1. Does the baby latch on well?
  2. How long does the baby nurse at one time?
  3. How frequently are you nursing the baby?
  4. How many wet diapers?
  5. How many stools?
  6. Are you having any irritation or pain from your nipples?
     Review all medications that mother may be taking (see Chapter 5). If mother expresses concerns about the nursing, observe a nursing session, give suggestions, and obtain a lactation consult from the hospital lactation resource.
B. If baby is bottle fed, review preparation and number of feedings, how much the baby is taking each time, number of wet diapers, and number of stools per day. Commercially prepared, iron-fortified formulas come in powder, concentrate, ready-to-feed. Do not dilute ready-to-feed. Follow directions for mixing concentrate and powder.
  1. Do not reuse bottle if more than 4 hours since opened.
  2. Mix formulas with bottled water for first month, continue to use bottled water if house is on well/unsure of water quality. Store mixed and open formula in refrigerator; do not feed formula that has been premixed and in the refrigerator longer than 24–36 hours. Specialized formulas have similar preparation directions; read labels. Goat's milk, whole cow's milk, rice milk have inadequate amounts of vitamins and minerals.
  3. Serve formula at room temperature. Do not microwave to heat. Do not let formula sit out to warm for more than 15–20 minutes.
  4. Clean technique is sufficient for mixing formulas. Clean off cans with soap and water before opening. Use hot soapy water and bottlebrush to clean nipples, bottles or clean in dishwasher.
  5. Hold infant in upright, semi-reclined position; burp every 1–2 oz. No bottle propping. Babies will suck and then rest during the entire feeding. Encourage mother to let her husband/partner feed the baby at least once during the day.
  6. No smoking or drinking hot beverages while holding baby. Limit noise in the immediate area when doing feeding, and focus on baby. Talk or sing to the baby.
  7. Infant should take in 90 of feeding in first 20 minutes. Two-week old infant takes 3–5 oz/feeding, 5–6 feedings/24 hours (90–120 cal/kg/day).

III. ELIMINATION

A. Bowel movements should be formed or soft with no green color. Infant should have 1–6 yellow pasty stools/24 hours. Breastfed infant may have upper range of frequency with less formed texture. Void every 1–3 hours or with each feeding and diaper change.

IV. SLEEP

A. Awake and alert for feedings, every 2–4 hours. Should nurse vigorously for 15–20 minutes, then fall back to sleep.
B. Babies should sleep in own cribs to decrease smothering or injury. Babies should sleep on their back in cribs to decrease incidence of sudden infant death syndrome (SIDS).

V. GROWTH AND DEVELOPMENT

A. Growth.
  1. Should regain birth weight by 2 weeks. Should gain 0.5–1 oz/day or approximately 2 lbs/month for next 5 months.
  2. Infant grows, on average, 1 in./month for first 6 months.
  3. Head circumference increases 0.5 cm/month in first year.
B. Development.
  1. Moves all 4 extremities, keep hands fisted, and has flexed posture.
  2. Has startle response to noises.
  3. May have a smile. May begin to look for "who is talking."
  4. May have "fussy" time of 1–2 hours/day, often in evening.
  5. Should have some supervised, "tummy" play time (15–20 minutes/session).
  6. Ask about behavior after feedings to determine any colic or reflux.

VI. SOCIAL DEVELOPMENT

A. Babies have specific sounds/cries for specific needs. They will fuss/cry 1–2 hours/day. Providing for infant's needs should stop the crying. Crying gradually decreases by 3 months of age.
B. Infant needs holding; touching; feeding; dry, clean diaper; warm, yet comfortable environment.

C. Discourage taking baby to public places or visiting relatives since infant has not been immunized. Sick adults should stay away from infant.
D. Encourage mother to rest when baby rests/sleeps. Determine if night times are "awake times for the pair" and the mother is not getting her sleep.

VII. IMMUNIZATIONS (SEE APPENDIX A)

A. If mother is HBsAg–, infant may not have received first hepatitis B vaccine in newborn nursery and will need to get it today or before 2 months of age. If infant received hepatitis B immunization in the nursery, he/she will need to get four hepatitis B immunizations.
B. Infant should not have fever or fussiness from the immunization.
C. Discuss importance of getting immunizations. Many parents are concerned about risks. One in eight parents in the United States refused at least one recommended vaccine for their child.

VIII. SAFETY/ANTICIPATORY GUIDANCE

A. Sleep position "back to sleep."
   1. Not safe for baby to sleep in adult bed.
   2. Discuss room temperature (comfortable), amount of clothing to put on baby (not to overdress infant).
   3. No pillows/toys in the crib that could potentially smother child.
   4. Federal motor vehicle safety tested and approved car seat: installed properly in backseat, facing backward in automobile. Contact local hospital, fire department, or local March of Dimes for car seat rental programs.
B. No smoking around infant.
C. Reassure parents they cannot spoil infant at this age.
D. Discuss sibling jealousy and possible regression of toddler. Encourage parent to spend "special time" with older sibling.
E. Discuss pet safety: Do not leave infant unattended near pet.
F. Discuss toys.
G. Discuss what to look for when choosing babysitter or daycare (e.g., handwashing, number of children, sick policy, feeding techniques).
H. One-piece pacifiers only, discuss appropriate use of pacifiers. Should not pin them on a string to baby's clothing, wash with soap and water if they fall out of the baby's mouth, do not lick or moisten it prior to giving to baby.
I. May give 1 oz of sterile water in 24 hours if stools are very hard. No corn syrup (Karo) for constipation.

J. No solids.
K. Remind parents of when and how to call healthcare provider. Review call-in phone policy and explain hours that are best to call office.
1. Breathing difficulties.
2. Seizures.
3. Irritability.
4. Poor feeding, vomiting.
5. No urine in 12 hours, black or decreased bowel movements.
6. Reddened, draining umbilical site.
7. Jaundice.
8. Rash or pustules not present on discharge.
9. Concerns.

BIBLIOGRAPHY

Car Safety Seats: A Guide For Families 2010. American Academy of Pediatrics Healthy Children website: http://www.healthychildren.org/English/safety-prevention/on-the-go/pages/Car-Safety-Seats-Information-for-Famiies-2010.aspx. Accessed June 2, 2011.

DeMichele AM, Ruth RA. Newborn Hearing Screening. Medscape Reference; 2010: http://emedicine.medscape.com/article/836646. Accessed June 2, 2011.

Diekema DS, and Committee on Bioethics of American Academy of Pediatrics. Clinical Report: "Responding to Parental Refusals of Immunization of Children" Reaffirmed policy on May 1, 2009. American Academy of Pediatrics website: http://aappolicy.aappublications.org/cgi/content/abstract/pediatrics; 115/5/1428. Accessed June 2, 2011.

Fouzas S, Mantagou L, Skylogianni SM, et al. (2009). Transcutaneous bilirubin levels for the first 120 postnatal hours in healthy neonates. *Pediatrics*. 2009;125(1):e52–e57. Retrieved from American Academy of Pediatrics website: http://www.pediatrics.org/cgi/content/full/125/1/e52. Accessed June 2, 2011.

Hagan JF, Shaw JS, Duncan P. (eds). *Bright Futures Guidelines for Health Supervision of Infants, Children, and Adolescents*. 3rd ed. American Academy of Pediatrics; 2008: http://brightfutures.aap.org/3rd_Edition_Guidelines_and_Pocket_Guide.html. Accessed June 2, 2011.

March of Dimes. *National Standard for Newborn Screening is Announced.* Published May 21, 2010: http://www.redorbit.com/news/health/1869169/national_standard_for_newborn_screening_is_announced/. Accessed June 2, 2011.

March of Dimes. Pregnancy and Newborn: Newborn Screening Tests. 2010: http://marchofdimes.com/pnhec/298_834.asp. Accessed June 2, 2011.

Medoff-Cooper B, Bakewell-Sachs S, Buus-Frank ME, et al. (Near Term Advisory Panel). The AWHONN near-term infant initiative: A conceptual framework for optimizing health for near-term infants. *JOGNN: Principles and Practice*. 2005;34(6):666–671.

Rauch D. Neonatal weight gain. MedlinePlus website: http://www.nlm.nih.gov/medlineplus/ency/article/007302.htm. Accessed June 2, 2011.

Recommended Immunization Schedule for Persons Aged 0 through 6 Years—United States 2010. Centers for Disease Control and Prevention website: http://www.cdc.gov/vaccines/recs/acip. Accessed June 2, 2011.

CHAPTER 7

One-Month Visit

Candace F. Zickler

Breathing difficulties, 786.09	Poor feeding, 783.3
Decreased bowel movements, 564	Seizures, 780.39
Irritability, 799.2	Vomiting, 787.03
No urine in 12 hours, 788.2	

I. GENERAL IMPRESSION

A. Parents and infant should be settling into routine and more comfortable with each other. Parent should be very attentive to the infant and have lots of questions. There should also be a sense that parent is comfortable with the infant. Parent is able to describe characteristics of infant's temperament. Mother should have someone identified that she can leave baby with for brief periods of time.

II. NUTRITION

A. Breastfeeding is to be encouraged. Determine if baby is satisfied after feedings, how frequently baby is nursing, how long a feeding takes, and any concerns mom has about continuing nursing. Ask about plans/arrangements to return to work.

B. Formula.

1. Mix formula with bottled water for first month, continue to use bottled water if house is on well/unsure of water quality. Have well water tested at local health department for small fee.

2. Store ready-to-feed and open formula bottles in refrigerator. Refrigerate no longer than 24–36 hours.

3. Specialized formulas have similar preparation directions; read labels. Goat's milk, whole cow's milk, rice milk have inadequate amounts of vitamins and minerals.

4. Serve formula at room temperature. Do not microwave to heat. Do not let formula sit out to warm for more than 15–20 minutes.
5. Clean technique is sufficient for mixing formulas.
   a. Clean off cans with soap and water before opening.
   b. Use hot soapy water and bottlebrush to clean nipples and bottles or clean in dishwasher.
6. Hold infant in upright, semi-reclined position; burp every 1–2 oz.
   a. No bottle propping.
   b. No smoking or drinking hot beverages while holding baby.
7. One-month old infant will take 4–6 oz/feeding and 5–6 feedings/24 hours (90–120 cal/kg/day).

III. ELIMINATION

A. Should have 1–6 yellow pasty stools/24 hours.
B. With each feeding, breastfed infant may have softer, formed/seedy stools.
C. Void every 1–3 hours or with each feeding.

IV. SLEEP

A. Awake and alert for feedings, every 2–4 hours. Baby will suck vigorously for 15–20 minutes, then fall back to sleep.
B. Babies should sleep in own cribs, not with parents, to decrease risk of smothering or injury.
C. Babies should sleep on back or side in cribs to decrease risk of sudden infant death syndrome (SIDS).
D. No pillows/toys that baby could get face against and smother.

V. GROWTH AND DEVELOPMENT

A. Growth. Weigh infant naked on infant scales. Compare weight to last visit. Calculate rate of gain since last visit. Measure length on length board and head circumference. Plot values on National Center for Health Statistics (NCHS) growth chart. Discuss your findings from the growth charts.
   1. Should gain 0.5–1 oz/day or approximately 2 lbs/month for next 4 months.

2. Infant grows, on average, 1 in./month for first 6 months.
3. Head circumference increases 0.5 cm/month in first year.
B. Development. Responds to human face and follows briefly with eyes. Is attentive to sound of parent's voice.
   1. May be able to lift head off bed if on tummy.
   2. May have a smile.
   3. Has positive red reflexes bilaterally and blinks to light. Tear ducts may have tears appear; tear ducts should be patent.
   4. Assess scalp for cradle cap and diaper area for dermatitis. Review how to care for baby's skin.
      Examine baby's mouth for teeth, intact palate, and presence of thrush. If bottle-feeding and thrush is found, discuss cleaning of pacifiers, nipples. If breastfeeding, review washing nipples before feedings, and applying antifungal (prescription) after feedings.
   5. Gently palpate abdomen looking for masses, and location of the liver.
   6. Observe movement of all 4 extremities, usually simultaneously. Has a flexed posture and keeps hands fisted.
   7. May cry but parents are learning what each cry means; crying ceases with needs being met. Cry gradually decreases by 3 months of age.
   8. May have "fussy" time of 1–2 hours/day, often in evening. Use "fussy" time as interaction time, not extra feeding.
   9. Baby may have symptoms of "colic" start around 2–3 weeks of age. Infant cries for prolonged periods, no specific cause or pathology identified. Infant requires additional comfort measures to quiet and settle.

VI. SOCIAL DEVELOPMENT

A. Parent should be assessed for sadness, depression, fatigue. Parent should show attentive, animated behavior toward baby. Listen carefully for frustration, potential for abuse/neglect.
B. Parents should hold, cuddle, and talk to infant when awake. Infant should have 15–20 minutes of "tummy time" with supervision, daily.
C. Discourage taking baby to public places or visiting relatives because no immunizations as yet.
D. Encourage mother to rest when baby rests/sleeps.
E. Baby is learning to "trust" parent and caretakers.

VII. IMMUNIZATIONS (SEE APPENDIX A)

A. If mother is HBsAg–, infant may not have received hepatitis B #1 in newborn nursery or at 2-week visit. Will need to get it today.
B. Discuss need for immunizations at next visit. Parents hear many negative remarks from friends and family and the Internet. But they do listen to a trusted healthcare provider.
C. Infants should not have fever or fussiness from immunization.

VIII. SAFETY/ANTICIPATORY GUIDANCE

A. Sleep position "back to sleep."
B. Protect baby from direct sunlight. Skin is very sensitive and they burn easily.
C. Not safe for baby to sleep in adult bed.
D. Temperature of room comfortable. Discuss type of clothing needed to dress infant for inside, outside, and for bed.
E. A Federal Motor Vehicle Safety Standards seat (FMVSS) should be installed properly in backseat, facing backward in their automobile. Contact local hospital, fire department, or March of Dimes chapter for car seat rental program.
F. No smoking around infant. Do not drink hot beverages when holding baby.
G. One-piece pacifiers only. Do not pin it to the clothing.
H. No corn syrup (Karo) for constipation. May give 1–2 oz of sterile water daily for infrequent or hard stools.
I. Infant still not old enough to be fed solid foods. Diet should be breastmilk or formula.
J. Obtain CPR training. Make sure smoke alarms are working and functional in the home.
K. Remind parents of when and how to call the healthcare provider.
1. Breathing difficulties.
2. Seizures.
3. Irritability, lethargy.
4. Poor feeding, vomiting, diarrhea (describe how stools would be if diarrhea).
5. No urine in 12 hours, black or decreased bowel movements.

BIBLIOGRAPHY

Car Safety Seats: A Guide For Families 2011. American Academy of Pediatrics Healthy Children website: http://www.healthychildren.org/English/safety-prevention/on-the-go/Pages/Car-Safety-Seats-Information-for-Families.aspx. Accessed July 20, 2011.

Diekema DS, and Committee on Bioethics of American Academy of Pediatrics. Clinical Report: "Responding to Parental Refusals of Immunization of Children" Reaffirmed policy on May 1, 2009. American Academy of Pediatrics website: http://aappolicy.aappublications.org/cgi/content/abstract/pediatrics; 115/5/1428. Accessed June 2, 2011.

Centers for Disease Control and Prevention. Growth Charts for Birth through 36 Months. CDC website: http://www.cdc.gov/growthcharts/clinical_charts.htm. Accessed June 2, 2011.

Hagan JF, Shaw JS, Duncan P, eds. *Bright Futures Guidelines for Health Supervision of Infants, Children, and Adolescents.* 3rd ed. American Academy of Pediatrics; 2008: http://brightfutures.aap.org/3rd_Edition_Guidelines_and_Pocket_Guide.html. Accessed June 2, 2011.

Recommended Immunization Schedule for Persons Aged 0 through 6 Years—United States 2010. Centers for Disease Control and Prevention website: http://www.cdc.gov/vaccines/recs/acip. Accessed June 2, 2011.

Task Force on Sudden Infant Death Syndrome. *The Changing Concept of Sudden Infant Death Syndrome: Diagnostic Coding Shifts, Controversies Regarding the Sleeping Environment, and New Variables to Consider in Reducing Risk.* American Academy of Pediatrics website: http://aappolicy.aappublications. org/cgi/content/full/pediatrics; 116/5/1245. Accessed June 2, 2011.

Tips and Tools: Safety for Your child; Birth to 6 Months. Retrieved from http://www.healthychildren.org/english/tips-tools/Pages/default.aspx. Accessed June 2, 2011.

Two-Month Visit

Candace F. Zickler

I. GENERAL IMPRESSION

    A. Parents should be enjoying their infant and taking joy from infant's accomplishments.

    B. Infant is more responsive with smiling and cooing.

    C. Parents should have many questions and be able to share stories of babies' activities.

II. NUTRITION

    A. Two-month old infant will take 6–8 oz/feeding, 4–6 feedings/24 hours (94–130 cal/kg/day). Feedings should be more predictable and infant should have periods when he/she sleeps for 3–4 hours at a time.

    B. Baby should take in 90 of feeding in first 20 minutes.

    C. Hold infant in semi-reclined position; burp every 1–2 oz.

    D. Specialized formulas have similar preparation directions; read labels. Goat's milk, whole cow's milk, rice milk have inadequate amounts of vitamins and minerals.

    E. Serve formula at room temperature. Do not microwave to heat. Do not let formula sit out to warm for more than 15–20 minutes.

    F. Clean technique is sufficient for mixing formulas.

        1. Clean off cans with soap and water before opening.

        2. Use hot soapy water and bottlebrush to clean nipples and bottles or clean in dishwasher.

G. No bottle propping. Pacifiers are used for non-nutritive sucking. Breastfeeding should be well established before starting infant on a pacifier, but babies who suck pacifiers are at decreased incidence of sudden infant death.

H. No smoking or drinking hot beverages while holding baby.

III. ELIMINATION

A. Should have 1–5 yellow pasty, but formed stools/24 hours.

B. Breastfed babies may have more stools than bottle-fed babies.

C. Void every 1–3 hours or with each feeding and diaper change.

IV. SLEEP

A. Babies sleep 16–18 hours/24 hours. Infant is developing sleep pattern. May sleep through night. May have longer awake periods during day.

B. Sleep cycles have both active and quiet sleep periods in equal proportions. Each sleep cycle lasts 50–60 minutes. Infants are less efficient with sleep and easily interrupted with noise. Should be alert for feedings, nurse vigorously for 15–20 minutes, and fall back to sleep/stay awake for short periods.

C. Babies should sleep in own cribs, not with parents, to decrease smothering injury to infant.
   1. Babies should sleep on back in cribs to decrease incidence of sudden infant death syndrome (SIDS).
   2. No pillows/toys that baby could get face against and smother.

V. GROWTH AND DEVELOPMENT

A. Growth. Plot length, weight, head circumference, and weight-for-height on the National Center for Health Statistics (NCHS) growth grids. Compare to last visit growth plots.
   1. Babies should gain 0.5–0.75 oz/day or approximately 2 lbs/month for the first 4–5 months.
   2. Infant grows, on average, 1 in./month for first 6 months.
   3. Head circumference increases 0.5 cm/month in first year.

B. Development.
   1. Holds head upright for short periods. Follows people and looks for voice.
   2. Responds to smiling with return smile.

3. Babbles and makes sounds with prompt of verbal cue.
4. Shows interest in what is happening in room.
5. Moves all 4 extremities, simultaneously.
6. May cry but parents are learning what each cry means. Crying ceases when needs are met.

VI. SOCIAL DEVELOPMENT

A. Baby learning to "trust" parent and caretakers to meet needs.
B. Family is settling into routines with infant.
C. Listen carefully for frustration, potential for abuse/neglect. Discuss child's unique temperament characteristics, relate to parents' feelings.
D. Parent should be assessed for sadness, depression, fatigue.
    1. Encourage mother to rest when baby rests/sleeps.
    2. Encourage mother to take breaks away from baby to do self-nurturing (needs designated sitter).
E. Take baby on selective, limited outings because infant is not fully immunized; will only receive first set today.
F. Ask about plans for returning to work. Discuss guidelines for selecting sitter/daycare.
G. May have "fussy" time of 1–2 hours/day, often in evening. Use "fussy" time as interaction time, not extra feeding. Cry gradually decreases by 3 months of age. Baby may have symptoms of "colic" (starts 2–3 weeks of age, ceases by 12 weeks). Infant cries for prolonged periods, no specific cause or etiology identified. Infant continues to grow well. Infant is alert and playful at other times. Infant may require additional comfort measures to quiet and settle and should be accepted as expected for age.
H. Should have some supervised, "tummy" play time while awake.
I. Encourage parent to actively talk, play with infant. Select age-appropriate toys.

VII. IMMUNIZATIONS (SEE APPENDIX A)

A. Infant will receive first set of immunizations today. Combinations are available that decrease number of injections. Parents trust providers to guide them in their decision to immunize their children. Need to discuss risks and benefits of immunizations and have parent sign consent. The following immunizations are best practice for 2-month-old infants.

1. Hepatitis B 2: After the birth dose, the hepatitis B series can be completed with either monovalent HepB or a combination vaccine containing HepB. Administer 4 doses of HepB to infants if combination vaccines with HepB are given after the birth dose.
2. DTaP #1 (diphtheria-tetanus-acellular pertussis). Minimum age of 6 weeks.
3. IPV #1 (inactivated poliovirus). Minimum age of 6 weeks.
4. Hib #1 (Haemophilus influenzae type b). Minimum age of 6 weeks.
5. PCV #1 (pneumococcal conjugate). Minimum age of 6 weeks.
6. RV (rotavirus vaccine). Minimum age of 6 weeks. Maximum age of 14 weeks and 6 days to start series.

B. Giving acetaminophen prophylactically after immunizations may decrease the response to the vaccine. Few infants run fevers after immunizations.

VIII. SAFETY/ANTICIPATORY GUIDANCE

A. Needs safe sleep position "back to sleep."
   1. Not safe for baby to sleep in adult bed.
   2. Discuss temperature of room, temperature of water, bathing safety guidelines.
   3. Discuss appropriate amount of clothing to keep baby comfortable in varied environments.
B. Never leave baby unattended near pet or sibling.
C. Keep hand on baby when on changing tables, sofas, avoid risk of falling.
D. Review need for car seat that is Federal Motor Vehicle Safety tested and approved, installed properly in backseat, facing backward in automobile. Contact local hospital, fire department, or March of Dimes chapter for car seat rental program.
E. No smoking around infant.
F. To treat constipation, advise giving extra water (no more than 1 oz/day).
G. No solids should be offered. Offer pacifier if acting "hungry" or going to nap.
H. Make sure smoke detectors are installed and functioning in home. Home should have working fire detectors, a fire evacuation plan, and periodic drills to ensure preparedness.
I. Limit sun exposure, use sunscreen with SPF rating of at least 15 if out for even 15 minutes of direct sun exposure. Protect babies by using hats and long sleeve shirts and pants.
J. Baby will be seen for regular appointment again at 4 months. Discuss skills infant will acquire and how to work with baby to learn them: babbling, cooing,

trying to roll over, and more. Discuss second set of immunizations, similar to what baby had at this visit.
K. Remind parents of when and how to call the healthcare provider.
   1. Breathing difficulties.
   2. Seizures.
   3. Irritability.
   4. Poor feeding, vomiting.
   5. No urine output in 12 hours, black/decreased bowel movements.
   6. Any fever.
   7. Praise the parents for all that they are doing for the infant.

BIBLIOGRAPHY

Back to Sleep, Tummy to Play. Healthy Child Care America; 2009: http://www.healthychildcare.org/pdf/SIDStummytime.pdf. Accessed June 2, 2011.

Car Safety Seats: A Guide For Families 2011. American Academy of Pediatrics Healthy Children website: http://www.healthychildren.org/English/safety-prevention/on-the-go/Pages/Car-Safety-Seats-Information-for-Families.aspx. Accessed July 20, 2011.

Centers for Disease Control and Prevention. *Growth Charts for Birth through 36 Months*. CDC website: http://www.cdc.gov/growthcharts/clinical_charts.htm. Accessed June 2, 2011.

Dowshen S. *Choosing Child Care*. KidsHealth from Nemours; 2007: http://kidshealth.org/parent/positive/amily/child_care.html. Accessed June 2, 2011.

Hagan JF, Shaw JS, Duncan P, eds. *Bright Futures Guidelines for Health Supervision of Infants, Children, and Adolescents*. 3rd ed. American Academy of Pediatrics;2008: http://brightfutures.aap.org/3rd_Edition_Guidelines_and_Pocket_Guide.html. Accessed June 2, 2011.

Oral Health Initiative: Protecting All Children's Teeth: Nonnutritive Sucking, Pacifiers. American Academy of Pediatrics; 2010: http://www.aap.org/oralhealth/PACT/ch8_sect1b.cfm. Accessed June 2, 2011.

Port Washington Fire Department. *E.D.I.T.H. Exit Drills in the Home*. http://www.pwfd.com/content/850_fs3.html. Accessed August 9, 2011.

Recommended Immunization Schedule for Persons Aged 0 through 6 Years—United States 2010. Centers for Disease Control and Prevention website: http://www.cdc.gov/vaccines/recs/acip. Accessed June 2, 2011.

Soloway KB. *Prophylactic Acetominophen could lower response to childhood immunizations*. Medscape Today; 2009: http://www.medscape.com/viewarticle/712540. Accessed June 2, 2011.

Task Force on Sudden Infant Death Syndrome. *The Changing Concept of Sudden Infant Death Syndrome: Diagnostic Coding Shifts, Controversies Regarding the Sleeping Environment, and New Variables to Consider in Reducing Risk*. American Academy of Pediatrics website: http://aappolicy.aappublications.org/cgi/content/abstract/pediatrics;116/5/1245. Accessed June 2, 2011.

Tips and Tools: Safety for Your child; Birth to 6 Months. Retrieved from http://www.healthychildren.org/english/tips-tools/Pages/default.aspx. Accessed June 2, 2011.

White J. *Overview of Infacnt Colic*. http://baby.about.com/od/healthandsafety/p/infant_colic.htm. Accessed June 2, 2011.

Four-Month Visit

Patricia Clinton

Dehydration, 276.5	Fever, 780.6
Diarrhea, 787.91	Vomiting, 787.03

I. GENERAL IMPRESSION

A. Four-month-old infant is generally well integrated into family unit, interacts with family members, is beginning to actively explore environment by making more purposeful movements.

B. Patterns of sleeping, eating, elimination are fairly well established.

II. NUTRITION

A. Caloric needs: 98–108 kcal/kg/day.

B. Breastfeeding.
   1. Recommended as sole source of nutrition.
   2. Infant easily distractible.
   3. Support mother in continuing to nurse throughout first year.
   4. Vitamin D supplementation recommended at 400 IU/day.

C. Formula feeding.
   1. Iron-fortified only.
   2. No cow's milk of any kind.

D. Introduction of solids.
   1. May begin after 4-month visit.
   2. Preference is to postpone until 6 months to minimize allergies.
   3. Introduce solids when tongue thrust diminishes, infant has good head control (see Chapter 10).

III. ELIMINATION

A. Voiding pattern.
1. Average 6–8 wet diapers/day.
2. Illness (fever, vomiting, diarrhea) associated with decreased voiding and concerns of dehydration.
B. Stooling pattern.
1. Breastfed infants generally have 1 stool/day to 1 stool every 7–10 days.
2. Consistency more important than frequency.
3. Stools should be soft, semiformed, odor not offensive.
4. Formula-fed infants generally have 1 or more stools/day, color varies by formula, may be more odiferous.

IV. SLEEP

A. Requirements.
1. Nighttime 9–12 hours; may still waken for nighttime feedings.
2. Naps 2–4 times/day; 30 minutes to 2 hours.
B. Environment.
1. Begin to establish consistent bedtime routine.
2. Put to bed drowsy but awake.
3. Room temperature should be temperate and not excessively warm.
4. Transitional object such as blanket may be comforting.
5. Room dim, may use night-light.
6. Cosleeping is family/culturally determined; encourage discussion, avoid being judgmental; safety should be focus.
7. Avoid bottles in bed.
C. Safety.
1. Put to bed on back. Once he/she rolls over, infant determines position during sleep.
2. Sleeping surface should be firm; avoid pillows, comforters. Slats 2 3/8 in. apart; corner posts 1/16 in. high.
3. Smoke-free environment.
4. Remove mobiles, Venetian blind cords, other hanging toys before infant learns to pull up in crib.

V. GROWTH AND DEVELOPMENT

  A. Growth.
    1. Infants should gain 0.5–1 oz/day or about 2 lbs/month; doubles birth weight between 4 and 6 months.
    2. Infants grow, on average, 1 in./month.
    3. Head circumference increases 0.5 cm/month.
  B. Development.
    1. Grasps objects, begins with raking motion.
    2. Brings hands together.
    3. Follows objects with eyes to 180°.
    4. Good head control. Lifts head and chest when prone.
    5. Bears weight on legs.
    6. Rolls from front to back.
    7. Rooting and palmar grasp disappear.
    8. Moro, Babinski, and tonic neck no longer as prominent, may disappear by 4 months.
    9. Begins to link event with action such as quieting when put in nursing position.
    10. Ability to wait begins to develop as infant learns to anticipate response from caregiver.
    11. Cooing, laughing, squealing. Vocalizes in variety of ways to initiate and sustain interaction.
    12. Beginning to listen when others speak.

VI. SOCIAL DEVELOPMENT

  A. Relationships.
    1. Recognizes primary caregiver.
    2. Variety of facial expressions such as smiling, surprise, fear.
    3. Enjoys being cuddled.
  B. Environment: conditions that foster trust, positive psychosocial feelings, development.
    1. Learning to trust caretakers.

2. Responsiveness to infant's needs and cues reinforces trust and does not result in spoiling.
3. Smiles are purposeful.

VII. IMMUNIZATIONS (SEE APPENDIX A)

A. Review immunization schedule: DTaP #2, Hib #2, IPV #2, PCV #2, RV #2, hepatitis B if not previously started.
B. Review immunization reactions.

VIII. SAFETY/ANTICIPATORY GUIDANCE

A. Always check bathwater temperature.
B. Never leave infant alone in tub or on changing table.
C. Use sunscreen of at least SPF 15 and avoid prolonged sun exposure.
D. Use car seat consistently. Never leave infant alone in car.
E. Avoid use of walkers.
F. Begin "baby proofing": outlet covers, door and drawer latches, safety gates. Remove cords, wires, string, plastic bags from baby's environment.
G. Maintain smoke-free environment.
H. If mother is returning to work, plan strategies for breastfeeding.
I. No honey or corn syrup (Karo).
J. Do not prop bottles. Do not put cereal in bottles.
K. Allow infant to self-regulate amount eaten: Watch for cues, e.g., turning head away.
L. Secure infant in highchair. Never leave infant alone in highchair.
M. Encourage floor "tummy" time so infant can begin to explore surroundings.
N. Talk, read, sing to infant.
O. Use variety of toys/other household objects to stimulate infant. Introduce infant to different textures in toys, objects.
P. Discuss infant's temperament and how it relates to sleep/wake activities.
Q. Begin exploring parental ideas about discipline.
R. Cleanse gums with soft cloth after feeding.
S. Increased drooling indicates functional salivary glands, not teething.
T. Stress handwashing by all caregivers.
U. Use of cool mist vaporizers for upper respiratory illness.
V. Review guidelines for calling healthcare provider, illness signs (i.e., fever, vomiting, diarrhea).

BIBLIOGRAPHY

Burns CE, et al. *Pediatric Primary Care: A Handbook for Nurse Practitioners.* 4th ed. Philadelphia, PA: W.B. Saunders; 2009.

Centers for Disease Control and Prevention. *2011 Recommendations and Guidelines: Childhood & Adolescent Immunization Schedules.* http://www.cdc.gov/vaccines/recs/schedules/child-schedule.htm. Accessed June 2, 2011.

Dixon SD, Stein MT. *Encounters with Children: Pediatric Behavior and Development.* 4th ed. St. Louis, MO: Mosby; 2006.

Hagan JF, Shaw JS, Duncan P (eds). *Bright Futures: Guidelines for Health Supervision of Infants, Children, and Adolescents.* 3rd ed. Elk Grove Village, IL: American Academy of Pediatrics; 2008.

Marcdante KJ, Kliegman RM, Jenson HB et al. (eds). *Nelson Essentials of Pediatrics.* 6th ed. Philadelphia, PA: Saunders; 2011.

Mindell JA, Owens JA. *A Clinical Guide to Pediatric Sleep: Diagnosis and Management of Sleep Problems.* 2nd ed. Philadelphia, PA: Lippincott Williams & Wilkins; 2009.

Ontario Society of Nutrition Professionals in Public Health. Pediatric Nutrition Guidelines for Primary Care Providers. Ontario, CA, 2008. http://www.osnpph.on.ca/pdfs/ImprovingOddsJune-08.pdf. Accessed June 2, 2011.

Porter RS, Kaplan JL. The Merck Manual Online: http://www.merck.com/mmpe/index.html. Accessed June 2, 2011.

Samour PQ, King K. *Handbook of Pediatric Nutrition.* 3rd ed. Sudbury, MA: Jones and Bartlett Publishers; 2005.

Six-Month Visit

Patricia Clinton

Breathing difficulties, 786.09	Rash, 782.1
Irritability, 799.2	Seizures, 780.39
No urine output in 12 hours, 788.2	

I. GENERAL IMPRESSION

A. Six-month-old infant is active, social person in family and with others although new people may be cause for some anxiety.

B. Parents are comfortable in their role, look forward to infant's new achievements.

II. NUTRITION

A. Caloric and nutrient needs.
   1. 95–105 kcal/kg/day.
   2. Iron stores may not meet needs; encourage iron-fortified cereals and formulas.
   3. Nutrient needs generally cannot be met from breastmilk or formula alone.

B. Breastfeeding.
   1. Continue to encourage breastfeeding through first year.

C. Formula feeding.
   1. Continue with iron-fortified formula.
   2. No cow's milk until after first birthday.

D. Solid foods.
   1. Should be offering solid foods by 6 months 2–3 times/day.
   2. Goal is to accustom infant to new textures and tastes.
   3. Introduce solids with spoon; do not put cereal in bottle.
   4. Begin with iron-fortified rice cereal; prepare with either breastmilk or formula.

     5. Progress from iron-fortified cereals to fruits and vegetables.

     6. Add new foods one at a time and start with 1–2 teaspoons.

     7. Meat not added until later in first year.

     8. Avoid feeding as a comfort measure.

  E. Eating habits/safety.

     1. No bottles in bed.

     2. Infants with strong family history of allergies avoid foods with high allergy potential (strawberries, eggs, etc.) until end of first year.

     3. No honey until after first year.

     4. Vary textures from pureed to fine grind.

     5. Eating is social time; include infant in family meals. Introduce cup. As infant's pincer grasp develops, may offer finger foods.

III. ELIMINATION

  A. Continues to have 6 wet diapers/day.

  B. Stool consistency and color change with intake of solid foods.

IV. SLEEP

  A. Should be sleeping through night; 9–12 hours.

  B. Naps in morning and afternoon from 30 minutes to 2 hours.

  C. Regular patterns are established although there may be occasional lapses.

  D. Continue to put to bed drowsy but awake. Encourage consistent bedtime rituals.

  E. Transitional objects continue to be important.

  F. Night feedings not needed.

V. GROWTH AND DEVELOPMENT

  A. Doubles birth weight between 5 and 6 months. Length increases 0.5 in./month. Growth may occur in spurts; always plot.

  B. Anterior fontanel still open, no overriding sutures palpated. Head circumference increases about 1 cm/month.

  C. Rakes objects. Grasps objects with hands. Transfers objects between hands.

  D. "Plays" with objects: drops, shakes, bangs.

E. Sits alone or with minimal support and no head lag.
F. Rolls over both directions.
G. Bears weight on legs.
H. Moro and tonic neck reflexes have disappeared.
I. Responds to name.
J. Babbles ("ba," "ga," "da"), laughs, squeals.

VI. SOCIAL DEVELOPMENT

A. Enjoys interacting with parents.
B. Expects that needs will be met and expresses frustration when they are not.
C. Separation anxiety emerges.
D. Begins to differentiate angry or friendly tone of others and respond accord ingly.
E. Uses gestures to gain attention (pointing, reaching).

VII. IMMUNIZATIONS (SEE APPENDIX A)

A. DTaP #3.
B. Hib (depending on which vaccine used).
C. IPV #3 (3rd dose anytime between 6 and 18 months).
D. PCV #3.
E. RV (not necessary if Rotarix administered at 2 and 4 months).
F. Influenza annually.

VIII. SAFETY/ANTICIPATORY GUIDANCE

A. Always check bathwater temperature. Never leave infant alone in tub or on changing table.
B. Use sunscreen of at least SPF 15 and avoid prolonged sun exposure.
C. Use car seat consistently. Never leave infant alone in car.
D. Avoid use of walkers.
E. Baby proof environment with outlet covers, door and drawer latches, safety gates. Remove cords, wires, string, or plastic bags from baby's environment. Avoid tablecloths; remove heavy/hot objects from tables that have tablecloths.
F. Maintain smoke-free environment, ensure smoke alarms in baby's home.

G. Do not leave alone in room with pets or siblings.

H. Monitor for small objects or toys especially if other young children present.

I. Keep bathroom door closed, toilet lid down, remove buckets with water.

J. Use protective enclosures around swimming pools, hot tubs, other water sites (ponds, fountains).

K. Provide poison control number to be placed by telephone; syrup of ipecac no longer recommended.

L. Play games such as "peek-a-boo." Encourage reading activities with picture books, infant board books.

M. Treat teething discomfort with oral massage, frozen wet washcloths, other cold hard objects for chewing, acetaminophen or ibuprofen. Discourage use of numbing gels because of likelihood of numbing entire oral cavity, suppressing gag reflex.

N. Assess fluoride source, supplement as necessary (see Appendix B).

O. Illness prevention.
   1. Review illness symptoms and interventions.
   2. Reinforce handwashing.
   3. Use of cool mist vaporizers for upper respiratory illness.

P. When to call health care provider:
   1. Breathing difficulties.
   2. Irritability.
   3. No urine output in 12 hours.
   4. Seizures.
   5. Rash.
   6. Concerns.

BIBLIOGRAPHY

Burns CE, et al. *Pediatric Primary Care: A Handbook for Nurse Practitioners.* 4th ed. Philadelphia, PA: W.B. Saunders; 2009.

Centers for Disease Control and Prevention. *2011 Recommendations and Guidelines: Childhood & Adolescent Immunization Schedules.* http://www.cdc.gov/vaccines/recs/schedules/child-schedule.htm. Accessed June 2, 2011.

Dixon SD, Stein MT. *Encounters with Children: Pediatric Behavior and Development.* 4th ed. St. Louis, MO: Mosby; 2006.

Hagan JF, Shaw JS, Duncan P, eds. *Bright Futures: Guidelines for Health Supervision of Infants, Children, and Adolescents.* 3rd ed. Elk Grove Village, IL: American Academy of Pediatrics; 2008.

Marcdante KJ, Kliegman RM, Jenson HB et al., eds. *Nelson Essentials of Pediatrics.* 6th ed. Philadelphia, PA: Saunders; 2011.

Recommendations for using fluoride to prevent and control dental caries in the United States. *Morb Mortal Weekly Rep.* 2001;50:RR-14.

Nine-Month Visit

Patricia Clinton

Breathing difficulties, 786.09	Rash, 782.1
Irritability, 799.2	Seizures, 780.39
No urine output in 12 hours, 788.2	Separation anxiety, 309.21

I. GENERAL IMPRESSION

    A. On the move! Need to explore critical for cognitive development.

    B. Rapidly gaining new motor/cognitive skills; 9-month olds present new challenges to parents.

    C. Separating from parents is difficult.

II. NUTRITION

    A. Caloric needs: 98–100 kcal/kg/day.

    B. Breastfeeding/formula feeding.

        1. Infant receiving most nutrients from solid foods.

        2. Continue to encourage breastfeeding through first year.

        3. If using formula, continue with iron-fortified product.

        4. Avoid cow's milk until after first year.

    C. Assess for risk factors, screen for iron-deficiency anemia if necessary.

        1. Watch for use of cow's milk, low-iron formulas, low intake of iron-rich foods.

        2. Supplement as necessary (see Chapter 32 for more on iron-deficiency anemia).

    D. Solids.

        1. Infant should be eating table food with family.

        2. Finely chopped meats may be introduced.

        3. Finger foods appropriate at this time as fine pincer grasp has developed.

        4. May take up to 10 offerings before infant accepts new food.

E. Eating habits/safety.
1. Offer liquids from cup.
2. Limit juice to 4–6 oz/day.
3. No honey or corn syrup (Karo) until after first year.
4. Offer solids 3–4 times/day.
5. Atmosphere should be relaxed, pleasant. Expect a mess!
6. Avoid foods that may cause choking: grapes, raisins, peanuts/peanut butter, popcorn, hard candy, carrots, celery, other hard vegetables/fruits.
8. Encourage infant to self-feed; provide infant with spoon.
9. Watch for infant cues to signal satiation.

III. ELIMINATION

A. Voiding pattern.
1. Stays dry for longer periods.
2. Usually voids after naps.
B. Stooling pattern.
1. Stools usually firm, dark.
2. Individual pattern established between 9 and 12 months.
3. Generally 1–2 stools/day (but may vary considerably between infants).

IV. SLEEP

A. Requirements.
1. Total sleep in 24 hours between 11 and 13 hours.
2. Night awakenings common but should be able to put self back to sleep.
3. Continues to nap in morning and afternoon.
B. Environment.
1. Bedtime rituals well established.
2. Room should remain dim and not overly warm.
C. Safety.
1. Avoid bottles in bed.
2. Lower crib mattress.
3. Remind parents about removing blind or drapery cords, hanging objects (especially mobiles), small objects in cribs.

V. GROWTH AND DEVELOPMENT

A. Physical.
   1. Growth is slower in second half of first year.
   2. Weight gains average 1 lb/month and length 1 in./month.
   3. Growth should be steady but pattern may vary from early infancy; growth spurts more common.
B. Motor.
   1. Fine.
      a. Pincer grasp developed. Able to pick up small objects.
      b. Begins to poke with index finger.
      c. Can drop, bang, throw objects.
      d. Can self-feed.
   2. Gross.
      a. Sits well.
      b. Creeping/crawling.
      c. May begin to pull up on furniture.
      d. Weight bearing when pulled to stand.
   3. Infant reflexes.
      a. Primitive reflexes should be absent.
      b. Parachute reflex emerges.
C. Cognitive.
   1. Object permanence more prominently developed.
   2. May look for objects and go after them.
D. Language.
   1. Combines syllables.
   2. Imitates speech sounds. Uses intonations.
   3. "Dada" and "mama" are nonspecific.
   4. Responds to name.

VI. SOCIAL DEVELOPMENT

A. Relationships.
   1. Beginning to indicate wants.
   2. May begin to wave "bye-bye."
B. Environment: conditions that foster trust and development of positive psychosocial feelings. Separation anxiety emerges. Stranger anxiety apparent.

VII. IMMUNIZATIONS (SEE APPENDIX A)

    A. Make up for missed immunizations.

    B. Influenza annually.

VIII. SAFETY

    A. Infant care activities.

        1. Always check bathwater temperature.

        2. Never leave infant alone in tub, changing table, highchair.

        3. Use sunscreen; avoid prolonged sun exposure.

    B. Environment.

        1. Use car seat consistently.

        2. Never leave infant alone in car.

        3. Avoid use of walkers.

        4. Reinforce "baby proofing": outlet covers, door drawer latches, safety gates. Remove cords, wires, string, small objects, plastic bags from baby's environment.

        5. Keep sharp objects out of reach.

        6. Maintain smoke-free environment; use smoke alarms.

        7. Do not leave alone in room with pets or young children. Keep litter boxes away from infant's environment. Feed pets in area away from infant; do not allow infant near pet when eating.

        8. Avoid tablecloths or remove heavy/hot objects from tables with table-cloths.

        9. Keep toilet lid down, remove buckets with water.

     10. Use protective enclosures around swimming pools, hot tubs, other water sites (ponds, fountains).

     11. Provide poison control number (to be placed by telephone); syrup of ipecac no longer recommended.

     12. Keep houseplants out of reach; remove any poisonous plants.

IX. ANTICIPATORY GUIDANCE

    A. Parent–infant interaction.

        1. Continue to encourage floor time for infant to provide opportunities to explore.

        2. Talk with infant while engaging in other activities (e.g., grocery shopping).

3. Continue singing and movement activities with infant. Play games such as "peek-a-boo."
4. Encourage reading activities with picture books, infant board books.
5. Foster infant's ability to self-soothe with transitional objects such as blanket, stuffed toy.

B. Discipline.
1. Discuss appropriate discipline measures aimed primarily at protecting infant from injury such as physical removal from danger.
2. Distraction most effective to redirect behavior.
3. Limited use of word "no."
4. Begin to think about rules: keep them few and simple.
5. Consistency is key to discipline.

C. Oral hygiene.
1. No bottles in bed.
2. Use soft toothbrush without toothpaste to clean teeth. Assess fluoride source and supplement as necessary (see Appendix B).

D. Illness prevention.
1. Review illness symptoms/interventions.
2. Reinforce importance of handwashing.
3. Use cool mist vaporizer for upper respiratory illness.

E. When to call healthcare provider:
1. Breathing difficulties.
2. Seizures.
3. Irritability.
4. No urine output in 12 hours.
5. Rash.
6. Concerns.

BIBLIOGRAPHY

Burns CE, et al. *Pediatric Primary Care: A Handbook for Nurse Practitioners.* 4th ed. Philadelphia, PA: W.B. Saunders; 2009.

Centers for Disease Control and Prevention. *2011 Recommendations and Guidelines: Childhood & Adolescent Immunization Schedules.* http://www.cdc.gov/vaccines/recs/schedules/child-schedule.htm. Accessed June 2, 2011.

Dixon SD, Stein MT. *Encounters with Children: Pediatric Behavior and Development.* 4th ed. St. Louis, MO: Mosby; 2006.

Hagan JF, Shaw JS, Duncan P (eds). *Bright Futures: Guidelines for Health Supervision of Infants, Children, and Adolescents.* 3rd ed. Elk Grove Village, IL: American Academy of Pediatrics; 2008.

Porter RS, Kaplan JL. *The Merck Manual Online:* http://www.merck.com/mmpe/index.html. Accessed June 2, 2011.

Mindell JA, Owens JA. *A Clinical Guide to Pediatric Sleep: Diagnosis and Management of Sleep Problems.* 2nd ed. Philadelphia, PA: Lippincott Williams & Wilkins; 2009.

Recommendations for using fluoride to prevent and control dental caries in the United States. *Morb Mortal Weekly Rep.* 2001;50:RR-14.

Samour PQ, King K. *Handbook of Pediatric Nutrition.* 3rd ed. Sudbury, MA: Jones and Bartlett Publishers; 2005.

Twelve-Month Visit

Patricia Clinton

Anemia, 280.9	No urine output in 12 hours, 788.2
Breathing difficulties, 786.09	Rash, 782.1
Irritability, 799.2	Seizures, 780.39

I. GENERAL IMPRESSION

A. Twelve-month visit heralds onset of toddlerhood.
B. Toddler's increasing mobility opens new worlds to explore and requires close supervision to prevent injuries.

II. NUTRITION

A. Caloric needs: 98–100 kcal/kg/day.
B. Breastfeeding/formula feeding.
    1. Breastfeeding may continue, but toddler is getting majority of nutrients from table food.
    2. If formula feeding, discuss switching to whole cow's milk.
C. Assess for risk factors, screen for iron-deficiency anemia if necessary.
    1. Birth weight < 1500 grams, result of use of cow's milk or low-iron formulas during first year, low intake of iron-rich foods, low socio-economic status.
    2. Supplement as necessary (see Chapter 32 for more on iron-deficiency anemia).
D. Solids.
    1. Offer infant variety of foods from all food groups.

2.   Offer liquids from cup.
3.   Limit juice to 4–6 oz/day. Limit whole milk to 16–24 oz/day.

E.   Eating habits/safety.
1.   Reinforce mealtime as family time.
2.   Three meals and two snacks/day appropriate; rule of thumb for serving size is 1 tablespoon/year of age.
3.   Toddler's attention span limits ability to sit for long periods.
4.   Foods should be chopped into small pieces. Avoid foods that may cause choking: grapes, raisins, peanuts, popcorn, raw vegetables.
5.   Encourage toddler to self-feed with spoon, cup.
6.   If breastfeeding, discuss interest in weaning to cup.
7.   If bottle feeding, weaning to cup should be started.
8.   Reassure parents that toddlers' eating patterns are inconsistent from meal to meal; think in terms of several days when reviewing recommended servings of foods.

III. ELIMINATION

A.   Voiding and stooling pattern.
1.   Regular patterns may be established but these continue to be involuntary.
2.   Discourage toilet training until closer to 24 months; toilet training dependent on complete myelinization of pyramidal tracts in spinal cord.

IV. SLEEP

A.   Requirements.
1.   12–13 hours total/day.
2.   1–2 naps/day.

B.   Environment.
1.   Continue bedtime rituals; consistency is key.
2.   Transitional objects continue to be important.
3.   Bedtime resistance and night wakings are common.
4.   Avoid naps late in day that may interfere with nighttime sleeping.

C.   Safety.
1.   Mattress should be in lowest position to prevent climbing out of crib.
2.   No bottles in bed.
3.   All cords, small objects, plastic bags, latex balloons removed.

V. GROWTH AND DEVELOPMENT

A. Physical.
1. Most toddlers will have tripled birth weight.
2. Overall growth slows; typically will gain 3–3.5 kg (6–8 lbs) in next year and gain about 12 cm (5 in.) in length.
3. Head circumference averages about 47 cm (18 in.); brain weight doubles its birth weight in first year.

B. Motor.
1. Fine.
   a. Pincer grasp well developed.
   b. Puts block in cup.
   c. Can hold crayon/pencil and make marks on paper.
2. Gross.
   a. Stands alone for a few seconds. May take some free steps.
   b. Cruising around furniture.

C. Cognitive.
1. Continues in Piaget's sensorimotor stage; actions more intentional.
2. Increasing mobility fosters exploration of environment.
3. Toddler observes other's actions, listens, touches/mouths objects.
4. Play more spontaneous and self-initiated.

D. Language.
1. Uses 1–2 words.
2. "Dada" and "mama" specific.
3. Imitates sounds.
4. Begins to respond to simple commands.
5. Understands "no," "hot."
6. When an object is named, will look for it.

VI. SOCIAL DEVELOPMENT

A. Relationships.
1. Anxious around strangers.
2. Emotions emerge such as anger, affection.

B. Environment: conditions that foster trust and development of positive psychosocial feelings.
1. Waves "bye-bye."
2. Plays games such as "pat-a-cake."

3. Indicates wants.
4. Imitates activity of others.

VII. IMMUNIZATIONS (SEE APPENDIX A)

A. HepB #3 if necessary.
B. Hib #4 between 12 and 18 months.
C. IPV #3 if necessary.
D. MMR between 12 and 15 months.
E. Varicella at 12 months or after.
F. PCV 12–15 months.
G. Influenza annually.

VIII. SAFETY

A. Toddler care activities.
1. Always check bathwater temperature; make sure hot water thermostat < 120°F (48.9°C).
2. Never leave toddler alone in tub, changing table, highchair.
3. Use sunscreen, avoid prolonged sun exposure.
B. Environment.
1. Switch to toddler car seat. Never leave toddler alone in car.
2. Never leave toddler alone outside.
3. Reexamine "baby proofing" from toddler walking perspective: outlet covers, door/drawer latches, safety gates. Remove cords, wires, string, small objects, plastic bags from toddler's environment.
4. Climbing follows walking; anticipate dangers on counters, tables, stairs.
5. Keep sharp objects out of reach.
6. Maintain smoke-free environment; use smoke alarms.
7. Do not leave alone in room with pets or young children. Feed pets in area away from toddler. Do not allow infant near pet when eating. Keep litter boxes away from toddler's environment.
8. Avoid tablecloths or remove heavy or hot objects from tables with tablecloths.
9. Keep toilet lid down, remove buckets with water.
10. Protective enclosures around swimming pools, hot tubs, other water sites (ponds, fountains).

11. Provide poison control number (to be placed by telephone). Syrup of ipecac no longer recommended.
12. Keep houseplants out of reach; remove any poisonous plants.

IX. ANTICIPATORY GUIDANCE

A. Parent–toddler interaction.
   1. Continue to talk, sing, tell stories to toddler.
   2. Parent should make it a habit to describe what she/he is doing with toddler (e.g., "this is how we put on socks").
   3. Play games such as naming things, body parts, people.
   4. Encourage reading activities with picture books, infant board books.
   5. Limit TV to 1 hour or preferably less per day.
   6. Toddlers explore; this includes genital area.
B. Discipline.
   1. Consistency reinforces trust.
   2. Discuss appropriate discipline measures aimed primarily at protecting infant from injury; cognitively, infant cannot appreciate danger or intent.
   3. Positive reinforcement to support appropriate behavior; distraction continues to be effective.
   4. Limit use of word "no."
   5. Spanking never appropriate.
   6. Occasionally gentle physical restraint (holding toddler) may be necessary to prevent injury.
   7. Decide on a few important rules and be consistent about enforcing them.
C. Oral hygiene.
   1. No bottles in bed.
   2. Assess for bottle mouth caries.
   3. Use soft toothbrush, small pea size amount of fluoridated toothpaste. Assess fluoride source, supplement as necessary (see Appendix B).
   4. Make appointment for first dental visit.
D. Illness prevention.
   1. Review illness symptoms and interventions.
   2. Reinforce importance of immunizations.
   3. Reinforce importance of handwashing.
   4. Use cool mist vaporizer for upper respiratory illness.
E. When to call healthcare provider:
   1. Breathing difficulties.

2. Seizures.
3. Irritability.
4. No urine output in 12 hours.
5. Rash.
6. Concerns.

BIBLIOGRAPHY

Burns CE, et al. *Pediatric Primary Care: A Handbook for Nurse Practitioners.* 4th ed. Philadelphia, PA: W.B. Saunders; 2009.

Centers for Disease Control and Prevention. *2011 Recommendations and Guidelines: Childhood & Adolescent Immunization Schedules.* http://www.cdc.gov/vaccines/recs/schedules/child-schedule.htm. Accessed June 2, 2011.

Dixon SD, Stein MT. *Encounters with Children: Pediatric Behavior and Development.* 4th ed. St. Louis, MO: Mosby; 2006.

Hagan JF, Shaw JS, Duncan P, eds. *Bright Futures: Guidelines for Health Supervision of Infants, Children, and Adolescents.* 3rd ed. Elk Grove Village, IL: American Academy of Pediatrics; 2008.

Porter RS, Kaplan JL. *The Merck Manual Online*: http://www.merck.com/mmpe/index.html. Accessed June 2, 2011.

Mindell JA, Owens JA. *A Clinical Guide to Pediatric Sleep: Diagnosis and Management of Sleep Problems.* 2nd ed. Philadelphia, PA: Lippincott Williams & Wilkins; 2009.

Ontario Society of Nutrition Professionals in Public Health. *Pediatric Nutrition Guidelines for Primary Care Providers.* Ontario, CA; 2008: http://www.osnpph.on.ca/pdfs/ImprovingOddsJune-08.pdf. Accessed June 3, 2011.

Recommendations for using fluoride to prevent and control dental caries in the United States. *Morb Mortal Weekly Rep.* 2001;50:RR-14.

Samour PQ, King K. *Handbook of Pediatric Nutrition.* 3rd ed. Sudbury, MA: Jones and Bartlett Publishers; 2005.

CHAPTER 13

Fifteen- to Eighteen-Month Visit

Susan G. Rains

Bow-legged, 736.42	Rash, 782.1
Developmental delay, 783.4	Separation anxiety, 309.21
Irritability, 799.2	Strabismus, 378.9
No urine output in 12 hours, 788.2	

The toddler is no longer an infant. The world is forever changed by the new ability to *move*, explore, and *control* the environment.

I. NUTRITION

 A. Requirements: Growth slows in toddlerhood, decreasing energy needs to 102 kcal/kg/day, 1.2 g of protein/kg/day, fluids to 115 mL/kg/day; growth may average only 4.5 lbs/year.

  1. Servings should be 1–2 tablespoons of each food for each year of life, or about ¼–⅓ of adult servings.

  2. Milk (whole until age 2) should be limited to < 24 oz/day (16 oz is adequate), due to lack of iron and interference with intake of other nutrients. Calcium requirements are 500 mg/day; vitamin D 200 iu/day.

  3. Limit fat to < 30% of diet; protein 15–20%, carbohydrates to 55%.

  4. Screen for anemia if appropriate: (large amounts of cow's milk/day, especially bottle; diet deficient in other iron-rich foods).

 B. Eating habits.

  1. Understanding toddlers.

   a. Lifelong eating habits, food preferences, and activity level have roots in the early self-feeding experiences of toddlers.

   b. They are able to recognize themselves as separate from others and need to explore independence by testing limits, including feeding limits.

    c. They recognize the newness and difference of foods and also crave the comfort of rituals.

    d. Toddlers often have appetite slumps or are sporadic eaters. If at daycare, they may only eat well at midday with the other children, so the parent rarely sees them eat! Or they may need 2 days to get all of the food groups in!

2. Promoting good habits: Now is the time to help your child develop healthy eating habits and make good choices. As they become more independent:

    a. Be a good role model. Eat meals as a family, without TV, at regularly scheduled times.

    b. Provide nutritious snacks 2–3 times/day, not as a reward; limit sugar.

    c. Allow choices and experimentation; do not force. Offer new foods several times in order to give the child an opportunity to learn to accept and to like it.

    d. Allow toddler to self-feed with hands or utensils. Use cup, not bottle.

    e. Limit fruit juice to 4–6 oz/day.

    f. Serve appropriately sized portions, examples:
- ½ piece of fresh or ¼ cup canned (preferably in its own juice) fruit.
- 2 tablespoons cooked vegetables.
- 1 tablespoon smooth peanut butter (thinly spread on cracker or bread).
- ½ egg, 2 tablespoons ground meat.
- ⅓ cup yogurt, ½ cup milk.
- 1–2 crackers, ¼–½ slice of bread.

3. Safe eating.

    a. Sit when eating; avoid eating in the car.

    b. Avoid screaming, fighting, tickling while eating.

    c. Avoid foods that can cause choking:
- Popcorn.
- Hot dogs, chunks of meat.
- Globs of peanut butter with or without bread.
- Large seeds, nuts, especially peanuts (or foods containing nuts).
- Hard candy, jelly beans.
- Large chunks of raw vegetables or fruits.
- Whole grapes.
- Chewing gum.
- Carrot sticks.

II. ELIMINATION: TOILET TRAINING

A. Attempting to toilet train a child younger than 24 months of age is generally unadvisable; however, most children begin to show some interest between the ages of 18–24 months.
   1. Parents are encouraged to watch the child for signs of readiness:
       a. Child is dry at least 2 hours at a time during the day or is dry after naps.
       b. Bowel movements become regular and predictable.
       c. Facial expressions, posture, or words reveal that the child is about to urinate or have a bowel movement. This is one of the most crucial signs—to be able to tell *prior to the incident*, not just after the event, which is an earlier skill.
       d. Child asks to wear grown-up underwear.
       e. Child asks to use the potty chair or toilet.
       f. Child seems uncomfortable with soiled diapers and wants to be changed.
       g. Child is able to follow simple directions.
       h. Child is able to walk to and from the bathroom and help undress.
   2. Parents are encouraged to introduce children to the "business" of toileting: allow to observe older children/parents when appropriate; obtain potty chair and allow to sit on it; allow to flush the toilet.
   3. Discourage parents from considering toilet training if the child is under stress—should not suppress their desire to use the potty, but should not pressure them in any way to train, nor be surprised if they regress. Stress factors include:
       a. New sibling arriving.
       b. Moving houses.
       c. Family crisis such as death, major illness.
   4. Encourage use of proper names for body parts and for products of elimination. Without making bowel movements sound "dirty" or "nasty," teach children that we do not play with feces.
   5. Pick a potty chair that offers foot support either in the chair itself or because it is low to the floor. Read books about pottying together with the child.
   6. Try to make pottying routine. Everyone generally goes first thing in the morning, before bed, before bath, after meals. Try for a few minutes, but don't fight about it as that undoubtedly will hinder the process.
   7. Positive reinforcement and sensing the child's readiness and pace of learning are essential for success.

III. SLEEP

A. Requirements.
   1. Averages 12 hours total/day.
   2. One to two naps/day; may have difficulty combining morning and afternoon naps.
B. Difficulty with sleep.
   1. Common, especially going to sleep and falling asleep.
   2. May be due to separation anxiety and independence issues.
C. Strategies to assist sleep.
   1. Bedtime rituals: standard sleep time, snack, quiet activity.
   2. Utilizing transitional objects such as special toy, blanket.
   3. Place child in bed while *awake*.
   4. Check on child at progressively longer intervals.
   5. Comfort, but do not feed, rock, place in bed with parent.
   6. Ideally, institute above strategies prior to child being able to climb out of crib.

IV. GROWTH AND DEVELOPMENT

A. Physical growth slows.
   1. Average increases in second year of life: 5 lbs, height 3″, OFC 1″.
   2. Anterior fontanel closes by 18 months.
   3. Head is in smaller proportion to the body.
   4. Physique duck-like: lordotic, pot-bellied, bow-legged.
   5. Vision binocular (true strabismus should be referred).
   6. 14 teeth averaged by 18 months.
   7. Immune system much better developed, but passive immunities from mother gone (especially if not breastfed) and just beginning increased exposure to antigens in environment.
B. Development.
   1. Physical. Utilizing newly developed locomotion skills and wanting to control the environment. Toddlers push and carry large objects; put themselves into spaces such as boxes, cabinets, and under tables; delight in repetitive throwing and retrieving; scribbling. Handedness is established.
   2. Speech. By 18 months understands much of language spoken to him, but commands very few words. Largest jump in language is in second half of second year.

3. Emotional/social. Toddlers strive for independence, i.e., autonomy, and are looking for admiration and positive reinforcement of newly found skills. Still experience dependency needs (separation anxiety) during this quest. Beginning body image development. Negativism is a part of individualization. May be becoming aware of gender.

4. Cognitive (intellectual). Toddlers are beginning to work on causality with an increase in physical abilities and memory development. Starting to see objects symbolically. Imagination begins.

   Note: Early signs of autism spectrum disorder (ASD), including atypical development in socialization and communication, are now detected by pediatric providers in children as young as 18 months. Consistently, those signs include decreases in frequency of gaze to the examiner's face, social smiles, and vocalizations to others.

C. Developmental milestones.

1. By 15 months: says 3–6 words; can point to a body part; understands simple commands; walks well; stoops; climbs stairs; stacks two blocks; feeds self with fingers; drinks from a cup; listens to a story; tells what he wants by pulling, pointing, or grunting.

2. By 18 months: Walks backwards; throws ball; says 15–20 words; imitates words; uses two-word phrases; pulls a toy along the ground; stacks three blocks; uses a spoon and cup; listens to a story, looking at pictures and naming objects; shows affection; kisses; follows simple directions; points to some body parts; scribbles.

D. Developmental delay—possible referral if not present by 18 months:

1. Walks upstairs with assistance.
2. Self-feeds with spoon at times.
3. Mimics actions of others.
4. Uses at least 6 words.

V. SOCIAL

A. Growth, development, and socialization of the child are demonstrated in play activities. The toddler progresses from the sensorimotor play of infancy to parallel play, incorporating imitation, fine and gross motor skills, and new language.

B. Appropriate toys for the toddler are: swing sets, sandboxes, play kitchens, play tools, musical and "talking" toys (especially interactive ones), riding toys (especially without pedals), push toys, balls, containers, telephones, mirrors, dolls and puppets, large crayons, and books. (Contact Reach Out and Read for information in setting up a literacy promotion program in clinics and offices: http://www.reachoutandread.org.)

C. The toddler's new mobility and drive for autonomy make discipline a new challenge for the parent and caregiver. Appropriate discipline guidelines for the toddler include offering choices when available, including following a "no" with a "yes;" keeping rules simple and few; removing objects about which there is constant disagreement; "catching the child being good;" and rewarding positive behaviors with verbal praise and physical affection. Time-out is not appropriate until 2.5–3 years.

D. Parents should be encouraged to help the child learn to express emotions such as joy, fear, anger, sadness, and frustration.

E. Dealing with temper tantrums.

1. Tantrums are a frequent occurrence in toddlers as the young child begins to establish independence and easily becomes frustrated in doing so. He also often does not have his every need met immediately (hunger and fatigue) and is even told "no" on occasion!

2. Parents should: Attend to hunger and sleep needs if possible to help allay underlying causes; stay calm, firm, and consistent; help allay frustrations by helping the child do/learn whatever it is that is frustrating them; distract the child by offering an alternate activity; quietly walk away.

3. Time out can be used with a toddler. One minute per year of age is recommended for time out. This may be too long for a toddler, however, and the adult may need to help them physically (and calmly) stay in time out, again, keeping all conversation to a minimum, to avoid reinforcing negative behavior by giving it attention. Many children quickly learn that they are able to acquire a parent's one-on-one attention with negative behavior, and often do not care if it is negative attention.

4. Do praise and give reinforcement for positive behaviors such as tantrums ceasing. Give choices if possible.

5. Spanking has no place in the discipline (which means teaching) of children. When spanking and hitting are used by parents, children often learn to use physical force to express anger and deal with conflict.

6. Signs of abnormal behaviors may include: Self-injurious behavior during a tantrum, consistent aggressive behavior toward others or destructive behavior toward objects > 50% of the time during a tantrum, high frequency of tantrums (> 5/day or > 10–20/month), tantrums > 25 minutes.

VI. SAFETY

A. Toddlers are at increased risk for injury due to increased locomotion and primitive cognition. Leading causes of death and injury and prevention strategies are listed.

B. Motor vehicles.
   1. Use federally approved car seat in backseat of vehicle. May face forward if older than 1 year and > 20 lbs. Child safety seat inspection: 1-866-SEAT-CHECK; seatcheck.org.
   2. Use bike helmet.
   3. Teach children pedestrian/vehicle safety.
   4. Never allow toddlers to play alone outside.

C. Poisoning.
   1. Use childproof caps on medications; keep medications and household poisons (including plants) out of reach or better locked.
   2. Have poison control number readily available for all caregivers. 1-800-222-1222. Never tell children medication is candy.
   3. Screen for lead risk.

D. Burns.
   1. Use caution in kitchen with young children present.
   2. Turn handles of cooking utensils away from outer edge of stove.
   3. Adjust hot water to 120°F.
   4. Keep matches/candles out of reach.
   5. Use sunscreen when children are exposed to sunlight.
   6. Keep sockets covered and cords out of sight.
   7. Have working smoke detector on every floor of the house.

E. Drowning.
   1. Supervise closely near any water, including buckets.
   2. Fence swimming pools.
   3. Close bathroom doors and put lid down on toilet.
   4. Utilize life preservers in addition to above.

F. Choking and suffocation.
   1. Do not give danger foods listed in nutrition section (including nuts, hot dogs, gum, hard candy).
   2. Only allow play with age-appropriate items (no small pieces).
   3. Discard old appliances/furniture or remove doors.
   4. Keep automatic garage door opener inaccessible.
   5. Select safe toy chests without heavy, hinged lid.

G. Falls.
   1. Confine play in fenced areas.
   2. Supervise all climbing play.
   3. Place gates at top and bottom of stairs.
   4. Lock windows, screens, doors.
   5. Keep crib rails up and mattress at lowest level.
   6. Keep bumper pads and large stuffed animals out of crib or playpen (child may climb on top).
   7. Dress in safe clothing that will not catch or drag.
H. Other injuries.
   1. Never leave children alone in a car or at home.
   2. Do not allow play near any machinery.
   3. Do not allow running with sharp objects, or with anything in the mouth.
   4. Teach children to avoid strange animals, especially ones that are eating.
   5. Avoid personalized clothing in a public place.
   6. Use safety glass and decals on large windows/doors.
   7. Remove guns from house.

VII. IMMUNIZATIONS

A. HIB #4 (if not previously given).
B. PCV #4.
C. IPV #3.
D. DTaP #4.
E. HepB #3 (if not previously given).
F. MMR #1 (if not previously given; may see moved to 15 months to increase immunogenicity).
G. Varivax (if not previously given; may see moved to 15 months to increase immunogenicity).
H. Influenza seasonally.

VIII. OTHER SCREENINGS IF RISK ASSESSMENT INDICATES

A. Dental (ensure fluoride source).
B. B/P: if high risk history.

C. Vision: prematurity < 32 weeks, family history of ophthalmologic problems (other than acuity).
D. Hearing: caregiver concern, postnatal infection, head trauma, family history, certain syndromes associated with hearing loss.
E. TB: exposure, born outside United States, HIV associated.

IX. ANTICIPATORY GUIDANCE

A. Primary responsibility of the PNP is to assist the parent in understanding and parenting this emerging person—the toddler—and his thoughts, behaviors, and needs, as well as attending to the parent's needs.
B. Social competence.
   1. Give individual attention, create opportunities for exploration and physical action.
   2. Encourage self-care, self-expression, choices.
   3. Limit number of rules, but consistently enforce them.
   4. Suggest acceptable alternatives.
   5. Keep discipline brief.
   6. Allow assertiveness within limits, but no hitting, biting, or aggressive behavior.
   7. Reassure once negative behavior has stopped.
   8. Delay toilet training.
   9. Expect genital curiosity.
C. Family relationships.
   1. Parent needs to take time for himself or herself and with partner.
   2. Pick up toddler, hold, cuddle, show affection.
   3. Listen, show respect and interest in activities.
   4. Encourage all family members to spend time playing with toddler.
   5. Help child express emotions.
   6. Keep family outings short.
   7. Do not expect child to share all toys.
   8. Help siblings resolve conflicts. Allow older children own space/things.
   9. Serve as role model for healthy habits and care.
D. Health promotion.
   1. Nutrition.
      a. Eat meals as family.
      b. Allow toddler to self-feed with hands and utensils and drink from cup, not bottle.

      c. Provide healthy choices, allow experimentation, and do not force eating.

      d. Give two to three snacks/day, not as a reward; limit sugar.

      e. Avoid choking foods.

  2. Oral health.

      a. Never put to bed with a bottle.

      b. Brush teeth (allow imitation, but parent must do the job well).

      c. Investigate level of fluoride in child's water.

      d. Encourage making appointment with dentist.

  3. Injury prevention (expanded list in safety section).

      a. Maintain smoke-free environment.

      b. Check smoke and carbon monoxide detectors.

      c. Check car seat use.

      d. Reexamine home to ensure it is childproof.

      e. Supervise toddler closely, especially near dogs, lawnmowers, streets, and driveways.

      f. Ensure water safety.

      g. Use sunscreen.

      h. Discuss first-aid procedures.

E. Community interaction.

  1. Assess needs of the family for appropriate referrals: financial assistance, Medicaid, housing, transportation.

  2. Refer child for appropriate developmental, physical, behavioral problems.

  3. Refer parent to support group if appropriate.

  4. Review childcare.

  5. Maintain community involvement by attending local activities.

BIBLIOGRAPHY

American Academy of Pediatrics Committee on Injury, Violence, and Poison Prevention. Poison treatment in the home. *Pediatrics*. 2003; 112:1182–1185.

American Heart Association. Dietary recommendations for children and adolescents: a guide for practitioners. *Pediatrics*. 2006;117(2):544–559.

Belden AC, Thomas NR, Luby JL. Temper tantrums in healthy versus depressed and disruptive preschoolers: Defining tantrum behaviors associated with clinical problems. *J Pediatrics*. 2008; 152:117.

Burns C, Brady M, Dunn A, et al. *Pediatric Primary Care*. 3rd ed. Philadelphia, PA: W.B. Saunders; 2004.

Centers for Disease Control and Prevention. Recommended childhood and adolescent immunization schedule. *Morb Mortal Weekly Rep*. 2003; 52:Q1–4.

Fox J, et al. *Primary Health Care of Children*. St. Louis: Mosby; 1997.

Gottesman MM. Nurturing the social and emotional development of children, a.k.a. discipline. *J Pediatr Health Care*. 2000;14:81–84.

Gottesman MM. Helping toddlers eat well. *J Pediatr Health Care*. 2002;16:92–96.

Green M, Haggerty R, Weitzman M, et al. *Ambulatory Pediatrics*. 5th ed. Philadelphia, PA: W.B. Saunders; 1999.

Haslam R. Screening scheme for developmental delay. In Behrman RE, Kliegman R, Jenson H, et al.: *Nelson Textbook of Pediatrics*. 17th ed. Philadelphia, PA: W.B. Saunders; 2004.

"HEAT: Early Childhood Parent Tips," Healthy Eating and Activity Together. Cherry Hill, NJ: National Association of Pediatric Nurse Practitioners and The Napnap Foundation. 2007.

Howell, DM. et al. Toilet training. *Pediatrics in Review*. 2010;31 262–263.

Joseph J, Hagan MD, eds. *Bright Futures: Guidelines for Health Supervision of Infants, Children, and Adolescents*. 3rd ed. Elk Grove, IL: American Academy Of Pediatrics; 2010.

Ozonoff S, et al. A prospective study of the emergence of early behavioral signs of autism. *J Am Acad Child Adolesc Psychiatry*. 2010;49:256.

Peterson S, Siquam-Grant M. Impact of adopting lower fat food choices on nutrient intake of American children. *Pediatrics*. 1997;100:e4.

Slade E, Winslow L. Spanking in early childhood and later behavior problems: a prospective study of infants and young toddlers. *Pediatrics*. 2004;113(5):1321–1330.

Vazquez M, LaRussa P, Gershon A, et al. Effectiveness over time of varicella vaccine. *JAMA*. 2004;291: 851–855.

Wardle J, Guthrie C, Sanderson S, et al. Food and activity preferences in children of lean and obese parents. *Intl J Obes Relat Metab Disord*. 2001;25:971–977.

.

CHAPTER 14

Two-Year Visit

Frances K. Porcher

Breathing difficulties, 786.09	Rashes, 782.1
Fever, 780.6	Seizures, 780.39
No urine output in 12 hours, 788.2	Temper tantrums, 312.1

I. GENERAL IMPRESSION

    A. Two-year old is very active, has good vocabulary, and is integral part of family.

II. NUTRITION

    A. Quadruples birth weight by age 2 years.

    B. Average 2-year-old weighs 12.5–13.5 kg (26–28 lbs), is 85–90 cm (34–35 in.) tall, has head circumference of 48–50 cm (19–19.5 in.).

    C. Requires approximately 102 kcal/kg.

    D. Needs approximately 1.2 g/kg of protein, 500–800 mg of calcium, 10 mg iron.

    E. Fluoride supplement is necessary if water supply contains < 0.3 ppm fluoridation (see Appendix B).

    F. Requires 2–3 servings of protein, 2–4 servings of fruit, 3–5 servings of vegetables, 6–11 servings of grains, and 2 servings of milk each day.

    G. Limit juice to 4–6 oz/day. Offer skim, 1%, 2% milk versus whole milk.

    H. Offer 5–6 smaller nutritious meals or snacks each day.

    I. Start limiting fat intake to ≈ 30% of daily calories.

    J. Child's serving is about ⅔ of a standard adult serving.

    K. Needs structured mealtime environment.

    L. Has unpredictable eating habits (likes one food one day but not next day).

    M. Usually eats only 1–2 foods at meal.

    N. Feeds self, loves finger foods.

    O. Complete set of 20 primary teeth (second molars may not erupt until age 3 years).

    P. Assess child's risk for hyperlipidemia.

III. ELIMINATION

A. Regular elimination pattern is usually established with soft, formed stool daily or every other day and several urinations/day.
B. Toilet training is major developmental task between ages 2 ½ and 3 ½ years.
C. Ready for toilet training if bowel movements are regular, child interested in toileting.

IV. SLEEP

A. Should be able to sleep all night and maintain one nap/day.
B. Important to have pleasant bedtime routine.
C. Not uncommon to experience nighttime sleep awakenings, bedtime difficulties.
D. May sleep in crib or small bed depending on child's size, climbing skills.

V. GROWTH AND DEVELOPMENT

A. Age of autonomy, egocentrism, negativism.
B. Gains 4.5–6.6 lbs and 2.5–3.5 in./year from ages 2–5 years.
C. Gross motor: runs without falling; kicks large ball; jumps; walks up/down stairs one step at a time.
D. Fine motor: stacks 5–6 blocks; makes/imitates horizontal/circular strokes with crayon/large pencil; manipulates/solves single-piece puzzle; can unravel, undo, untie.
E. Language: 50% of speech is understandable by stranger; has at least a 20-word vocabulary; uses 2-word phrases; understands more than says; understands and uses "I" and "you"; clearly verbalizes wants; follows 2-step commands.
F. Fears bodily harm (limit intrusive procedures, approaches).
G. Increasingly independent, loves to explore.
H. Negativity, temper tantrums often become an issue (hence, the "terrible twos").
I. Time-out measures (no longer than 2 minutes/episode) recommended rather than hitting or spanking for discipline.
J. Consistency with discipline measures important (discipline for same behavior tomorrow as today).
K. Lots of love, reassurance needed.

VI. SOCIAL DEVELOPMENT

A. Increasingly independent, curious (exploring, climbing, hiding).
B. Active and delightful but testy and frustrating at times as child learns to become social.
C. Frustration manifested as temper tantrums.
D. Differentiates self from others but still needs frequent parental reassurance.
E. Common to experience stranger anxiety (will hide head in parent's arms/ behind legs).
F. Engages in parallel play (plays alongside peers, not with them).
G. Imitates adult activities/tasks (e.g., sweeping, dusting, shaving, combing hair).
H. Often develops fears (e.g., fear of going down toilet with flushing).
I. Needs positive behavior reinforced frequently (praise good behaviors).

VII. IMMUNIZATIONS (SEE APPENDIX A)

A. Bring up to date.
B. Consider varicella vaccine if no reliable history of disease or if not previously given.
C. Consider hepatitis A vaccine if indicated by geographical area of residence.
D. Consider tuberculin skin test (PPD) if meets risk criteria.

VIII. SAFETY

A. Install and periodically check smoke alarms.
B. Ensure crib slats are no more than 2 3/8 in. apart.
C. Avoid crib mobiles due to risk of strangulation or choking.
D. With small bed, ensure mattress is close to floor to minimize injury if child falls out of bed.
E. Encourage use of potty chair that sits directly on floor rather than toilet.
F. Remove dangling objects such as blind cords, curtain draws.
G. Supervise play and do not allow toys with small or sharp parts.
H. Supervise eating: Do not allow foods that may lead to choking (popcorn, peanuts, marshmallows, wieners, raw vegetables).
I. Use childproof lids on all medications; store medications in locked cabinet.
J. Keep household cleaning products out of reach.
K. Use gates and fences where appropriate to prevent falls.

L. Supervise in kitchen (turn pot handles away from edge of stove, store knives out of sight).

M. Supervise around water; set hot water thermostat to < 120°F (48.9°C).

N. Use child-approved sunscreen with at least SPF 15.

O. Use child safety seats approved for child's weight at all times in motor vehicles. (If weighs at least 20 lbs, use forward-facing car seat in middle of backseat; never place car seat in front seat of vehicle with a passenger airbag.)

P. Teach stranger safety.

IX. ANTICIPATORY GUIDANCE

A. Nutrition.
   1. Will eat variety of all food groups. Will eat larger servings.
   2. Still likes finger foods, but can use child-sized fork, spoon.
   3. Continues to drink skim, 1%, 2% milk (no more than 2–3 cups/day). Avoid flavored milk and soda.
   4. Encourage to drink water especially if playing outside in heat.
   5. Encourage to wash hands before eating.
   6. Brushes teeth with fluoridated toothpaste and parents' assistance.
   7. Needs dental check up.

B. Elimination.
   1. Daytime and nighttime bowel movement control established by age 3 years.
   2. Daytime urine control established by age 3 years. May still experience nighttime urination.
   3. Needs to be encouraged to wash hands after toileting and blowing nose.

C. Sleep.
   1. Continues to need regular bedtime routine.
   2. Needs 10–12 hours of sleep at night (does usually awaken).
   3. Usually continues to have one daytime nap.
   4. Should sleep in own bed.
   5. May experience nightmares.

D. Growth and development.
   1. Rate of growth slowing down.
   2. Gross motor: jumps in place, kicks ball, throws ball overhand, rides tricycle, climbs everything.
   3. Fine motor: copies circle and cross, dresses self, feeds self using small fork, washes and dries hands, can put on T-shirt, may be able to dress self without help.

4. Language: at least 50% of speech is understandable, uses sentences, can carry on a conversation of 2–3 sentences, uses prepositions, may use adjectives, may be able to identify 4 colors, identifies friend by naming, identifies 4 pictures by naming, knows own name, age, gender.

E. Social.
   1. Parallel play still prevails; unlikely to share toys.
   2. Should not view more than 1 hour television/video per day.
   3. Needs daily physical activities (outdoors if possible).
   4. Curious about body parts, may start exploring (use correct terms for body parts).
   5. Needs positive reinforcement of good behaviors.

F. Safety.
   1. Needs supervision while playing, eating, when around water.
   2. Continues to need child safety seat or restraint appropriate to child's weight.
   3. May be able to learn own telephone number.

G. Immunizations: if current, should not need any until age 4 years.

H. When to call healthcare provider:
   1. Breathing difficulties.
   2. Seizures.
   3. No urine output in 12 hours.
   4. Rashes.
   5. Fever.
   6. Concerns.

I. Sibling rivalry.
   1. Defined as jealousy that develops between brothers and sisters as they compete for parental time, attention, love, and approval.
   2. Often occurs following arrival of second child in family.
   3. Older child often becomes aggressive, acts out, or regresses.
   4. Prevention is key. Discuss new baby during pregnancy, allow firstborn to help make decisions, including preparations for new baby, move older child to new bed months before arrival of new baby.
   5. After baby arrives, spend one-on-one time with older child, listen to how older child feels, let child know they are special, try not to compare two siblings, and do not play favorites.
   6. Passive noninterventions recommended for minor squabbles between older siblings such as ignoring the conflict or allowing children to resolve the conflict themselves.
   7. Encouraging articulation of disagreements recommended for more significant conflicts in older children such as allowing siblings to express emotions and problem solve with parental support.

8. Parental intervention recommended in situations involving physical or verbal abuse—do not allow older sibling to hit new baby; avoid yelling; separate children if necessary and discuss actions after everyone has calmed down.

BIBLIOGRAPHY

Anderson, JE Sibling rivalry: When the family circle becomes a boxing ring. *Contemporary Pediatrics.* 2006; 23:2.

Hagan JF, Shaw JS, Duncan P, eds. *Bright Futures: Guidelines for Health Supervision of Infants, Children, and Adolescents.* 3rd ed. Elk Grove Village, IL: American Academy of Pediatrics; 2008.

Story M, Holt K, Sofka D, eds. *Bright Futures in Practice: Nutrition.* 2nd ed. Arlington, VA: National Center for Education in Maternal and Child Health; 2002.

CHAPTER 15

Three-Year Visit (Preschool)

Betsy Atkinson Joyce

Night terrors, 307.46

Nightmares, 307.47

I. GENERAL IMPRESSION

A. Preschooler can behave one moment and want to please the parent, but can also be unreasonable and resistant to being examined.
B. Pay attention to evidence of tooth cavities, eye alignment, evidence of bruising or other injuries that may indicate neglect, inadequate supervision, or abuse.

II. NUTRITION

A. Needs 1000–1100 calories/day or 100 kcal/kg/day.
B. Three small meals, 2 snacks, 16–24 oz of milk.
C. Seven grains, 3 vegetables, 2 fruits, 2 meats.
D. Eats with a fork or spoon.

III. ELIMINATION

A. Toilet trained for daytime, occasional accidents.
B. Regular pattern for bowel movements.

IV. SLEEP

A. Requires 10–12 hours of sleep a night.
B. One nap/day (usually).
C. Arouses several times a night.
D. May have night terrors or nightmares.

1. Night terrors: occur early after going to bed.
   a. Partial arousal from very deep sleep, screams, thrashes during the terror, returns to sleep without fully awakening.
   b. Will have no memory of incident in morning.
2. Nightmares: occur usually during the second half of night.
   a. Scary dream followed by complete awakening, crying and fearful after awakening; parent should reassure child.
   b. May have trouble falling back to sleep.
   c. Remembers and may talk about it in the morning.

V. GROWTH AND DEVELOPMENT

A. Continues to follow individual growth chart curve.
B. Pelvis straightens.
C. Graceful and agile with good posture.
D. Physical.
   1. Height: grows 2–4 in./year.
   2. Weight: gains 4–6 lbs.
   3. Head: grows about 1 in./year.
   4. Blood pressure averages 100/60.
   5. Heart rate range is 73–137.
   6. Respiratory rate approximately 22–25.
   7. Twenty primary teeth; growth is mainly under the gums.
E. Gross motor.
   1. Alternates feet when going up stairs.
   2. Rides tricycle.
   3. Dresses self, may need help with buttons.
   4. Puts on shoes.
   5. Climbs, jumps, hops.
F. Fine motor.
   1. Holds crayon with fingers.
   2. Copies circle and cross.
   3. Draws a person with two body parts.
G. Language.
   1. Approximately 900 words by age 3; up to 1500 by age 4.
   2. 85–90 of speech understandable by people outside the family.
   3. Knows name, gender, age.
   4. Longer sentences; puts 2–3 sentences together.
   5. Uses plurals, pronouns, some prepositions (under, on, in, out).

6. Understands concepts of big/little, up/down.
7. Can tell you some colors
8. Can name a friend

VI. SOCIAL DEVELOPMENT

A. Can separate easily from parents if they want to.
B. Can take turns.
C. Helps with simple chores.
D. Needs other children to play with in order to learn socialization.
E. Discipline method: continue with time out.

VII. IMMUNIZATIONS (SEE APPENDIX A)

A. No scheduled immunizations at this visit.
B. Check for currency, only need if immunizations were delayed or new vaccines have come out since 2.5-year visit.

VIII. SAFETY/ANTICIPATORY GUIDANCE

A. Share meals as family if possible, but otherwise child should eat first and get down from table.
B. Do not get in food fights. Offer food; if does not eat, child gets down and no food or milk until next meal.
C. Improve (if necessary) nutritional quality of meals and snacks; limit fast food to less than once a week.
D. Promote toilet training if not already accomplished.
E. Limit TV viewing to 1–2 hours/day.
F. Promote active play. Indoor: have imagination station with safe, active toys; outdoor: play with balls, jump ropes, games, etc.
G. Consistent discipline: use as a way to learn rules, not just punishment; set limits, because if child knows limits, she/he can relax.
H. Find ways to praise child.
I. Encourage choices; link with consequences.
J. Realize need for constant vigilance, supervision, patience.
K. Safety-proof house (if not already done); reinforce safety issues.
L. Use car seat. Continue to keep in backseat of car.

   M. Practice water safety.

   N. Use sunscreen of SPF 15 or higher.

   O. Wear helmet when riding tricycles, scooters, or other toys with wheels.

   P. Teach gun safety. Keep guns out of reach, locked, unloaded. Store ammunition and guns separately.

   Q. Teach about "good touch/bad touch."

   R. Promote dental health; visits to the dentist and brushing 2 times a day.

BIBLIOGRAPHY

Berkowitz, CD. *Berkowitz's Pediatrics: A Primary Care Approach.* 3rd ed. Elk Grove Village, IL: American Academy of Pediatrics; 2008.

Burns CE, Brady MA, Dunn AM, et al., eds. *Pediatric Primary Care.* 4th ed. Philadelphia, PA: Elsevier Health Sciences; 2008.

Dixon SD, Stein MT. *Encounters with Children: Pediatric Behavior and Development.* St. Louis, MO: Mosby; 2006.

Hagan JF, Shaw JS, Duncan P, eds. *Bright Futures: Guidelines for Health Supervision of Infants, Children, and Adolescents.* 3rd ed. Elk Grove Village, IL: American Academy of Pediatrics; 2008.

Kleinman RE, ed. *Pediatric Nutrition Handbook.* 6th ed. Elk Grove Village, IL: American Academy of Pediatrics; 2009.

Polen EU, Taylor DR. *Journey Across the Life Span: Human Development and Health Promotion.* Philadelphia: F.A. Davis; 2007.

Puckett, MB. et al. *The Young Child: Development from Prebirth Through Age Eight.* 5th ed. Upper Saddle River, NJ: Prentice Hall; 2008.

CHAPTER 16

Six-Year Visit (School Readiness)

Pamela Meador Nickell

ADD, 314	Night terrors, 307.46
ADHD, 314.01	Nightmares, 307.47
Behavioral problems, 312.9	School phobia, 300.23
Bowel incontinence, 787.6	Urinary incontinence, 788.39
Emotional immaturity, 300.9	

I. GENERAL IMPRESSION

A. Six-year old will be attending school perhaps for first time and is quite excited about it. The 6-year old is becoming much more independent.

II. NUTRITION

A. Caloric and nutrient needs.
   1. 90 kcal/kg/day divided into three meals with two nutritious snacks.
   2. Limit junk food, nonnutritious foods.
   3. Refer to My Plate for serving size, food group recommendations (see Appendix E).
   4. Encourage family meals as often as possible.
B. Oral hygiene.
   1. Semiannual dental visits.
   2. Regular tooth brushing twice/day.
   3. Fluoride supplement in diet or drinking water (see Appendix B).
   4. Discourage thumb sucking.

III. ELIMINATION

A. Most 6-year olds are toilet trained but may have occasional accidents.

    B. Frequency of bowel movements varies. Obtain parental input for what is normal for child; 1–3 times/day to 1 time every 2–3 days is acceptable.

    C. Normal urine volume should be similar to adult: 650–1500 mL/day.

    D. Urination frequency approximately 5–6 times/day.

    E. Approximately 5–7% have problematic enuresis.

    F. Occasional incontinence due to miscues/deep sleep not uncommon.

IV. SLEEP

    A. 8–12 hours/night.

    B. Encourage consistent bedtime routine.

    C. Occasional nightmares are normal.

    D. Night terrors/sleepwalking may emerge.

V. GROWTH AND DEVELOPMENT

    A. Average weight gain/year: 1.8–2.7 kg (4–6 lbs) for both boys and girls.

    B. Average linear growth/year: 5 cm for both boys and girls.

    C. Well-established vocabulary.

    D. Can follow three-step directions.

    E. Moving from magical thinking to concrete operations.

    F. Mastered skills:

        1. Personal.

            a. Independent in dressing, hygiene; feeds self, monitoring only as needed.

            b. Can recite address, phone number.

        2. Fine motor.

            a. Can draw/copy shapes.

            b. Can draw a man with 6 parts.

            c. Can print some letters, numbers.

        3. Language.

            a. Can articulate needs but semantics may be incorrect.

            b. Recognizes most letters of alphabet.

            c. Can define at least 7 words.

            d. Can identify some opposites.

        4. Gross motor.

            a. Can balance on each foot for 6 seconds.

            b. Can heel–toe walk forward and backward.

            c. Rides tricycle without problems.

VI. SOCIAL DEVELOPMENT

   A. The child is beginning to move from family relationships as primary focus to peer relationships as primary focus.

   B. Continues to use play to develop skills, competencies, and learn about his world.

   C. Social cooperation, morality, critical thinking, and self-concept are developing.

   D. Demonstrates cooperative play.

   E. Team/group activities encouraged (arts programs, organized clubs/sports, etc.); regular exercise encouraged.

   F. Making friends is primary social goal; developing "best friends."

   G. Developing conflict resolution skills.

VII. IMMUNIZATIONS (SEE APPENDIX A)

   A. Recommended:
      1. DTaP #5 if not done previously.
      2. IPV #4 if not done previously.
      3. MMR #2 if not done previously.
      4. PPD #1 if not done previously.
      5. Varicella.
      6. Influenza annually.

   B. Catch-up.
      1. Hepatitis B series.
      2. Varicella.
      3. Pneumococcal vaccine.
      4. MMR.
      5. DTaP.

   C. High-risk children.
      1. Influenza (yearly).
      2. Hepatitis A series.
      3. Pneumococcal pneumonia vaccine.
      4. PPD (yearly).
      5. Meningococcal.

VIII. SAFETY

   A. Motor vehicle.
      1. Consistent use of appropriate safety restraints in motor vehicles.

2. Knows appropriate pedestrian safety rules.
3. Riding a motorcycle is discouraged. However, consistent helmet use when passenger on motorcycle.

B. Sports/recreation.
   1. Consistent use of appropriate protective equipment for all activities (biking, rollerblading, sports, boating, etc.).
   2. Ensure appropriate safety instruction provided for all activities.
   3. Obtain swim lessons.
   4. Ensure safety of sports/play areas and proper supervision provided.
   5. Use sunscreen of SPF 15 or higher.
   6. Discourage use of mini-bikes and ATVs.

C. Household.
   1. Never leave child without appropriate supervision.
   2. Teach appliance safety and monitor use.
   3. Teach hazardous materials/medication safety. Keep out of reach and monitor use.
   4. Teach fire safety. Develop family plan.
   5. Teach gun safety. Keep guns out of reach, locked, unloaded. Store ammunition and guns separately.

D. Social.
   1. Teach phone number, address.
   2. Teach use of 911.
   3. Teach stranger safety.
   4. Teach about "good touch/bad touch."

IX. ANTICIPATORY GUIDANCE

A. Preventive care.
   1. Annual physical.
   2. Semiannual dental visits.
   3. Immunizations on schedule.

B. Home.
   1. Establish family rules and remain consistent in enforcement.
   2. Avoid corporal punishment for breaking rules.
   3. Limit TV viewing to 1 hour/day.
   4. Enforce good personal hygiene.
   5. Avoid punishment for urinary or bowel incontinence.
   6. Encourage family meals.
   7. Encourage continued reading to and with child.

8. If parents work, ensure appropriate, safe supervision is provided before and after school.
9. Encourage responsibility for age-appropriate chores.
10. Develop fire safety plan for home.
C. Family/community.
1. Encourage and praise school activity, accomplishments.
2. Encourage socialization with peer groups in organized and unorganized activities.
3. Encourage consistent exercise; ensure proper supervision for all activities.
4. Discourage "hurried child syndrome"; no more than 1–2 activities/week.
5. Reinforce school/bus rules; encourage parents to become actively involved in school/community parent groups.
6. Encourage parents to teach/model moral behavior, good citizenship ("Do unto others as you would have them do unto you.").
D. Safety.
1. Ensure proper motor vehicle restraints consistently used.
2. Encourage swim lessons.
3. Reinforce proper bicycle use, rules, and use of helmet.
4. Reinforce use of proper safety equipment for all activities including sunscreen SPF 15 or higher applied 30 minutes before going outdoors.
5. Reinforce proper pedestrian rules.
6. Reinforce proper gun safety and storing of ammunition separately.
7. Reinforce "good touch/bad touch" concepts.
8. Teach "just say no" concepts.
9. Reinforce how to use telephone to call 911 in an emergency.
10. Ensure child knows address and phone number.
11. Reinforce age-appropriate child-proofing in residence and use of smoke detectors.
12. Reinforce fire safety; ensure family has plan for evacuation.
13. Don't leave child without proper supervision.
14. Discourage mini-bike and ATV use.

X. SCHOOL READINESS

A. Physical readiness.
1. Has met developmental milestones in cognitive, gross and fine motor areas.
2. Cognitive, visual, hearing deficits addressed.

B. Emotional readiness.
   1. Able to separate easily from parent.
   2. Dresses without supervision.
   3. Toilet trained.
   4. Follows instructions.
C. Screening and assessment tools.
   1. Physical exam including full neurologic evaluation.
   2. Vision and hearing screening.
   3. Developmental testing (draw a man and Denver II recommended for ease of administration).
D. Anticipatory guidance.
   1. Encourage and reinforce positive parental attitudes regarding school.
   2. Prepare parent and child for separation, change in routine.
   3. Have parent obtain list of school/classroom rules and review.
   4. Have parent tour school and meet teacher prior to first day of school.
   5. Prepare parent for child's potential fear/anxiety.
   6. Prepare family to advocate for child in positive, supportive manner.
E. Potential concerns.
   1. School phobia.
   2. Lack of expected intellectual ability/progress.
   3. ADD/ADHD.
   4. Emotional immaturity.
   5. Behavioral problems related to classroom.

BIBLIOGRAPHY

Burns CE, et al. *Pediatric Primary Care: A Handbook for Nurse Practitioners.* 4th ed. Philadelphia, PA: W.B. Saunders; 2009.

Dixon SD, Stein MT. *Encounters with Children: Pediatric Behavior and Development.* 4th ed. St. Louis, MO: Mosby; 2006.

Hagan JF, Shaw JS, Duncan P, eds. *Bright Futures: Guidelines for Health Supervision of Infants, Children, and Adolescents.* 3rd ed. Elk Grove Village, IL: American Academy of Pediatrics; 2008.

Pulcini J. Assessing school readiness. In: Fox J, ed. *Primary Health Care of Infants, Children and Adolescents.* 2nd ed. St. Louis: Mosby; 2002.

Seven- to Ten-Year Visit (School Age)

Elizabeth Godfrey Terry

Appendicitis, 541	Myopia, 367.1
Asthma, 493.9	Night terrors, 307.46
Attention deficit hyperactivity disorder, 314.01	Nightmares, 307.47
Osgood-Schlatter's disease, 732.4	Puberty, V21.1
Breast enlargement, 611.79	Ringworm, 110.9
Chickenpox, 052	Rubella, 056.9
Cystic fibrosis, 277	Scabies, 133
Emotional disturbances, 313.3	School phobia, 300.23
Encopresis, 787.6	Scoliosis, 737.3
Enuresis, 788.3	Separation anxiety, 309.21
Epiphyseal separations, 732.9	Sexual abuse, 995.83
Eruption of a tooth, 520.6	Sickle cell anemia, 282.6
Heart disease, 429.9	Sleep apnea, 780.57
Heart murmurs, 785.2	Sleep disturbances, 780.5
Impetigo, 684	Sleepwalking, 307.46
Learning disorders, 315.2	Substance abuse, 305.9
Legg-Perthes disease, 732.1	Urinary tract infections, 599
Measles, 055.9	Voice change, 784.49
Menstruation, 626.9	Wet dreams, 608.89
Mumps, 072.9	

I. OVERALL IMPRESSION

    A.   Early school agers are in routine of being in school, learning; now gaining skills to get along with many different personalities.

II. NUTRITION

A. Caloric and nutrient needs.
   1. Three full meals and 1–2 snacks a day.
   2. Consumes 1600–2400 calories/day; needs vary depending upon amount of activity and development. Or: female 1200–1600 calories (4–8 years 1200 calories; 9–13 years 1600 calories); male 1400–1800 calories (4–8 years 1400 calories; 9–13 years 1800 calories). Calorie estimates based on a sedentary lifestyle. Increased physical activity will require additional calories: by 0 to 200 kcal/day if moderately physically active and by 200 to 400 kcal/day if very physically active.
   3. Refer to My Plate for serving size, food group recommendations (see Appendix E).
   4. Whole grains preferred over refined-grain products; at least half the grains should be whole grains.
   5. Sweetened beverages and naturally sweet beverages, such as fruit juice, should be limited to 8 to 12 oz/day.
   6. Need at least 800–1200 mg of calcium/day.
   7. Introduce and offer fish regularly, especially oily fish such as salmon, broiled or baked, and sardines. Avoid fish high in mercury content. Remove skin from poultry prior to serving. Offer more meat alternatives, such as legumes (beans) or tofu.
   8. Serve fresh, frozen, or canned vegetables and fruits at every meal.
B. Willing to try variety of foods from major food groups.
C. Appetite varies according to growth, activity.
D. May have big appetite during growth spurt and then cut back.
E. Good internal cues regarding appetite. Parents choose types of food and beverages served and child chooses how much to eat.
F. Beginning steps toward obesity may start if child is not allowed to listen to internal cues.
G. 19.6% of children ages 6–11 are obese. Excess caloric intake and physical inactivity strongly associated with obesity.
H. Consider daily children's multivitamin if child is not consuming enough servings to get essential nutrients.

III. ELIMINATION

A. Enuresis occurs in 10% of 7-year-olds and 5% of 10-year-olds.

1. Children with this condition should receive complete exam to rule out underlying conditions such as urinary tract infections.
2. Children with sleep apnea at greater risk for enuresis.

B. Encopresis affects 1.5% of young school children.

IV. SLEEP

A. Need 10–11 hours/night.
B. Encourage and emphasize need for regular and consistent sleep schedule and bedtime routine.
C. Make bedrooms conducive to sleep—keep TV and computers out of bedroom.
D. Occasional nightmares or sleep disturbances such as night terrors, sleep walking.
E. May have fear of dark or of being alone (separation anxiety).
F. Emotional disturbances such as stress, anxiety, leading to insomnia.
G. Difficult bedtime behavior may develop.
H. Snoring, daytime sleepiness may be symptoms of sleep apnea.

V. GROWTH AND DEVELOPMENT

A. Musculoskeletal.
1. Calculate and plot BMI once a year. BMI between 85th and 95th percentile for age and sex is considered at risk for overweight. Close supervision by healthcare provider may be considered.
2. Development not as rapid.
3. As body size increases, body fat relatively stable, giving slimmer appearance than preschool years.
4. Average height increase: a little over 2 in./year.
5. The closer to puberty, greater the chances for increased growth.
6. Tends to be an increased growth rate between 6 and 8 years of age that may be accompanied by appearance of small amount of pubic hair.
7. If unusually short/tall for age, may need to consider possibility of growth disorder.
8. Appetite tends to vary due to growth fluctuations, but child should not be losing weight.

      9. Orthopedic problems of this age group:
        a. Fractures, sprains, strains.
        b. Epiphyseal separations, dislocations.
        c. Scoliosis.
        d. Avascular necrosing lesions of epiphysis.
           • Legg-Calve-Perthes disease.
           • Osgood-Schlatter disease.
    10. Motor skills improve in strength, balance, coordination.
B. Skin.
    1. Hair may become a little darker, skin becomes more adult like.
    2. Scabies, impetigo, ringworm can be problems at this age.
C. Teeth.
    1. Should be able to brush teeth by themselves, may still require some assistance.
    2. Brush with fluoride toothpaste after each meal but at least twice a day; floss once a day.
    3. Water supply should contain adequate fluoride, if not, consider fluoride supplement (see Appendix B).
    4. Eruption of permanent teeth occurs in order in which primary teeth are lost.
    5. Dental visits twice a year for exams, cleanings.
    6. Sealants as recommended.
    7. Problems with dental decay can peak during these years as well as periodontal diseases, often due to poor hygiene.
D. Eyes: visual acuity of 20/20 although about age 8 may begin to have myopia with no overt signs except school difficulty.
    1. Evaluate regularly for visual acuity and ocular alignment (approximately every 1–2 years) at primary healthcare visits. Screening examinations should be done at routine school checks or after the appearance of symptoms. Screening emphasis should be directed to high-risk children, such as those with positive family history. Any child who does not pass screening test should have an ophthalmological examination.
    2. Children with presumed or diagnosed learning disabilities should undergo a comprehensive pediatric medical eye examination to identify and treat any undiagnosed vision impairment. Referrals should be made for appropriate medical, psychological, and educational evaluation and treatment of the learning disability.
E. Ears: problems decrease due to further development of eustachian tubes and nasopharynx, although ear infections can still be frequent in younger school ager.

1. Consider hearing screening if history of frequent ear infections or concerns about speech development.
F. Throat: tonsillar tissue continues to enlarge, reaching its peak from 8–12 years when it levels off, begins to recess.
G. Immune system: continues to mature; allergic conditions more common.
H. Hematopoietic system: abnormal hemoglobin/hematocrit levels should not be attributed to dietary intake. Etiology should be established for any hemoglobin below 11.5 g.
I. Heart.
   1. Murmurs are often heard in these years.
   2. Any doubt of etiology requires referral to pediatric cardiologist.
   3. Circulation.
      a. Average pulse rate:
         • Age 8: 78.
         • Age 10: 74.
      b. Average blood pressure:
         • Age 8: 105/60.
         • Age 10: 111/66.
      c. Cholesterol screening for children with a family history of high cholesterol or heart disease, whose family history is unknown, or who have other factors for heart disease including obesity, high blood pressure, or diabetes. Screening should take place after age 2 but no later than age 10.
J. Respiration rate.
   1. Age 8: 22 breaths/minute.
   2. Age 10: 20 breaths/minute.
K. Gastrointestinal system.
   1. Liver function is mature but still growing in size.
   2. Appendix: open lumen and increased size increases risk of blockage, inflammatory reaction (appendicitis).
L. Genitourinary system.
   1. Urinary tract infections can be common, especially in girls; often asymptomatic at this age.
M. Nervous system: essentially mature by age 10.
   1. Begins puberty.
      a. Girls.
         • Breast budding can begin as early as age 8; others not until 13, with the average being around age 10.
         • Puberty before age 8: girl should be evaluated for precocious puberty (twice as frequent in females as in males).

- Peak growth period (height, weight, muscle mass, etc.) occurs 1 year after puberty has begun.
- Menstruation usually begins 2 years after onset of puberty, on average just before age 13.

   b. Boys.

- Peak growth period occurs about 2 years after onset of puberty.
- Begin puberty about 1 year later than girls.
- First sign of puberty in boys is enlargement of testes, thinning and reddening of scrotum. This occurs on average at age 11, but may occur anytime between 9 and 14 years of age.
- Puberty before 9: boy should be evaluated for precocious puberty.

  2. Secondary sex characteristics.

   a. Girls.

- Breast enlargement: 8–13 years.
- Axillary hair: 11–13 years.
- Pubic hair: 10–12 years.
- Menarche: 10–16 years.

   b. Boys.

- Genitalia enlargement: 9–13 years.
- Axillary hair: 12–14 years.
- Facial hair: 11–14 years.
- Pubic hair: 12–15 years.

N. Language.

  1. Although better able to express emotions and ideas, may talk in abstract terms without fully comprehending meaning of such speech.

  2. Learning to communicate clearly with friends.

VI. SOCIAL DEVELOPMENT

A. Needs to master balance of feelings in dealing with successes, failures.

  1. Self-concept (body self, social self, cognitive self) affects child's ability to be successful.

B. Successful accomplishments are of high priority for child in order to build positive self-image. Should feel successful with most day-to-day skills, activities, and chores.

C. Making friends is one of most important mid-childhood tasks.

  1. Average number of friends: about five.

  2. Sibling friendships may replace outside friends or need for them.

3. Selects friends of similar temperament, interests.
4. Often focus on "best friend" relationship, which can be more satisfying than large group.
D. Increasingly seeks peer for companionship.
E. Cliques may begin to form.
F. Parents and teachers are important significant others and will influence behavior, self-concept.
   1. Encourage parents to share unscheduled spontaneous time with their child; time to be together, to listen, and to talk.
G. School issues.
   1. School phobia.
   2. Learning disorders.
   3. Attention deficit hyperactivity disorder.
   4. Bullying.
   5. After school care and activities.
   6. Dealing with fears, disappointments, and stress.
   7. Parent–teacher communication.

VII. IMMUNIZATIONS (SEE APPENDIX A)

A. Influenza vaccine.
   1. Annual trivalent seasonal influenza immunization is recommended for all children 6 months of age and older.
   2. Especially recommended for children with high-risk conditions such as asthma, diabetes, or neurological disorders.
   3. Live-attenuated influenza vaccine is acceptable alternative to inactivated influenza vaccine for healthy persons 2–49 years of age.
   4. Children 9 years of age and older need only 1 dose.
   5. Children < 9 years need a minimum of 2 doses of 2009 pandemic H1N1 vaccine. If H1N1 not received during last year's flu season, 2 doses of seasonal influenza vaccine needed this year.
   6. Children < 9 years who have never received the seasonal flu vaccine before will need 2 doses.
   7. Children younger than 9 years who received seasonal flu vaccine before the 2009–2010 flu season need only 1 dose this year if they received at least 1 dose of the H1N1 vaccine last year. They need 2 doses this year if they did not receive at least 1 dose of the H1N1 vaccine last year.
   8. Children < 9 years who received seasonal flu vaccine last year for the first time but only received 1 dose should receive 2 doses this year.

     9. Children younger than 9 years who received a flu vaccine last year, but for whom it is unclear whether it was a seasonal flu vaccine or the H1N1 flu vaccine, should receive 2 doses this year.

   10. Children who need 2 doses should receive the second dose at least 4 weeks after the first dose.

B. Varicella vaccine.

    1. Children ages 7 through 18 years without evidence of immunity should receive 2 doses if not previously vaccinated or the second dose if only 1 dose has been administered.

    2. For children ages 7 through 12 years, minimum interval between doses is 3 months—but accepted as valid if the second dose was given at least 28 days after the first dose.

C. Measles, mumps, rubella (MMR): Children not previously vaccinated should receive 2 doses or the second dose for those who have received only 1 dose, with at least 28 days between doses.

D. Hepatitis A vaccine: recommended for children over 23 months of age who live in areas where vaccination programs target older children or who are at an increased risk for infection or for whom protection is desired; can begin vaccine at any visit with the 2 doses being given at least 6 months apart.

E. Hepatitis B vaccine: The 3-dose series should be given to those not previously vaccinated.

F. Pneumococcal vaccine (PPSV): To be given to children with certain underlying medical conditions, including a cochlear implant. A single revaccination should be given after 5 years to children with functional or anatomic asplenia or an immunocompromising condition.

G. Meningococcal conjugate vaccine (MCV4).

    1. Recommended for children ages 2 through 10 years with persistent complement component deficiency, anatomic or functional asplenia, or certain other conditions placing them at high risk.

    2. Recommended for children previously vaccinated with MCV4 or MPSV4 who remain at increased risk after 3 years (if first dose administered at age 2 through 6 years) or after 5 years (if first dose administered at age 7 years or older).

H. Human papillomavirus vaccine (HPV): May be given in a 3-dose series to males ages 9 through 18 years to reduce their likelihood of acquiring genital warts.

VIII. SAFETY/ANTICIPATORY GUIDANCE

A. Nutrition.
  1. Offer nutrient-dense foods that include a wide variety of fruits, vegetables, whole grains, and nonfat or low-fat dairy foods.
  2. Stress importance of parents being good role models. Child who sees parent enjoying a wide variety of nutritious foods is more likely to want them.
  3. Encourage a healthy breakfast daily.
  4. Encourage reading food labels when shopping especially noting calories from fat, type of fat, sodium, cholesterol, vitamins, minerals, and serving size. Child can help to read the labels.
  5. Encourage family meals at home. Children who eat meals with family at home have a better quality diet.
  6. Offer healthy ways of eating when eating out is necessary and remind parents to be mindful of portion sizes.
  7. Encourage parents to closely supervise but involve child in family food preparation. Children are more likely to eat foods that they help prepare.
  8. Encourage family use of USDA's Food Guide for Kids
  9. Child may need multivitamin if not eating enough to get essential nutrients if an erratic eater or on a highly selective diet. Most healthy children eating well-balanced diet do not require supplementation.
  10. Some children may still be picky eaters at this age so may have to slightly adjust portions or food groups in order ensure adequate intake; may eat more at snack times than at regular meals.
  11. Healthy snacks 1–2 times a day can include:
    a. Fresh, canned, frozen vegetables or fruits. Keep cut-up veggies such as celery sticks, cucumber slices, or broccoli in the refrigerator. Try frozen grapes or bananas for fun treat.
    b. Cold skim or 1% milk with whole-grain sugar-free cereal, peanut butter sandwich, or crackers with hummus.
    c. Fruit smoothie made with fresh fruit, skim milk, ice, and a dash of vanilla or cinnamon.
    d. Non fat or low-fat yogurt or cheese.
    e. Air-popped or unbuttered popcorn.
    f. Baked tortillas or pretzels with salsa.
    g. Chocolate skim milk made at home to control the amount of sugar.
    h. Low-fat frozen yogurt, fruit juice bars (without added sugar).

12. Encourage healthy eating behaviors including no snacking in front of TV. Parents should model these behaviors.

B. Sleep.

1. Stay consistent in routine activities such as daily mealtimes, playtimes, bedtime, wake-up time.

2. Avoid caffeine/other stimulants; limit food, drink before bedtime.

3. An hour or so before bedtime, begin a relaxing routine such as warm bath then a story in quiet bedroom.

4. Bed should only be used for sleeping, not for watching TV or homework. TVs and computers should be kept out of bedrooms.

5. Children who are overtired/have interrupted sleep may be more likely to have sleep disturbances such as night terrors.

C. Growth and development.

1. Musculoskeletal.

a. Need an hour or more of a variety of age-appropriate daily physical activities including team/individual sports, family activities, free play, walking, bicycling, chores, walking up and down stairs. Parents should model, prioritize, and promote regular physical activity.

b. Limit total amount of screen time (TV, computer) to < 2 hours a day.

c. As they approach puberty, children tend to put on a little more weight, which is normal.

d. Increases in BMI percentiles should be discussed with parents but in nonjudgmental, blame-free manner.

e. Because fractures are common in this age group, children should wear appropriate protective sports gear but also consume adequate calcium to decrease risk of fractures.

2. Skin.

a. 30 minutes before going outside, on both sunny and cloudy days, thickly apply broad-spectrum UVA-UVB sunscreen with SPF 15+ to all exposed areas of body, especially ears, nose, face, neck, shoulders, hands, and feet.

b. Suggest using sunscreen or sunblock with zinc oxide or titanium dioxide for areas that easily burn.

c. Reapply sunscreen every 2 hours and after swimming or sweating heavily, regardless of whether sunscreen is waterproof.

d. Use cool, comfortable clothing, especially clothes with a tight weave, to cover the body and protect from the sun.

e. Wear a wide-brimmed hat to shield head, face, ears, and neck.

f. Encourage sun avoidance between 10 a.m. and 4 p.m. when UV rays are the strongest. Seek shelter, shade, or umbrellas when out during those times. Remind that UV rays reflect and bounce back from sand, water, concrete, and snow so even in shade sun protection is needed.

3. Teeth.
   a. Dental visits twice a year for exams, cleaning.
   b. Brush teeth at least twice a day with tartar-control, fluoride toothpaste; floss once a day.
   c. Still may need some help with brushing.
   d. Verify water source for adequate fluoride.
   e. Care of baby teeth as important as permanent teeth. Early loss of baby teeth due to caries or accidents can lead to spacing issues with premature rupture of permanent teeth resulting in orthodontic issues.
   f. Discuss importance of wearing mouth guards, helmets while playing sports.
4. Eyes.
   a. Wear sunglasses with 100% UVA-UVB protection whenever outside, in car.
   b. All youth in organized sports should be encouraged to wear appropriate eye protection and especially when engaged in high-risk sports and activities such as basketball, baseball/softball, lacrosse, hockey, paintball, BB gun, or when around yard debris. Mandatory protective eyewear for athletes who are functionally one-eyed and for athletes whose ophthalmologists recommend eye protection after eye surgery or trauma.
   c. Warn about dangers of fireworks to eyes; enjoy fireworks displays put on by professionals.
5. Puberty.
   a. Encourage honest, age-appropriate discussions about sex with child using accurate terminology and listening carefully to child's questions so parent only gives as much information as child requires.
   b. Concerns of girls about puberty:
      • Menstruation.
      • Breast development.
   c. Concerns of boys about puberty:
      • Voice change.
      • Wet dreams.
      • Involuntary erections.
      • Breast enlargement.
      • One testicle lower than other.
6. Cognitive and social development.
   a. Very sensitive to views of others.

    b. Appreciate having rules.

    c. Begin to have strong internal gauge of right and wrong.

    d. Friendship and teamwork are important parts of this stage of development.

    e. Eager for more independence but frustrated by what they cannot accomplish since they are still in the process of mastering skills. Important to have sense of achievement, accomplishment to build strong self-esteem.

    f. Encourage an appropriately challenging academic schedule and a balance of extracurricular activities. This is determined by child's unique needs, skills, and temperament.

    g. Encourage exploration of activities and interests in a balanced way without the pressure of having to excel in everything.

    h. Encourage parents to promote child activities that are fun, increase self-confidence, and involve friends.

D. Safety.

  1. Auto.

    a. Children should be properly secured at all times while traveling in car.

    b. Children should ride in booster seats until the vehicle safety belts fit correctly, when they are 4 ft 9 in. tall. This may not be until they are 8 to 12 years of age. Can move to safety belt when child can place his/her back firmly against vehicle seat back cushion with knees bent over vehicle seat cushion. Lap belt must fit low and tight across upper thighs. Belt should rest over shoulder and across chest.

    c. Shoulder belt should never be placed under arm or behind child's back.

    d. Children younger than 12 years should never ride in front seat.

    e. Keep all doors locked while in motion.

    f. Never leave young children alone in car.

    g. Children should not ride in truck beds or any other area of vehicle that does not have seat and seat belt.

    h. Children lack judgment, coordination, reflexes to drive other motorized vehicles such as mopeds, snowmobiles, mini-bikes, ATVs.

  2. Bicycle safety. Children who ride bikes should:

    a. Wear helmets at all times. Helmets should meet safety standards of the Consumer Product Safety Commission (CPSC; www.cpsc.gov). Helmets should fit properly; parents may want to bring them in to check for proper fit. Parents should wear helmets as well to serve as a good role model.

    b. Know basic road rules such as obey all traffic signs/lights, stop and look both ways at intersecting points such as driveways/streets, ride in single file or on bike paths, ride in same direction as traffic.
    c. Should not wear loose-fitting clothing, strings, ties that could get caught in bike chain or parts.
    d. Wear shoes with laces tied.
    e. Should not wear earphones while riding.
3. Skateboard safety: children should always wear helmet and never ride near traffic.
4. Water safety.
    a. Never allow child to swim alone or play unsupervised in or by water—even for a moment.
    b. Child should learn to swim and take lessons from qualified instructor.
    c. Backyard swimming pools should be enclosed with high, locked fence on all sides. Fences should be at least 4 ft high on all sides.
    d. Diving should not be allowed until underwater depth has been determined and checked for hazards.
    e. No swimming near boats, fisherman, unsupervised open water.
    f. Children should always wear a life jacket when in a boat.
    g. Parents should know how to perform CPR.
5. Fire and burn accidents.
    a. Install smoke detectors, on all floors and particularly in or near sleeping areas.
    b. Keep fire extinguishers in kitchen, other areas where fire could start.
    c. Have family fire plan in place; practice regular fire drills.
    d. Discourage playing with matches, etc.
    e. To avoid scalding burns from water, heaters should never be set > 120°F (48.9°C).
6. Home alone: most children are not old enough until age 11 or 12. Child should be learning safety, security, emergency guidelines (calling parent, neighbor, 911) in preparation for emergencies or for when the time comes that the child is old enough to be left alone for short times such as after school.
7. Gun safety: guns, ammunition need to be stored and locked separately. Child needs to know to stay away from and alert parent should he encounter a gun at a friend's house or elsewhere.
8. Bullying: children of this age can sometimes be the target of bullies. Child needs to know strategies for dealing with bullying. Strong friendships should be encouraged to avoid being bullied.

9. Sexual abuse.
   a. Most sexual abuse occurs between the ages of 8 and 12.
   b. In 80% of these cases, abuser is known to child.
   c. Reinforce "good touch/bad touch" concepts and awareness of possible scenarios that may occur. Promote abuse-prevention programs at school and encourage parents to listen carefully to child who might have a concern, particularly of a sexual nature.
10. Substance abuse.
    a. Begins with experimentation and casual use, often under peer pressure.
    b. Problem drinking often begins in grade school.
    c. Prevention of substance abuse needs to begin before adolescence.
    d. Secondhand smoke is a serious health hazard for children. Increases risk of developing asthma, bronchitis, middle-ear disease, pneumonia, wheezing and coughing spells, behavioral/cognitive problems.
    e. Children whose parents smoke are more than twice as likely to smoke themselves than are children of nonsmokers.
11. Media.
    a. In addition to < 2 hours of screen time per day and keeping TVs and computers out of bedrooms, remind parents about the importance of careful selection, watching together, and discussing programs their children watch.
    b. Encourage parents to be knowledgeable about online and social media.
    c. Keep computers in a central area of the house where computer activities can be monitored. Parents may want to consider purchasing online programs that allow them to monitor computer activity.
    d. Encourage parents to talk often with their children about online and social media safety and responsibility.
    e. Encourage parents to set a good example by limiting their own viewing time and engaging in other healthy activities.

BIBLIOGRAPHY

American Academy of Ophthalmology. *Policy Statement: Frequency of Ocular Exams.* Revised and approved. November 2009: http://www.aao.org/about/policy/upload/Frequency-of-Ocular-Exams-2009.pdf. Accessed June 4, 2011.

American Association for Pediatric Ophthalmology and Strabismus and the American Academy of Ophthalmology. *Policy statement: Vision Screening for Infants and Children.* Revised and approved, March 2007: http://www.aao.org/one_passthru.cfm?link=URL&target=http://one.aao.org/asset .axd?id=2efe6879-b631-4878-b878-18bc1679114c. Accessed June 4, 2011.

American Academy of Pediatrics and American Academy of Ophthalmology. *Joint Statement: Protective Eyewear for Young Athletes.* Revised and approved October and November 2003: http://www.aao.org/about/policy/upload/Protective-Eyewear-for-Young-Athletes.pdf. Accessed June 4, 2011.

American Academy of Pediatrics. *Policy Statement: Dietary Recommendations for Children and Adolescents: A Guide for Practitioners.* February 2006: http://aappolicy.aappublications.org/cgi/content/full/pediatrics;117/2/544. Accessed June 4, 2011.

American Academy of Pediatrics. *Policy Statement: Prevention of Pediatric Overweight and Obesity.* Reaffirmed October 2006: http://aappolicy.aappublications.org/cgi/content/full/pediatrics;112/2/424. Accessed June 4, 2011.

American Academy of Pediatrics. *Policy Statement: Recommended Childhood and Adolescent Immunization Schedule, United States, January 2010.* http://aapredbook.aappublications.org/resources/IZSchedule7-18yrs.pdf. Accessed June 4, 2011.

American Dietetic Association. Nutrition guidance for healthy children ages 2 to 11 years. *J Am Dietetic Assoc.* 2008;108(6):1038–1047.

American Dietetic Association. Total diet approach to communicating food and nutrition information. *J Am Dietetic Assoc.* 2007;107(7):1224–1232.

Bennett HJ. *Waking Up Dry: A Guide to Overcoming Bedwetting.* Elk Grove Village, IL: American Academy of Pediatrics; 2005.

Brooks LJ, Topol HI. Enuresis in children with sleep apnea. *J Pediatr.* 2003;142(5):515–518.

Council on Communications and Media. Media violence. *Pediatrics.* 2009;124:1495–1503.

Daniels SR, Greer FR, and the Committee on Nutrition. Policy statement on lipid screening and cardiovascular health in childhood. *Pediatrics.* 2008;122(1):198–208.

Dietz WH, ed. *American Academy of Pediatrics Guide to Your Child's Nutrition.* New York, NY: Random House; 1999.

Ginsburg KR, and the Committee on Communications and the Committee on Psychosocial Aspects of Child and Family Health. The importance of play in promoting healthy child development and maintaining strong parent-child bonds. *Pediatrics.* 2007;119:182–191.

National Association for Sport and Physical Education: www.naspeinfo.org.

National Highway Transportation Safety Association: www.nhtsa.dot.gov/Safety/CPS.

National Sleep Foundation: Sleep in America: www.sleepfloundation.org.

Ogden C, Carroll M. *Prevalence of obesity among children and adolescents: United States, trends 1963–1965 through 2007–2008.* Centers for Disease Control and Prevention; 2010: www.cdc.gov/nchs/data/hestat/obesity_child_07_08/obesity_child_07_08.htm. Accessed June 4, 2011.

Schor EL, ed. *American Academy of Pediatrics, Caring For Your School-age Child, Ages Five to Twelve.* New York: Bantam Books; 2004.

CHAPTER 18

Eleven- to Thirteen-Year Visit (Preadolescent)

Mary J. Alvarado and Beth Richardson

Acne, 706.1	HIV, 042
Coronary artery disease, 414	Peripheral vascular disease, 443.9
Depression, 311	Physical abuse, 995.54
Emotional abuse, 995.51	Scoliosis, 737.3
Goiter, 240.9	Sexual abuse, 995.53

I. GENERAL IMPRESSION

    A. Preadolescence is time of rapid change and emotional turbulence.

    B. Need support, understanding, caring from adults in particular, which is not usually what they receive.

II. NUTRITION

    A. Nutritional requirements.

        1. Increased energy and protein requirement due to rapid growth.

        2. Require 2200–3000 calories/day.

        3. To meet increased need, increase milk and dairy products to 4 servings/day, bread group servings to 9 servings/day.

        4. One-fourth of daily calories is typically consumed in snacks; encourage fruit, cheese, milk beverages, raw vegetables, nuts.

        5. Diet should consist of 10–15% protein, 25–30% fat, 50–60% carbohydrates.

        6. Needs 8–15 mg of iron/day; iron is most commonly deficient nutrient.

        7. A well-balanced diet does not require supplementation; irregular eating patterns and/or high-calorie/low-nutrient snacking may lead to deficiencies requiring multivitamin.

  B. Nutritional assessment.
      1. Calculate and plot body mass index (BMI) (see Appendix D).
      2. Evaluate 24-hour recall.
      3. Examine intake, eating patterns; ask about special diets or supplements.
      4. Assess for eating disorders.
      5. Monitor athletes' increased need for calories; advise on appropriate dietary changes.
      6. Provide guidance about nutrition annually.
      7. Refer to nutritionist if indicated.

III. ELIMINATION

  A. Expect consistent pattern of elimination.
  B. Changes may occur with irregular eating patterns, illness, diets, stress, eating disorders.
  C. Check understanding of normal elimination and methods employed to deal with problems.

IV. SLEEP

  A. Question about amount of sleep; at least 8 hours/night.
  B. Age and activity level.
  C. Monitor for any difficulties, ability to cope.
  D. Advise on sleep hygiene if necessary.

V. GROWTH AND DEVELOPMENT

  A. Physical.
      1. Early adolescence is marked by rapid physical change. Tempo of adolescent development is variable and may be influenced by gender, health, socioeconomic status, genetics. Predictable sequence of events occurs over 2–6 years from onset, which on average is age 9–11 for girls and age 10–12 for boys. The preadolescent may prefer to be examined with parent out of the room.
      2. Perform complete physical exam with attention to the following:
         a. Document height, weight, and BMI annually (see Appendix D).
         b. Assess and document Tanner stage of pubertal development annually.

    c. Monitor blood pressure annually.

    d. Screen cholesterol once in this age group if following risk factors exist:
- Parent with serum cholesterol > 240.
- Family history unknown.
- Parent/grandparent with stroke, peripheral vascular disease, coronary artery disease, sudden cardiac death younger than 55 years.

    e. Palpate thyroid gland; goiter may present in this age group.

    f. Examine spine for development/progression of scoliosis during rapid growth.

    g. Assess for presence/severity of acne.

    h. Ask about sexual activity; screen sexually active teens for sexually transmitted infections (STIs), evaluate risk for acquiring HIV.

B. Emotional.

    1. Rapid physical changes of early adolescence lead to increased self-consciousness and focus on external characteristics.

    2. Adolescent feels everyone is looking at him/her and questions if he/she is normal.

    3. Reassure about normal findings in the physical exam.

    4. Explain that each individual progresses through physical changes of adolescence in same sequence but at his/her own pace.

    5. Ask about friends, family, school. Is there a best friend? A supportive adult? Monitor self-esteem.

    6. Ask about moods. Emotional lability is normal. Assess for excessive stress or depression.

    7. Ask about physical, emotional, or sexual abuse.

    8. Discuss safe use of Internet and online social networks. Remind to use caution when sharing personal information, photos, and videos by Internet and phone.

C. Intellectual.

    1. Adolescent begins to transition from concrete to abstract thinking; timing is variable. Some develop higher level thinking in early adolescence, some later or not at all. Individual may be able to think abstractly about algebra but not about decision making regarding risky behaviors. Abstract thinking gives adolescent better ability to reason and see other points of view.

    2. How is school performance? Ask about academic, athletic, personal goals. May still have impractical/unrealistic ideas.

    3. What are responsibilities at home? Early adolescents should be encouraged to take on new responsibilities with supervision.

    4. Ask about extracurricular activities. Encourage involvement in groups that interest him/her. Increasing communication skills help with

problem solving. Group discussions help adolescents learn to express themselves.

5. Advise to keep TV viewing, computer time, video games to < 2 hours/day. These activities interfere with opportunities to engage in communication with peers, family.

VI. SOCIAL DEVELOPMENT

A. Early adolescents begin to develop greater independence from parents, family.

B. Establishment of reliable relationships with peers, other adults is important developmental task.

C. New peer group, which is usually same sex, provides opportunity to test, evaluate values/behaviors. It allows for sense of belonging, self-worth and affords opportunity to build social competence.

D. Recognize that hairstyles, clothing, music preferences, piercing are expressions of individuality; often mirror others in peer group.

E. Preoccupation with own appearance is typical. Help parents anticipate greater privacy need.

F. Encourage variety of school/community activities to allow wider exposure to peers/interests.

G. Testing authority may occur. Encourage families to clearly establish and enforce guidelines for appropriate behavior. Identify consistent caring adult with whom adolescent is comfortable communicating.

H. Question about friends, peer groups, adult role models. Social isolation is not normal.

I. As with other areas of development, individuals progress at variable rates and often oscillate between dependence/independence.

VII. IMMUNIZATIONS

A. Immunizations should be given according to recommended childhood immunization schedule (see Appendix A):

1. Hepatitis B: complete or initiate series.

2. MMR: give second dose now if not already administered.

3. Tetanus toxoid (Tdap): recommended at age 11–12 if at least 5 years since last dose. Subsequent doses every 10 years throughout adulthood.

4. Varicella: give if not previously immunized or unreliable history of disease. If 13 years or older, give 2 doses 4 weeks apart.

5. Mennigococcal: (MCV).
6. HPV: recommend initiating series for males and females.
7. Influenza: recommend annually at start of flu season.

VIII. SAFETY

A. Unintentional injury is main cause of death and disability in this age group.
   1. Counsel about accident prevention: seat belts, helmets, proper sports equipment, water-safety instruction, CPR.
   2. Instruct that firearms should be locked up, ammunition kept separate.
   3. Educate about dangers of drug use, both ingested and inhaled. Provide strategies to resist negative peer pressure.
   4. Discuss date rape prevention.
   5. Assess for depression. Adolescents at high risk for suicide: those with chronic illness or extreme stress (i.e., overachievers), athletes, those who feel unwanted.
   6. Assess for physical, emotional, sexual abuse.

IX. ANTICIPATORY GUIDANCE

A. Promotion of health.
   1. Review pubertal development of same and opposite sex.
   2. Explain menstruation and its management to females.
   3. Advise to get 8 hours of sleep every night.
   4. Encourage moderate to vigorous exercise for 30–60 minutes at least 3 times a week.
   5. Instruct to eat 3 nutritious meals/day. Snack on healthy foods such as fruits, vegetable, nuts, low-fat dairy. Choose foods rich in calcium, iron.
   6. Encourage maintaining healthy weight through exercise, appropriate eating habits.
   7. Remind to schedule dental exam every 6 months. Brush teeth twice a day. Floss daily.
   8. Educate about acne management.
   9. Provide safety instruction, avoidance of substance abuse and gang involvement.
B. Social development.
   1. Encourage participation in school activities.
   2. Advise to take on new responsibilities in home, school, community.

3. Clarify parental limits, consequences of unacceptable behavior.
4. Educate about safe use of the Internet and how to avoid exploitation.
C. Mental health.
   1. Encourage teens to consider their strengths and talents.
   2. Recommend talking with trusted adult/health professional if teen feels sad or helpless often.
   3. Advise against alcohol, drug use. Discuss strategies to resist negative peer pressure.
   4. Evaluate for potential abuse, counsel on avoiding date rape, gang involvement, abusive relationships.
D. Sexuality.
   1. Counsel on sexual abstinence. Encourage to identify supportive adult to provide accurate information. Invite adolescent to call the office for advice/information as needed. Explain confidentiality policy.
   2. If sexually active, discuss contraceptive methods, STI prevention. Counsel on abstinence.
   3. Educate about protection against STIs and pregnancy as indicated.

BIBLIOGRAPHY

Elster A, Kuznets N. *Guidelines for Adolescent Preventive Services*. Baltimore, MD: Williams & Wilkins; 1994.

Fisher J, Wildey L. Developmental management of adolescents. In: Burns C, et al., eds., *Pediatric Primary Care: A Handbook For Nurse Practitioners*. 3rd ed. Philadelphia: W.B. Saunders; 2004.

Fox J, ed. *Primary Health Care of Infants, Children, and Adolescents*. 2nd ed. St. Louis: Mosby; 2002.

Green M, Palfrey J, eds. *Bright Futures: Guidelines For Health Supervision Of Infants, Children, and Adolescents*. 2nd ed. Arlington, VA: National Center for Education in Maternal and Child Health; 2002.

Neinstein L. *Adolescent Health Care: A Practical Guide*. 4th ed. Philadelphia, PA: Lippincott Williams & Wilkins; 2002.

CHAPTER 19

Fourteen- to Eighteen-Year Visit (Adolescent)

Mary Lou C. Rosenblatt

Abdominal pain, 789	Hallucinations, 780.1
Acanthosis nigricans, 701.2	Hyperlipidemia, 272.4
Anemia, 285.9	Hypertension, 401.9
Anxiety, 300	Insomnias, 780.52
Catalepsy, 300.1	Iron-deficiency anemia, 280.9
Constipation, 564	Narcolepsy, 347
Delayed sleep phase syndrome, 780.5	Obesity, 278
Depression, 311	Obesity, morbid, 278.01
Diabetes, 250	Peristalsis of colon, 787.4
Diabetes, family history of, V18	Poor nutrition, 269.9
Drug abuse, 305.9	Sleep apnea, 780.57
Dysmenorrhea, 625.3	Sleep deprivation, 780.5
Eating disorders, 307.5	Snoring, 786.09
Enlarged tonsils, 474.11	Thyroid disease, 246.9

I. GENERAL IMPRESSION

 A. This well visit is an opportunity to provide health care for individual who is faced with many developmental challenges on road to adulthood.

 B. Introduce yourself and your role to teen and parent. Explain that you need information from both parent and teen and will spend some time just with teen to check on his/her concerns.

 C. Be knowledgeable of your state's confidentiality and consent statutes and explain how that will be handled in practice. Assure both teen and parent that your first goal is wellbeing of teen.

 D. Listening skills are especially important with teens. Show interest in their concerns and address them. "Hear" pauses, hesitation, body language, and validate your understanding of meaning of nonverbal communication with teen.

E. Be nonjudgmental and gather information before giving advice.

F. Have supply of well-written and informative handouts on variety of issues.

G. Involve parents by finding out what advice they give on sensitive subjects, such as substance abuse and sex. Interaction between parent and teen will give feedback on what is discussed in home and how open they are with each other. Encourage both parent and teen to talk about these subjects together.

H. Ask about responsibilities teen has at home. Many parents advance privileges based on teen's ability to take care of his/her chores. This can also support fair negotiations that take place in family.

I. Use tool such as HEADSSS assessment to take snapshot of teen's life and identify problem areas to focus on during acute visits. HEADSSS assessment: Ask open-ended questions about home, education, activities, drug use and depression, sexuality, suicide, and safety.

J. Have resources available if issues such as drug abuse, school problems, physical/sexual abuse, depression, sexual activity, pregnancy are present.

K. If an undesired behavior that is identified through screening can be dealt with during primary care office visit, state desired behavior, offer health information detailing risks of undesired behavior, benefit of change, and alternatives. If teen can commit to change, set goal and timeframe, offer support and resources, set up follow-up time.

II. NUTRITION

A. History.
1. Ask for 24-hour diet recall.
2. Are any foods/food groups avoided and why?
3. Is milk consumed? Skim, 2%, whole?
4. Is meat eaten? What types?
5. What fruits, vegetables does teen eat? How much juice is consumed?
6. Trying to gain or lose weight? How?
7. Are meals skipped? Is breakfast eaten?
8. Are meals eaten on run or sitting down with family?
9. What types of "junk" foods are consumed? How much?
10. How often does he/she eat at fast food restaurants? What foods?
11. Does teen watch TV and snack?
12. How much soda is consumed? Regular or diet?
13. What types of exercise is teen involved in?

14. Does teen spend time thinking about how to be thin?
15. Has he/she tried dieting, diet pills, laxatives, vomiting to control weight?
16. Does teen ever eat in secret?
17. Is teen dieting to fit into weight class for sports?
18. Are any nutritional supplements taken?

B. Teaching.
   1. Use My Plate (see Appendix E) to encourage healthy eating practices, daily requirements of protein, calcium, vitamins, fiber.
   2. Recognize that teen is likely making more choices on own, can start to read labels, becomes conscious of nutritional value.
   3. Skipping breakfast may make it harder to concentrate in school and lead to more hunger after school, possibly poor nutritional choices.
   4. Skipping meals may lead to more hunger, poor food choices.
   5. Encourage teen to talk with parent about planning meals, snacks.
   6. Encourage trying new foods.
   7. When limiting soda, drink more water, avoid excessive calories from juice products.
   8. Discuss sources of calcium.
   9. 5–8% of teen girls have iron-deficiency anemia.
   10. Teens risk dental decay with high-sugar diets, poor dental hygiene.
   11. 13–15% of children and adolescents are estimated to be overweight.
   12. Teach behavioral techniques for weight management, such as goal setting, self-monitoring, positive reinforcement, problem solving, social support.
   13. Incidence of eating disorders has increased and is estimated to affect 7% of male adolescents and 13% of female adolescents. Eating disorders can be associated with depression, substance abuse, low self-esteem.
   14. Discourage rapid weight gain/loss to fit into weight class for sports.
   15. Discourage major weight/dietary restrictions during growth spurt.

C. Physical exam.
   1. Chart height, weight, body mass index (BMI); review growth curves with teen.
   2. BMI at or above 95th percentile is considered overweight/obese. For obese teens, BMI is objective measure that is useful in motivating them to recognize their risks of developing heart disease, diabetes.

D. Labs.
   1. Screen hematocrit at beginning or ending puberty visit or both to check for anemia due to rapid growth, poor nutrition, menstrual losses.
   2. Glucose if there is family history of diabetes, symptoms of diabetes, or obesity and *Acanthosis nigricans.*

        3. Cholesterol for adolescents with heart disease, hypertension, diabetes or if there is family history of heart disease or hyperlipidemia.

E. Treatment plan.

    1. Encourage healthy eating practices.

    2. Encourage good exercise habits.

    3. For teens just starting to exercise, start slow, for example, walking for 20 minutes 3 times/week, so they can build up their exercise tolerance.

    4. For teens with special diets, such as vegetarian diets, be prepared to assess dietary content, give advice/referral resource to offer nutritional guidance, support.

    5. For obese teens, offer support and encouragement. When motivated, they may be ready for weight-loss program. Suggest starting by keeping daily food diary to look for problem areas in diet. Behavioral techniques, mentioned earlier, may be enough for some teens to get started with healthier eating practices. In supportive environment, family involvement may help to cut down excess intake. Some teens benefit from professional weight-loss programs. Refer morbidly obese patients to medical weight-loss program.

    6. When eating disorders are suspected, careful assessment and monitoring are needed. Denial is common and should not offer reassurance. Patients require nutritional, medical management as well as mental health assessment and referral. Referral to eating disorder program will offer comprehensive approach to assessment and management.

III. ELIMINATION

A. Teens are normally independent in their elimination practices.

B. Constipation.

    1. Infrequent and/or difficult passage of feces.

    2. Common cause of abdominal pain.

C. History.

    1. What are bowel habits?

    2. When was last bowel movement? Hard and dry? Any abdominal pain?

    3. How long has constipation been a problem?

    4. Is fiber present in teen's diet?

    5. What is fluid intake?

    6. Does teen avoid public or school restrooms?

    7. Does schedule allow time to use bathroom?

    8. Have laxatives or stool softeners been tried? How often?

9. Ask about other signs of thyroid disease, such as menstrual disorder, dry skin, brittle hair, lethargy, and weight gain.
D. Teaching.
   1. Describe gastrocolic reflex (peristalsis of colon induced by entrance of food into empty stomach).
   2. Describe bowel function and need for fluid and fiber to keep stool moist and moving through GI tract.
E. Physical exam for suspected constipation.
   1. Firm loops of bowel may be palpable on thin patients.
   2. Rectum is typically filled with hard stool.
   3. Passage of hard stool may cause anorectal pain or bleeding.
F. Labs.
   1. Abdominal film may be needed in case of abdominal pain, after ruling out other systems as sources of pain.
   2. Make sure female patients are not pregnant before sending for X-ray.
G. Treatment plan for constipation.
   1. Encourage drinking plenty of water.
   2. Help teen plan on how to add fiber to diet.
   3. Encourage good toilet habits, such as right after meals.
   4. Consider use of stool softener.
   5. In addition to the above, sitz baths may help anal fissure heal.
   6. Follow up in 1–2 weeks.

IV. SLEEP

A. Teenagers need 9–10 hours of sleep per night. Most teens do not get it.
B. Sleep history.
   1. Does teen feel rested or tired?
   2. What are concerns about sleep? Frequency? Duration?
   3. What are usual bedtimes and wake-up times?
   4. Are naps taken? If so, do they interfere with sleep later that night?
   5. Has family complained about teen's snoring?
   6. Does teen fall asleep in class? Other times?
   7. What are school hours?
   8. What are after-school activities?
   9. Does teen have job? How many hours?
   10. How many hours are spent on homework?
   11. Does teen care for child or have other household responsibilities?
   12. Is there family history of sleep disorders?

13. Is teen depressed, sad, moody?
14. Are stimulants (coffee, tea, soda, OTC medications, illicit drugs) used to stay awake longer?
15. Does teen have TV, radio/stereo, computer, phone in bedroom? Are these in use when trying to go to sleep and delaying bedtime?

C. Teaching.
1. Insomnias are most frequent sleep disorder during adolescence.
2. Insomnias involve problems falling asleep, staying asleep, waking too early.
3. Delayed sleep phase syndrome is inability to fall asleep at appropriate time, but if left to fall asleep naturally would fall asleep late, get up late. These teens will be sleepy if awakened to attend school.
4. Teens may be motivated to stay up late, sleep late. If teen can awaken by his/her own motivation but not for school, this may be form of school refusal.
5. Insomnia may occur due to stress, anxiety, poor sleep habits.
6. Excessive daytime sleepiness can be caused by chronic sleep deprivation, usually due to busy schedule.
7. Sleep apnea may be associated with obesity; symptoms include snoring, apneic periods during sleep, nighttime waking, and daytime sleeping.
8. Narcolepsy is uncommon disorder that has an onset of 10–25 years of age. Components include sleep attacks, catalepsy, sleep paralysis, and/or hallucinations. There is evidence of genetic component.

D. Physical.
1. Does teen appear alert?
2. Does teen appear sad or depressed?
3. Note blood pressure and pulse.
4. Is teen obese?
5. Is teen comfortable and able to breathe through both nostrils?
6. Are tonsils enlarged?

E. Lab.
1. To rule out sleep apnea, consider sleep study if teen/family reports snoring, frequent wake ups, apneic periods, daytime sleep.

F. Treatment plan.
1. Have teen track sleep patterns for 1–2 weeks.
2. Any question of depression needs assessment.
3. Have teen/parent look at schedule and commitments. Are there ways to decrease workload for overloaded teen?
4. Cut down on caffeine products, including OTC stimulants.
5. Cut out nap time.

6. Use bedroom for sleep only and put TV, computer, etc., elsewhere.
7. Teach relaxation techniques.
8. Identify stressors and write them down. If stressors are complex, consider counseling.
9. Stick to regular schedule of bedtime and waking up.
10. Encourage weight loss for obese teens.
11. Refer teens with nasal breathing problems/enlarged tonsils to ENT specialist.
12. Refer teens with difficult sleep problems, including those who do not do well with above plan, to sleep clinic.

V. GROWTH AND DEVELOPMENT

A. While some teens are able to state concerns, others may hope you will mention possible concerns for them, such as height, weight, pubertal development. Comfortable way to start such conversation may be "Some teens worry about being shorter (or taller, heavier, thinner) than their friends. I wonder if you have any concerns about this . . . "
B. Use growth charts to help see progress over time, relate their parameters to their blood relatives or point out what future growth is likely.
C. Tanner or sexual maturity rating (SMR) also may be reassuring.
D. For development outside of expected range, evaluate for medical cause.
E. Height.
   1. 33–60% of adult bone growth occurs during adolescence.
   2. 20–25% of final adult height occurs in puberty.
F. Weight: 50% of ideal adult body weight is gained during adolescence.
G. SMR: By middle adolescence most teens are in latter classes of Tanner or SMR scales. Spermarche occurs at about SMR 2.5. Menarche usually occurs at SMR 3 or 4. Using SMR can help teen to see where he/she is in puberty and what can be expected without having to compare himself/herself to friends.
   1. Menstrual history.
      a. Age at menarche?
      b. Frequency, duration, quantity of menstrual periods?
      c. Last menstrual period (LMP)?
      d. Dysmenorrhea and treatments used?
H. Psychosocial developmental tasks.
   1. Increased independence from parents, inviting conflicts over control.
   2. Peer group involvement intensifies. Conformity with peer values. Less time for family. Teams, clubs, gangs may become important.

3. Interest in dating, sexual experimentation. Preoccupation with romantic fantasy. Sexual orientation more evident to peers.
4. Identity and individuality grow. Increased acceptance of body image, more established ego and sexual identity. Increased intellectual abilities, emotional feelings. Vocational ideas more realistic.
5. Sense of omnipotence and immortality that may lead to high-risk behaviors.
6. Improved ability with abstract thought.

VI. SOCIAL DEVELOPMENT

A. Family.
    1. Who are family members living with teen?
    2. What is level of communication between members?
    3. What are supports? Conflicts?
    4. What are house rules? Who makes them?
    5. What are teen's responsibilities?
    6. Is there a curfew?
    7. Does teen drive family car? What supervision is given?
B. School.
    1. What is teen's school performance? Any recent changes?
    2. What does teen like or dislike about school?
    3. How does teen relate to classmates? To teachers?
    4. Are there learning problems? Has teen been evaluated by school?
    5. Are there behavior problems? How have those been addressed?
    6. What is educational/vocational plan?
    7. Has teen dropped out of school?
    8. Is he/she planning to get a GED?
    9. If chronic illness, is there teaching plan in place for missed days?
C. Peers.
    1. Who are teen's friends?
    2. Is there a best friend?
    3. Is there a trusted adult to talk to?
    4. Does teen prefer to be with friends or alone?
    5. What are interests and activities of peer group?
    6. Does parent know teen's friends?
D. Interests.
    1. What are teen's activities? Hobbies?

      2.   Does teen have a job? How many hours? Safety hazards on job?

      3.   Does teen like to read?

      4.   Does teen enjoy sports? Exercise?

E. Dating.

      1.   What are house rules about dating?

      2.   What advice have parents given about dating?

      3.   Is teen thinking about dating?

      4.   Does he/she have romantic feelings about anyone?

          a. Is this person male or female?

          b. If these feelings are for same-sex person, does teen feel support from parents? Friends? Community?

F. Sexual history.

      1.   Is teen thinking about sexual relationship or has he/she had sexual relations?

      2.   Able to talk with parent about being sexually active?

      3.   Aware of risks of sexual activity (emotional, sexually transmitted infections [STIs], pregnancy)?

      4.   Vulnerable to these risks?

      5.   Reason for being sexually active? Does teen feel pressured?

      6.   Specific sexual behaviors (vaginal/anal intercourse or oral-genital sex)?

      7.   Teen's age at first intercourse?

      8.   Number of lifetime partners?

      9.   How old is current partner? Is there more than one partner now?

     10. Are condoms used? Hormonal contraception? Spermicides?

     11. Does teen know how to use male/female condom?

     12. Does teen know about emergency contraception (EC)? Does teen who only uses condoms have prescription for EC?

     13. Any history of or current symptoms of STIs?

     14. Any history of pregnancy? Pregnancy scares? LMP?

     15. History of pregnancy termination? If so, how is teen coping?

     16. For teen parents, what are stresses? Support?

     17. Does teen feel safe in current relationship?

     18. In dating situations, has teen been hit or pushed? What did she/he do?

G. Substance use.

      1.   Does teen know risks of substance use?

      2.   Do any friends smoke cigarettes, drink alcohol, use inhalants, marijuana, other drugs?

      3.   Does teen smoke cigarettes, drink alcohol, use inhalants, marijuana, other drugs?

4. If teen does use substances, use screen such as CAGE (Cut down, Annoyed, Guilty, Eye-opener) to obtain more information (have resource available to teen who needs substance abuse treatment):

C: Do you think you should cut down your use of _____?

A: Do you get angry or annoyed when people tell you that you should cut down your use of _____?

G: Do you feel guilty about your use of _____?

E: Do you use this substance as eye-opener to get going in morning?

5. Does teen drink alcohol or use other drugs when driving?
6. Does teen attend parties where alcohol is served?
7. What plans are there to get home safely? Does teen have to deal with parents for this type of situation?

H. Antisocial behavior.
   1. Does teen skip school?
   2. Has he/she had trouble with the law?
   3. Does teen belong to or associate with a gang?

VII. IMMUNIZATIONS (SEE APPENDIX A)

A. May not have completed recommended vaccinations.
B. Immunization status can be reviewed at each visit.
   1. TD: booster usually given between 11 and 12 years but before 16 years, then every 10 years.
   2. MMR: 2 doses needed before school entry.
   3. Hepatitis B: recommended for all adolescents, especially those at risk (sexually active, injection drug abusers, work-related exposure to blood/body fluids). Routine vaccination of infants began in 1991; may be in need of immunization. Two-dose regimen for 11- to 15-year-olds; 3-dose regimen for others.
   4. Varicella: needed if there is no history of varicella disease. If history is unclear, vaccine is well tolerated, more cost effective than serologic testing in most cases. Two doses given more than 4 weeks apart needed if 13 years of age or older.
   5. Influenza: recommended for teens with chronic illness (i.e., asthma, sickle cell disease, HIV, etc.) or those living with persons with impaired immunity. Can be given to others who want immunity. Cannot be given to individuals with egg allergy.

6. Hepatitis A: vaccination recommended for those living in high-risk areas; 2 doses needed, at least 6 months apart.
7. *Neisseria meningitidis*: vaccination recommended in many states for college freshmen living in dormitories.

VIII. SAFETY

A. Self-protection.
   1. Does teen have any self-defense skills?
   2. Is teen aware of surroundings when in public?
   3. Does teen travel with friends?
   4. Has teen been victim of any attack in past? Any fear of someone threatening harm currently? Are parents/authorities aware?
   5. Does teen feel safe in school?
   6. Can teen walk away from conflict if she/he feels fear/anger?
   7. Does teen get into fights regularly?
   8. Is teen exposed to violence in home, community, media?
   9. Does teen have access to gun? What are rules for gun safety?
   10. Does teen carry a weapon? Why?
B. Injury prevention.
   1. Does teen wear seat belts?
   2. Does teen wear a helmet?
   3. Does teen plan to take driver's education classes?
   4. Does teen drive at night or with friends?
   5. Does teen use alcohol/other drugs?
   6. Does teen routinely take risks?
   7. Has teen had injuries in past?
   8. Does teen use power tools/lawn equipment?
C. Suicide prevention.
   1. Does teen or family worry about teen being depressed?
   2. Has teen lost pleasure in usual interests?
   3. Weight loss or gain?
   4. Sleep problem: too much or too little?
   5. Increased/decreased activity level?
   6. Daily fatigue?
   7. Feelings of worthlessness, excessive/inappropriate guilt?
   8. Decreased concentration or ability to make decisions?

9. Asking teen about mood can be done at every visit and is especially important if teen visits frequently or if physical complaints do not seem to make sense.
10. Recurrent thoughts of death or suicide? (If teen is suicidal, have resources, such as ability to escort to emergency department for psychiatric evaluation, immediately available.)

IX. ANTICIPATORY GUIDANCE

A. Many opportunities to give advice exist during history and physical exam.
B. Giving information in nonjudgmental way allows teen to make up his/her own mind about how to improve his/her health.
C. Puberty: Acknowledge where individual is regarding pubertal development and how development is likely to proceed.
D. Health care.
    1. Have yearly physical exam.
    2. See dentist twice/year, practice good dental hygiene.
    3. Keep up with routine vision care.
    4. Discuss use of sunscreen and skin cancer prevention.
E. Injury prevention.
    1. Wear seat belt when traveling in car.
    2. Wear helmet when riding bike, skates, scooter, motor bike/cycle.
    3. Wear appropriate protection when engaging in sports.
    4. Drowning prevention includes learning how to swim, not swimming alone, never abusing substances while doing water activities, entering unknown depths feet first.
    5. When operating equipment such as power tools, lawn mowers, tractors, know safety rules and use appropriate safety equipment.
    6. Leading causes of death and injury of young drivers are inexperience, risk taking (speeding, dares), distraction (driving with friends, talking on cell phones), driving at night. Parents who recognize these risks can outline safety plan (curfew, supervision, no driving with peers until parent feels teen is ready, contracting for no substance abuse) for young driver going through "rite of passage."
    7. Ask parents to remove guns from home. If not an option, guns/ammunition need to be stored separately, in locked boxes. Especially important for parents of depressed teens to realize risk guns pose to their teen.
    8. Learn CPR.

F. Self-exam.
  1. Teach females self-administered breast exam. Use breast model to show how lumps may feel. Reassure teen that most lumps in her age group are not cancer.
  2. Teach males self-administered testes exam. Reinforce that concerns are okay to talk about. Teach warning signs for testicular tumors, torsion, and epididymitis.
G. Nutrition.
  1. Eat breakfast.
  2. Eat a low-fat diet.
  3. Watch junk food, soda consumption.
  4. Use My Plate (see Appendix E) to evaluate diet.
  5. Encourage maintenance of healthy weight.
H. Exercise.
  1. Do aerobic exercise 3 times/week.
  2. Look for ways to increase exercise opportunities in daily life.
I. Peer pressure and self-esteem.
  1. Pick good friends who are interested in positive activities.
  2. Look at best qualities and feel good about them.
  3. Participate in activities because of desire to, not because everyone else is doing so.
  4. Figure out personally important goals, make sure friends derail.
J. Body modification: tattoos and piercings.
  1. Reasons for getting a tattoo range from expressing independence to being part of a group. Some teens may be self-described "risk takers" who may also engage in drug use and sexual activity.
  2. Parental consent may be required in some locales.
  3. Advise teens that tattoos should be considered permanent because removal is expensive, time consuming, and may leave a scar.
  4. Tattoos and piercings may become infected. Advise teens to research sterile practices of the tattoo/piercing establishment. Post-care hygiene needs to be strictly followed.
  5. Teens should not get a tattoo or piercing if they are upset or intoxicated.
  6. Alternatives such as temporary tattoos or magnetic piercing look-a-likes may satisfy a passing need.
K. Stress reduction.
  1. Encourage setting aside time to rest and gather thoughts.
  2. Get plenty of sleep at night.
  3. Eat varied, nutritious diet.

4. Encourage physical activity.
5. Teach deep breathing and counting to 10 if feeling stressed or angry.
6. Keep lines of communication open with parent/guardian.
7. Get help from adult in teen's life if teen has much stress.
8. Try to keep open communication with family.
9. Have resources available for depressed teens.
10. Arrange emergency evaluation for suicidal intent/severe depression.
L. Substance abuse.
1. Do not smoke cigarettes or marijuana.
2. Do not drink alcohol, use inhalants, other drugs.
3. Do not drive if intoxicated. Have teen make plan with parents about what to do if out and driver providing ride becomes intoxicated.
4. Point out risks of substance use including health consequences, accidents, school performance, impact on family/friends, legal implications, gateway to other drug use.
5. Make sure athletes are aware of risks of performance-enhancing drugs.
M. Sex.
1. Consider benefits of abstinence, such as ability to focus on personal and academic goals, less complicated breakups, STI prevention.
2. Consider risks of sexual activity, such as emotional stress, pregnancy, STIs.
3. Discuss how to deal with issues important to individual teen: sex drive, peer pressure, older partners, partners who refuse to use protection, desire to have baby.
4. If teen decides sexual activity is right for him/her, advise use of condoms and make sure teen knows how to leave room at top of male condom for ejaculate and that female condoms can cover part of external genitalia.
5. Be frank about risks of STIs, especially HIV and other viral infections.
6. Educate about all types of appropriate birth control.
7. Make sure teens are aware of emergency contraception and how to obtain it.
8. For sexually active teens, screen for STIs.
9. For sexually active females, perform yearly Pap smear.
10. Encourage teen to talk with adult in his/her life about sex if able.
11. If teen identifies as minority sexual identity (gay, lesbian, bisexual, transgendered) make sure teen has resources, support.
12. If teen is pregnant, outline options and encourage parental involvement.

BIBLIOGRAPHY

Behrman RE, Kleigman RM, Jenson HB. *Nelson Textbook of Pediatrics*. 18th ed. Philadelphia, PA: W.B. Saunders; 2007.

Dixon SD, Stein MT. *Encounters with Children: Pediatric Behavior and Development*. St. Louis, MO: Mosby; 2006.

Goldenring JM, Cohen E. Getting into adolescent heads. *Contemp Pediatr*. 1998;5:75-90.

Jellinek M, Patel BP, Froehle MC, eds. *Bright Futures in Practice: Mental Health, Vol I, Practice Guide*. Arlington, VA: National Center for Education in Maternal and Child Health; 2007.

Joffe A, Blythe MJ, eds. *Handbook of Adolescent Medicine*. Philadelphia, PA: Hanley and Belfus; 2009.

Neinstein LS. *Adolescent Health Care: A Practical Guide*. 5th ed. Baltimore, MD: Lippincott Williams & Wilkins; 2007.

Rosen D, and The Committee on Adolescence. Clinical report: Identification and management of eating disorders in children and adolescents. *Pediatrics*. 2003;111(1):204-211.

Schwimmer JB. Managing overweight in older children and adolescents. *Pediatr Ann*. 2004;33(1):39-44.

Sheehan K. Intentional injury and violence prevention. *Clin Pediatr Emerg Med*. 2003;4(1):12-20.

Song EH, Martel S, Anderson JE. Decorating the "human canvas": Body art and your patients. *Contemp Pediatr*. 2002;19(8):86-102.

Common Childhood Disorders

Dermatologic Problems

Peggy Vernon

Acne, 706.1	Papule, 709.8
Blackhead, 706.1	Pustules, 686.9
Comedone, 706.1	Skin nodule, 782.2
Hyperpigmentation, 709	Whitehead, 706.2

I. ACNE

A. Etiology.
  1. Acne vulgaris is a disorder of the pilosebaceous follicles.
  2. Hormonal stimulation increases the growth of the sebaceous follicles.
  3. Excess sebum, keratinocytes, and bacteria accumulate, causing follicular plugging and inflammation.

B. Occurrence.
  1. 40% of children 8 to 10 years of age will develop early lesions.
  2. The highest incidence of acne is during the adolescent years, with 85% of all adolescents experiencing some form of acne.
  3. 10% of adults in their 30s, 40s, and 50s continue to experience acne.
  4. There is a familial tendency to the disorder.

C. Clinical manifestations.
  1. The primary lesions are the open and closed comedones.
     a. The open comedone, or blackhead, is an obstruction of the follicle that is filled with stratum corneum cells. The black color is due to compacted melanocytes.
     b. The closed comedone, or whitehead, is the result of swelling of the follicular duct below the epidermis.
  2. The accumulation of sebum and keratin cause the follicle wall to rupture into the dermis, causing inflammatory acne, or papules and pustules—the inflammatory reaction to sebum, fatty acids, and the bacteria.
     a. *Propionibacterium acnes* distend the follicle, causing leakage around the comedone.

      b. Lesions developing in the lower portion of the follicle create warm, tender nodules and cysts. These lesions may result in scars, which in turn can develop into keloids.

      c. Inflammatory acne lesions may resolve with postinflammatory hyperpigmentation, which usually clears after several months.

  D. Physical findings. The highest concentration of sebaceous glands occurs on the face, chest, back, and shoulders. A variety of lesions appear simultaneously, presenting with a variety of comedones, papules, pustules, and nodules. Acne appears to be more severe in winter months, and females report a premenstrual hormonal correlation. The severity of acne is determined by the quantity, type, and distribution of lesions.

  E. Diagnostic tests. Acne is a visual diagnosis. History should include family history, other medical disorders, duration of acne, products used, and previous treatments—over-the-counter as well as prescription medications. Physical examination should include grade of acne according to type and location of lesions. See Table 20-1. Laboratory testing is indicated only if adrenal or gonadal function are in question.

  F. Differential diagnosis.

    1. Tuberous sclerosis.

    2. Nevus comedonicus.

    3. Miliaria of the newborn.

    4. Flat warts.

    5. Molluscum contagiosum.

Table 20-1 Grading Scale for Acne Severity

Scale	Definition
0	None: skin is clear
1	Few comedones
2	Mild comedones, few papules, minimal erythema
3	Comedones, papules, pustules, erythema
4	Moderate comedones, greater number of papules, pustules extending over wider area of face, chest, shoulders, back, increasing erythema
5	Comedones, increasing number of papules, pustules, nodules with erythema
6	Comedones, papules, pustules, nodules, cysts; scarring may or may not be present with hyperpigmentation

Table 20-2 Treatment of Acne

Types of acne	Lesions	Initial treatment	If not improving
Comedonal (706.1)	Open or closed comedones	Benzoyl peroxide 5% gel qd (if mild) *OR* trettinoin (Retin A) 0.0025% cream qd (if moderate) *OR* adapalene 0.1% gel	Combine benzoyl peroxide with tretinoin *OR* increase strength to 0.05%.
Mild papulo (709.8), pustular (686.9)	Red papules, few papules	Benzoyl peroxide 5-10% qd *OR* adapalene 0.1% gel *OR* azelaic acid bid (if mild) *OR* topical antibiotic bid *OR* erythromycin 3% with 5% benzoyl peroxide qd-bid (if moderate) *OR* clindamycin 1% with 5% benzoyl peroxide qd-bid	Increase benzoyl peroxide to bid *OR* combine benzoyl peroxide with tretinoin (for comedones). Substitute topical antibiotic bid (for inflammatory).
Moderate to severe papulo (709.8), pustular (686.9)	Red papules, many papules	Benzoyl peroxide 5% *AND* tretinoin 0.025% *OR* adapalene 0.1% gel *OR* azelaic acid (if comedonal) *OR* topical antibiotic bid (if not comedones) *AND* oral antibiotic bid	Increase strength of treatment or refer to dermatologist.
Nodulcystic, scarring, or unresponsive	Red pustules, cysts, and nodules	Oral antibiotics bid *AND* tretinoin 0.05% qd *OR* adapalene 0.1% gel *AND* benzoyl peroxide 10% gel bid (if comedonal)	Refer to dermatologist for oral isotretinoin.

G. Treatment. Goals of treatment include altering keratinization, counteract excess sebum production, decrease the production of *P. acnes*, and minimize scarring. Treatment choices depend on the severity of acne. See Table 20-2.

H. Follow up. Acne patients should be evaluated every 3 to 6 months for compliance, treatment progress, and worsening of the disorder. Dermatology referral should be considered for patients who are not 50% improved on topical medications and oral antibiotics after 6 months, or those who are developing scarring from acne lesions. Patients treated with isotretinoin are monitored monthly. The development of the iPLEDGE Program requires providers, patients, and pharmacists to access the program monthly to monitor for pregnancy, blood donation, and contraceptive counseling, as isotretinoin is teratogenic.

I. Complications. Lack of patient motivation, inappropriate treatments, and inappropriate expectations complicate acne treatment. Psychologic effects of acne include poor self-esteem, depression, and problems with interpersonal relationships. Resistance to treatment, especially oral antibiotics, also complicate treatment.

J. Education. Proper use of medications as well as cleansers, moisturizers, and make-up are important to encourage compliance. Although no evidence indicate dietary restrictions are helpful, a well-balanced diet including adequate intake of water is important in treatment. It takes weeks to months to treat acne, and occasionally the disorder will worsen with treatment. Compliance is crucial.

II. BITES

A. Animal bites.
1. Etiology and occurrence. Cat and dog bites, as well as other animal bites, are common injuries.
2. Clinical manifestations. Bite wounds may be infested with *S. aureus*, streptococci, and other oral flora bacteria. Approximately one-third of animal bites contain anaerobic bacteria. It is difficult to predict which wounds will become infected.
3. Physical findings and complications. Injuries include lacerations, crushing injuries, deep puncture wounds, as well as bone, tendon, muscle, and neurovascular tissue damage from deep bites. Secondary infection can lead to cellulitis.
4. Diagnostic tests. Wound cultures identify infectious agents. X-ray and MRI studies reveal bone, vascular, and nerve damage.
5. Differential diagnosis. Identify laceration and puncture wounds from other sources.
6. Treatment. Culture wounds before cleansing and debridement. Antibiotics for infected wounds, management of bone, tendon, nerve, and vascular wounds by appropriate specialists. If suturing is necessary, observe closely for infection. Hospitalization and reconstructive surgery

as indicated. Tetanus booster if indicated. Rabies prophylaxis if indicated. Psychological management.

7. Education. Teach children not to provoke any animal. Provide adequate adult supervision of children. Report stray animals to animal control officials.

B. Human bites.
1. Clinical manifestations. Human bite wounds harbor both anaerobic and aerobic bacteria, as well as *S. aureus* and Haemophilus, with a higher incidence of infections and complications than other bites. Human bites include occlusional wounds when teeth are sunk into the skin, and clenched-fist injuries when a tooth penetrates a joint or bone.
2. Diagnostic tests. Radiographic and surgical evaluation if a joint or bone is penetrated. Bacterial cultures for anaerobic and aerobic bacteria.
3. Treatment. Irrigation decreases risk of infection. Debridement of wound edges, appropriate antibiotic treatment (Augmentin, Erythromycin) and immunization if indicated.
4. Complications. Residual disability are frequent after clenched-fist injuries, including abscess, osteomyelitis, tendonitis, tendon rupture, and stiffness of the joint.

C. Atopic dermatitis/eczema.
1. Etiology. Eczema is a chronic disorder characterized by exacerbations and remissions. There is a strong family history of allergies and asthma.
2. Occurrence. Atopic dermatitis, or eczema, is the most common skin disorder seen in children, affecting 10–15% of all children; 30–80% percent of atopic patients continue to experience flares during their lifetime.
3. Physical findings. Atopic dermatitis is characterized by intense pruritus, erythema, scale, and excoriations. The borders are diffuse. Crusting and oozing are common in infants. Thickened skin (lichenification) from persistent scratching and rubbing may be present. Distribution is on the scalp, face, and extensors in infants, on the neck and flexor folds in children, and on the hands and feet in adolescents and adults.
3. Diagnostic tests. Atopic dermatitis is a clinical diagnosis based on careful history and clinical examination. A potassium hydroxide (KOH) scraping will exclude fungal infections.
4. Differential diagnosis. Tinea, seborrheic dermatitis, psoriasis, scabies, and molluscum contagiosum.
5. Treatment. Goals of treatment include controlling itching with antihistamines, hydrating the skin with lukewarm tub soaks followed by application of emollient moisturizers, (Eucerin, Aquaphor) alleviating

inflammation with topical corticosteroids, maintaining remission with immunomodulators such as Elidel and Protopic, and treating secondary bacterial infections with appropriate topical and systemic antibiotics. Bleach baths kill microbes that cause infection in children with atopic dermatitis. Add ¼ cup of bleach to a bath tub of lukewarm water and allow the child to soak for 10 minutes, followed by adequate moisturizers. Identifying and treating allergens helps control flares.

5. Follow up. Failure to respond to treatment requires referral to a dermatology specialist. Referral to an allergist may be necessary for evaluation and management of allergies.

6. Complications. Secondary bacterial infections from excoriations include Group A beta-hemolytic streptococci and staphylococcus. Patients with atopic dermatitis have a higher incidence of viral infections, including herpes simplex, molluscum contagiousum, and warts.

7. Education. There is no cure for atopic dermatitis. It is characterized by exacerbations and remissions. Teach proper use of antihistamines, topical corticosteroids, and immunomodulators, as well as bathing followed by application of moisturizers. Identify aggravating factors such as stress, allergies, weather change, and infections.

III. BURNS

A. Etiology and occurrence. Burns can be caused by thermal, chemical, or electrical agents. The majority of burns are thermal, and the minority of burns are chemical. Most burns are minor and can be managed on an outpatient basis.

B. Clinical manifestations. Burns are classified by depth of injury. Superficial or first-degree burns involve only the epidermis. Partial thickness or second-degree burns involve damage to the epidermis and varying depths of the dermis. Full thickness or third-degree burns involve the epidermis, the dermis, and the subcutaneous fat. Third-degree burns are painless. The size of the burn is measured by the percent of total body surface area (TBSA) involved. The rule of nines estimates the TBSA. See Figure 20-1.

C. Physical findings. Physical examination includes the TBSA, distribution, and depth of involvement.

D. Diagnostic tests. Bacterial cultures for suspected infection. Laboratory evaluation for serious burns includes complete blood count (CBC), serum electrolytes, serum glucose, blood urea nitrogen (BUN), creatinine, and urinalysis.

Figure 20-1 Rule of nines.

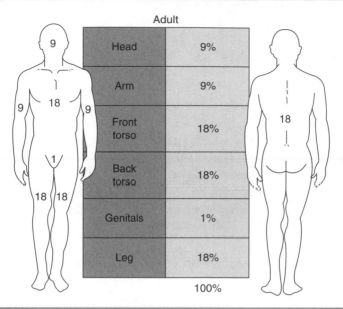

Adult

Head	9%	
Arm	9%	
Front torso	18%	
Back torso	18%	
Genitals	1%	
Leg	18%	
	100%	

E. Differential diagnosis. Careful history will determine the type of injury and degree of burn. Other diseases include scalded skin syndrome and Ritter's disease.

F. Treatment. Management depends on the classification of the burn. Electrical and chemical burns usually require hospital observation. Injuries with associated upper airway injury, fractures, abuse, or severe pain also should be hospitalized. Outpatient treatment includes maintenance of proper nutrition. Superficial burns are treated with cool compresses and pain management. Partial thickness burns are treated with daily cleansing, debridement of devitalized tissue, application of silver sulfadiazine cream, bacitracin, or gentamycin ointment, and a thin guaze dressing, as well as appropriate pain management.

G. Follow up. Treatment should continue for 1 to 2 weeks, or until wounds are healed. Assessment for infection should continue.

H. Complications. Local infection and inflammation, as well as neurologic and vascular compromise.

I. Education. Home and environmental safety issues should be addressed, first-aid measures, proper use of sunscreen to prevent sunburn of the affected areas. The extent of scarring is difficult to predict, depending on the severity and extent of the burn, whether grafting was needed, and skin color.

IV. DIAPER DERMATITIS

A. Etiology. Diaper dermatitis is an inflammation of the skin in the diaper area due to breakdown of the skin's natural barrier.
B. Occurrence. Diaper dermatitis is perhaps the most common skin disorder seen under 2 years of age. If not properly controlled, diaper dermatitis can recur regularly until toilet training is complete.
C. Clinical manifestations. Causes of diaper dermatitis include irritant secondary to prolonged contact with urine and feces, *Candida albicans*, bacterial infections including impetigo secondary to staphylococcus or streptococcus, and psoriasis.
D. Physical findings.
   1. The most prevalent form of diaper dermatitis is irritant dermatitis. Usually confined to the buttocks, perineal area, and medial thighs, sparing the interiginous areas. Contributing factors are prolonged time between diaper changes, harsh soaps, improper moisturization, use of barrier ointments, and excessive heat in warm climates.
   2. Candidal diaper dermatitis should be suspected when a diaper rash does not respond to topical treatments. It is a common occurrence with the use of oral antibiotics.
   3. Characterized by erythema on the buttocks, suprapubic area, and medial thighs with raised edges with sharply demarcated margins with pinpoint satellite lesions surrounding the borders.
   4. Impetigo is characterized by flaccid vesicles and bullae on the lower abdomen, medial thighs, and buttocks.
   5. Psoriasis is a violaceous plaque with adherent silvery-white scale. Borders are sharply demarcated.
E. Diagnostic tests. Microscopic examination with KOH will reveal budding yeasts with hyphae in Candidal infections. Bacterial culture of a vesicle or crust will diagnose bacterial infection. See Table 20-3.
F. Treatment.
   1. Irritant diaper dermatitis is treated with frequent diaper changes, cleansing the skin with a mild cleanser, drying the skin, and applying a barrier such as petrolatum or Aquaphor. Air drying between changes is also helpful.

Table 20-3 Diagnosis and Treatment of Diaper Dermatitis (691.0)

Type	Cause	Presentation and location	Other characteristics	Treatment
Irritant contact dermatitis (692.9)	Related to wearing diapers; contact with urine and feces	Chapped, shiny, erythematous, parchment-like skin with possible erosions on convex surfaces; creases spared	Peak at 9-12 mo; may progress to involve creases; skin may be dry	Frequent diaper changes, gentle cleansing; greasy lubricant; sitz bath, air dry; hydrocortisone for inflammation
Candidiasis (112.9)	Related to wearing diapers; a superinfection with *Candida*	Shallow pustules, fiery red	Satellite lesions, oral thrush; recent antibiotics or diarrhea; occurs at any age	Antifungal cream plus same measures as for contact dermatitis
Miliaria (705.1) or intertrigo (695.89)	Related to wearing diapers; due to heat and occlusion	Discrete vesicles or papules (miliaria); erythematous, scaly, maceration in skin folds	Sweat retention or friction associated	Self-limited (miliaria); avoid precipitation factors; care as for contact dermatitis
Seborrhea (706.3)	Exaggerated by wearing diapers; overgrowth of *Malassezia* yeast in areas of sebaceous gland activity	Greasy, erythematous scales; well circumscribed in creases of skin, groin; spared convex surfaces	Onset at 3-4 weeks of age. Also occurs on face or body; often superinfected with *Candida*	Ketoconazole is treatment of choice, or hydrocortisone

2. Candidal rashes should be treated with topical antifungal medications. Avoid topical corticosteroid ointments, including combination antifungal and corticosteroid medications to reduce the possibility of atrophy in an occluded area. Resistant infections should be treated with appropriate oral antifungal medications.
3. Bacterial infections should be treated with appropriate antibiotics. Infections that include a large proportion of the diaper area are best treated orally. Isolated areas may be treated appropriately with topical antibiotics, such as Mupirocin.
4. Psoriasis is a chronic condition. Topical steroid ointment should be applied twice daily for 2-week periods. Ointments such as petrolatum or Aquaphor can be used at diaper changes. Watch for psoriatic plaques in other areas, as well as psoriatic arthritis.

G. Complications. Resistant infections.
H. Education. Parents should be taught proper skin cleansing, frequent diaper changes, and proper use of barriers to prevent contact of urine and stool with skin.

V. RASHES

A. Allergic, contact: See Atopic Dermatitis.

VI. INFESTATIONS: PEDICULOSIS

A. Etiology and occurrence. Pediculosis or lice are spread from human to human, and epidemics are common in schoolchildren. Pediculosis corporis is often found in crowded living conditions and areas of poor personal hygiene.
B. Clinical manifestations and physical findings. Nits (louse eggs) are found in the hair on the scalp. Pediculosis corporis begins as small papules with secondary lesions developing from scratching, resulting in crusted papules and ulcerations.
C. Diagnostic tests. White nits are obvious on the hair shaft. A hair may be plucked and microscopic examination will reveal nits. Pediculosis corporis is diagnosed by examination of the seams of the clothing, which reveals the louse.
D. Differential diagnosis. Atopic dermatitis or other eczematous dermatitis, as well as scabies.

E. Treatment. Remove nits with a fine-tooth comb after soaking in vinegar or over-the-counter products such as Nix Crème Rinse, Rid, and Acticin. A second application of these agents is recommended in 7–10 days. Shaving the affected area is not necessary. Also can use dryer sheets to remove nits.
F. Complications. Atopic dermatitis secondary to pruritus and reaction to nits and eggs. Treat with appropriate topical corticosteroids and antihistamines.
G. Education. Proper use of topical medications and proper use of nit comb. Application of gasoline is not an accepted treatment and must be avoided.

VII. SCABIES

A. Etiology and occurrence. An infestation caused by *Sarcoptes scabiei*. Usually spread by skin-to-skin contact among household members and by sexual contact. The fertilized female mite burrows in the stratum corneum, laying eggs and feces which create irritation and pruritus.
B. Physical findings. Pinpoint vesicles and erythematous papules in S-shaped pattern. Finger webs, flexor wrists, areola, umbilicus, waist-band area, groin, and axilla are common sites of lesions. Children and adults rarely have lesions above the neck. Infants can manifest lesions on the palms and soles. Incubation from infestation to onset of symptoms is usually 1 month, with nocturnal itching most intense.
C. Diagnostic tests. Mineral oil applied to the vesicle, scraped with a No. 15 blade and placed on a slide with a cover slip reveals mites, eggs, or feces on microscopy.
D. Differential diagnosis. Insect bites, atopic dermatitis, drug eruptions.
E. Treatment. Permethrin is the treatment of choice. It has not been proven safe in infants younger than 2 months, or in pregnant or lactating women, therefore precipitated sulfur ointment is used for 3 nights. All household contacts should be treated. Treat pruritus with appropriate antihistamines, and secondary dermatitis with appropriate corticosteroids.
F. Follow up. Treatment failures, usually secondary to noncompliance, improper application of scabicide, or reinfection.
G. Complications. Secondary atopic dermatitis and bacterial infection.
H. Education. Proper application of scabicide. Mites can survive for 2 to 5 days on inanimate objects such as clothing and stuffed animals. Proper laundering should be taught.

VIII. LYME DISEASE

A. Etiology and occurrence. A systemic infection caused by the spirochete, *Borrelia burgdorferi*. Successful transmission requires 48–72 hours. It is found in the northeastern and midwestern United States, and can occur in any season, although most prevalent during the warmer months.

B. Clinical manifestations. Flulike symptoms including malaise, arthralgias, headache, fever and chills precede development of the rash.

C. Physical findings. A red macule or papule at the site of a tick bite 2–30 days after infection. The lesions expand to form annular erythematous lesions, generally with central clearing. The center of the lesion becomes darker, vesicular, hemorrhagic, or necrotic. Common sites are thigh, groin, trunk, and axilla.

D. Diagnostic tests. History, including exposure to tick bite, is important. Enzyme-linked immunosorbent assay (ELISA) and Western blot analyses for *B. burgdorferi* are recommended by the U.S. Centers for Disease Control and Prevention.

E. Differential diagnosis. *Tinea corporis*, urticaria, granuloma annulare, erythema annulare.

F. Treatment. Doxycycline 100 mg 2 times/day for 21 days, amoxicillin 500 mg 3 times/day for 21 days, ceftriaxone 500 mg 2 times/day for 21 days; azithromycin or erythromycin are second-line treatments for pregnant patients or those unable to tolerate above treatments.

G. Education. Educate patients on proper use of insect repellents, and to wear long pants, socks, and long-sleeved shirts in endemic areas.

IX. ROCKY MOUNTAIN SPOTTED FEVER

A. Etiology and occurrence. Rocky Mountain spotted fever, a prototype for all tick-borne spotted fevers, is caused by *R. rickettsii*. It occurs primarily in the southeastern and south central United States. All ages are susceptible; however, it is most common in children younger than 15 years of age. The incidence is highest in mid-summer, and lowest in winter.

B. Clinical manifestation and physical findings. A history of tick bite is common in more than 80% of cases. A prodrome of low-grade fever, headache, malaise, joint or muscle pain, and anorexia may precede the illness, which is sudden, consisting of sweating, chills, severe aches, vomiting, and diarrhea. The most common clinical findings are rash, edema, and fever. The rash may appear soon after the onset of symptoms, first on the ankles and feet, and spreading to the wrists, hands, trunk, and head. Discrete, rose-colored macules, blanching on pressure, soon become popular or purpuric. The resolving rash may desquamate with resulting hyperpigmentation. Nonpitting edema is frequent, with periorbital edema common in children. Conjunctivitis, pharyngitis, photophobia, CNS symptoms including confusion, delirium, seizures, and coma are common.

C. Diagnostic tests. Generally no rise in antibody titer is detected until the second week of the disease. An enzyme linked immunosorbent assay (ELISA) assay if IgM and IgG to *R. rickettsii* is sensitive and specific is indicated. Tissue direct and indirect immunofluorescence may identify rickettsiae.

D. Differential diagnosis. Viral exanthems, drug eruption, varicella, disseminated gonococcal infection, and Lyme disease.

E. Treatment. Doxycycline or tetracycline are the drugs of choice. Alternative treatment for those unable to treat or with history of allergies to these drugs include chloramphenicol. Supportive treatment for fever and myalgias.

F. Follow up. Close follow up for complications persisting beyond 1 year after acute infection for neurologic and nonneurologic disabilities.

G. Complications. Death is associated with older patients, those with delay in treatment, or undiagnosed disease. Untreated disease death rate is 25%. Other complications include neurologic disorders including hearing loss, peripheral neuropathy, bladder and bowel incontinence, cerebellar dysfunction, language disorders.

H. Education. Avoidance of tick bites and prompt removal of ticks. No vaccine is available.

X. MOLLUSCUM CONTAGIOSUM

A. Etiology. Molluscum contagiosum is a virus caused by a poxvirus infecting the epidermis, causing white papules. The center of the lesions are filled with keratinous material.

B. Occurrence. Molluscum contagiosum is common in infants and toddlers, and most adults are immune.

C. Clinical manifestations and physical findings. One- to 6-mm discrete umbilicated papules are seen usually in the interiginous areas. Occasionally, larger lesions up to 15 mm may be found. Incubation period is 2–7 weeks. Children are contagious as long as lesions are present. Lesions may resolve spontaneously, but this may take years.

D. Differential diagnosis. Warts, closed comedones, epidermal cysts. Blisters may be confused with molluscum contagiosum.

E. Treatment. Papules may be removed by curette or incision and drainage, however, this procedure is painful and may result in scarring. Treatment with liquid nitrogen, cantharidin, potassium hydroxide, or podophyllin applied to the central umbilication is less traumatic. Topical treatment at home with imiquimod cream is an alternative.

F. Complications. Secondary impetigo. Atopic dermatitis. Scarring.

G. Follow up. Office visits every 2 weeks for treatment will control spread of lesions.

H. Education. Lesions are benign but highly contagious.

XI. WARTS

A. Etiology. Warts are benign virus-induced tumors caused by human papillomavirus (HPV). More than 76 subtypes have been identified and are associated with specific cutaneous and mucous membrane location.

B. Occurrence. Transmission is by direct contact, and infection can occur by autoinnoculation, especially in interiginous areas. Immunocompromised patients are at increased risk.

C. Clinical manifestations and physical findings. Verrucous papules appear as solitary lesions or may be grouped, confluent, flat, or pedunculated. They may appear anywhere on the body, but occur most often on the extremities, interrupting the dermal ridges.

D. Diagnostic tests. No testing is necessary.

E. Differential diagnosis. Plantar warts may be differentiated from calluses by the interruption of dermal ridges. Common and filiform warts present no diagnostic challenge. Flat warts are often confused with closed comedones, lichen planus, and molluscum contagiosum.

F. Treatment. Multiple therapeutic modalities are available for treatment, including liquid nitrogen, cantharidin, electrodessication, laser therapy, candida and bleomycin injection, and excision. It is unlikely the warts will resolve with a single treatment except excision, and recurrence is high. Warts frequently resolve spontaneously, and good clinical judgment should be exercised when considering various therapies versus cautious observation. Multiple salicylic acid treatments are available over the counter, as well as prescription retinoids, podophyllin, and imiquimod cream. Cimetidine 30–40 mg/kg/day in combination with other treatment modalities is effective for resistant warts. See Table 20-4.

G. Follow up. Close follow up every 2 weeks.

Table 20-4 Treatment of Viral Warts

	Treatment		
Type of wart	First choice	Alternative	Response rate (%)
Common (078.1)	Cryotherapy	Salicylic acid paint	60–90
Periungual (078.1)	Imiquimod cream	Cantharidin	60
Flat (178.1)	Retinoic cream	Imiquimod cream	50
Filiform (078.1)	Surgery	Cryotherapy with forceps	50
Plantar (078.19)	Salicylic acid plaster	Imiquimod cream	60
Venereal (078.19)	Podophyllin or Condylox	Imiquimod cream	90

H. Complications. Proliferation of warts resulting in pain or difficulty with daily tasks. Social anxiety and social isolation due to cosmetic embarrassment requires more aggressive treatment.

I. Education. The recalcitrant nature of warts should be emphasized, as well as the need for multiple treatments. Genital warts in infants and toddlers should be evaluated for the possibility of sexual abuse.

XII. FIFTH DISEASE (ERYTHEMA INFECTIOSUM)

A. Etiology and occurrence. Erythema infectiosum (fifth disease) is caused by human parvovirus B19.

B. Clinical manifestations and physical findings. Fifth disease begins with intense red cheeks ("slapped cheeks") and spreads to involve arms, legs, and trunk with a macular red lacy exanthem. Although initially lasting less than 1 week, with heat exposure the exanthem can recur for up to 4 months.

E. Diagnostic tests. Serum obtained within 30 days of onset of rash will confirm the presence of immunoglobulin M (IgM) B19 antibodies

F. Differential diagnosis. Drug eruptions and other morbilliform eruptions can be differentiated by the classic lacy rash of fifth disease.

G. Treatment. There is no specific treatment nor are there specific control measures, other than avoid exposure to pregnant women and those who are immunocompromised. The disease is no longer contagious once the skin eruption occurs.

H. Complications. Hydrops fetalis may result in pregnant women who have not developed antibodies. Immunocompromised children may develop persistent infection. Patients with transient anemias may develop aplastic crisis and severe anemia.

I. Education. Inform of the likelihood of recurrence with heat exposure, including exercise and sun exposure. Avoid pregnant women and immunocompromised individuals, and those with chronic anemias.

XIII. SEBORRHEIC DERMATITIS

Atopic dermatitis, 691.8	Psoriasis, 696.1
Candida infection, 112.9	Scale, 782.8
Contact dermatitis, 692.9	Seborrhea dermatitis, 690.1
Infantile seborrhea dermatitis, 690.12	Tinea, 110

A. Etiology. Seborrheic dermatitis is an inflammatory disorder characterized by yellow-waxy scales in the scalp, eyebrows, auricular areas, and interiginous areas. These are areas of active sebaceous glands. *Malasezia furfur* is a yeast found on normal skin but highly prevalent in seborrheic dermatitis.

B. Occurrence. Usually appears in infancy and continues through adolescence and adulthood. More common in males. Affects 2–5% of the population.

C. Clinical manifestations. Greasy scales with well-defined borders, thick adherent symmetrical plaques distributed in the scalp, face, chest, and diaper area.

D. Differential diagnosis. Candidiasis, tinea, psoriasis, perioral dermatitis, as well as discoid lupus erythematosus.

E. Treatment. Removal of scalp scale with mineral oil and a fine tooth-comb provides relief. Shampoos containing selenium sulfide, pyrithione zinc, or ketaconazole can be used on the scalp as well as a face and body wash twice weekly as needed. Mild topical corticosteroids used sparingly control pruritus and erythema. In children older than 2 years of ages, topical immunomodulators may be used in place of topical steroids.

F. Education. This disorder waxes and wanes, therefore patients should be educated to restart therapy at the first sign of recurrence.

XIV. ERYTHEMA TOXICUM NEONATORUM

Erythema toxicum, 778.8	Pyoderma, 686
Herpes simplex, 054.9	Skin disorder, 709.9

A. Etiology. A common benign, self-limited eruption in the healthy, full-term newborn. Correlated with birth weight and gestational age, and seldom seen in preterm infants.

B. Occurrence. 30–70% full-term newborns, affecting sexes and races equally.

C. Clinical manifestations. One- to 2-mm discrete, pale yellow papules and pustules surrounded by erythematous wheal, predominantly on the face, trunk, and proximal extremities.

D. Diagnostic tests. Clinical appearance. Microscopic examination with Gram stain or Wright stain of pustular contents shows predominance of eosinophils.

E. Differential diagnosis.

Congenital cutaneous candidiasis, 112.9	Miliaria rubra, 705.1
Cytomegalovirus, 771.1	Scabies, 133
Group A streptococcal infection, 041.01	Superficial staphylococcal infection, 041.11
Herpes simplex, 054.9	

F. Treatment. No treatment necessary.

G. Education. Reassure parents that this is transient and benign. Post-inflammatory hyperpigmentation may follow but resolves within weeks to months.

XV. PITYRIASIS ROSEA

Pityriasis rosea, 696.3	Psoriasis, 696.1

A. Etiology. Common, benign, self-limited rash characterized by solitary salmon-colored "herald patch" which precedes exanthema by 1 to several weeks. Lesions usually asymptomatic. Human herpes virus types 6 and 7 have been implicated but not proven in etiology.

B. Occurrence. 10–35 years. Rare under 2 years of age. Most common in fall and spring of the year.

C. Clinical manifestations. Herald patch 1–10 cm followed by smaller, salmon-colored plaques with a fine collarette of scale, follows skin lines in a "Christmas tree configuration." Headache, malaise, and pharyngitis precedes rash in < 5% of cases.

D. Physical findings. Lesions on the trunk most common, in the axillae, posterior trunk, inguinal areas. Less common on the arms and legs. The face and head typically spared.

E. Diagnostic tests. Usually a clinical diagnosis based on history and clinical appearance. A KOH may be performed to rule out tinea.

F. Differential diagnosis.

Inea versicolor, 111	Tinea corporis, 100.5
Psoriasis, 696	

G. Treatment. No treatment is necessary, as this condition is self-limited. If lesions are pruritic, mild topical corticosteroids applied sparingly to affected areas as well as antihistamines control itching.

H. Education. Stress the benign nature of the exanthema. Post-inflammatory hyperpigmentation in pigmented skin can occur, and should be protected from sun exposure. Hyperpigmentation will resolve with time. It is uncommon for pityriasis rosea to recur.

BIBLIOGRAPHY

Burkhart CN, et al. *Visual DX: Essential Pediatric Dermatology.* Philadelphia, PA: Lippincott Williams & Wilkins; 2010.

Burns C, Barber N, Brady M, et al. *Pediatric Primary Care: A Handbook for Nurse Practitioners.* 4d ed. St. Louis, MO: Mosby; 2009.

Buttaro T, Trybulski J, Bailey P, et al. *Primary Care: A Collaborative Approach.* St. Louis, MO: Mosby; 1999.

Fitzpatrick T, Johnson R, Wolff K, et al. *Color Atlas and Synopsis of Clinical Dermatology.* 4th Ed. New York, NY: McGraw-Hill; 2001.

Goodheart H. *Goodheart's Photoguide of Common Skin Disorders.* Philadelphia, PA: Lippincott Williams & Wilkins; 2003.

Habif T. *Clinical Dermatology.* 3rd ed. St. Louis, MO: Mosby; 1996.

Kane KS-M, et al. *Color Atlas and Synopsis of Pediatric Dermatology.* 2nd ed. New York, NY: McGraw-Hill; 2009.

Schachner L, Hansen R. *Pediatric Dermatology.* 3rd ed. St. Louis, MO: Mosby; 2003.

Schalock, PC, et al. *Lippincott's Primary Care Dermatology.* Philadelphia, PA: Lippincott Williams & Wilkins; 2011.

Weston W, Lane A, Morelli J. *Color Textbook of Pediatric Dermatology.* 3rd ed. St. Louis, MO: Mosby: 2002.

Please see the end of the book for color images of dermatological conditions.

Eye Disorders

Frances K. Porcher

I. ALLERGIC CONJUNCTIVITIS

    A. Definition. Conjunctivitis: inflammation or infection of bulbar and/or palpebral conjunctiva.

    B. Etiology.

        1. Allergens such as pollen, molds, animal dander, smoke, dust.

    C. Occurrence.

        1. Common in all age groups.

        2. Often seasonal.

        3. May have had recent upper respiratory infection.

    D. Clinical manifestations.

        1. Watery, red eyes.

        2. Itching or burning bilaterally.

        3. Excessive tearing.

    E. Physical findings.

        1. Diffuse conjunctival hyperemia.

        2. Boggy conjunctiva.

        3. Stringy, mucoid discharge.

        4. May see concurrent asthma, atopic dermatitis, or allergic rhinitis.

    F. Diagnostic tests.

        1. None.

        2. Culture if conjunctivitis is persistent or does not respond to treatment.

G. Differential diagnosis.

Conjunctivitis, bacterial, 372.3	Corneal abrasion, 918.1
Conjunctivitis, viral, 077.99	Nasolacrimal duct obstruction, 375.56

    1. Bacterial or viral conjunctivitis.
    2. Nasolacrimal duct obstruction.
    3. Corneal abrasion.
H. Treatment.
    1. Eliminate offending agent.
    2. Systemic oral antihistamine (Claritin, Zyrtec).
    3. Topical ophthalmic mast-cell stabilizer (Cromolyn, Alomide).
    4. Topical ophthalmic antihistamine/mast-cell stabilizer combination (Patanol).
    5. Artificial tears.
    6. Cool, wet compresses.
I. Follow up.
    1. Routine follow up not necessary.
    2. Return if fails to improve in 2–3 days or worsens.
J. Complications.

Allergic reaction to medication, 995.5
Secondary bacterial infection, 041.9

    1. Allergic reaction to medication.
    2. Secondary bacterial infection.
K. Education.
    1. Avoid rubbing eyes.
    2. Use meticulous handwashing.
    3. Avoid wearing eye makeup until resolved.
    4. Avoid use of contact lenses until resolved.
    5. Will last about 10–14 days.

II. BACTERIAL CONJUNCTIVITIS

Conjunctival hyperemia, 372.71
Conjunctivitis, bacterial, 372.3
Otitis media, 382.9

A. Etiology.
   1. Haemophilus influenzae.
   2. Streptococcus pneumoniae.
   3. Moraxella catarrhalis.
B. Occurrence.
   1. Common in school-age children.
   2. Accounts for 80% of pediatric acute conjunctivitis.
C. Clinical manifestations.
   1. Red eyes.
   2. Purulent discharge, with matted eyelids on awakening.
   3. May complain of gritty sensation in eye.
   4. Usually starts unilaterally, becoming bilateral.
D. Physical findings.
   1. Diffuse and marked conjunctival hyperemia.
   2. Purulent or mucopurulent discharge.
   3. May see concurrent otitis media (especially with H. influenzae).
E. Diagnostic tests.
   1. Culture in infants younger than 1 month of age, multiple cases in a day-care/school; unless conjunctivitis is persistent or does not respond to treatment.
F. Differential diagnosis.

Blepharitis, 373	Corneal ulcer, 370
Chlamydial conjunctivitis, 077.98	Herpes simplex, 054.43
Conjunctivitis, viral, 077.99	Nasolacrimal duct obstruction, 375.56
Corneal abrasion, 918.1	Neisseria gonorrhoeae conjunctivitis, 098.4

   1. Viral conjunctivitis.
   2. Chlamydial conjunctivitis (refer to ophthalmologist).
   3. Neisseria gonorrhoeae conjunctivitis (refer to ophthalmologist).
   4. Nasolacrimal duct obstruction.
   5. Blepharitis.
   6. Corneal abrasion or ulcer (refer to ophthalmologist).
   7. Herpes simplex (refer to ophthalmologist).
G. Treatment.
   1. One year of age, newer generation ophthalmic fluoroquinolones.
      a. Levofloxacin (Quixin).

       b. Moxifloxacin (Vigamox).

       c. Gatifloxacin (Zymar).

    2. Younger than 1 year of age.

       a. Tobramycin (Tobrex) ophthalmic solution or ointment.

       b. Erythromycin ophthalmic ointment.

    3. Cool, wet compresses.

H. Follow up.

    1. No routine follow up necessary.

    2. Recheck if fails to improve in 2–3 days or worsens.

I. Complications.

Blindness, 369

Systemic infection, 038.9

---

    1. Systemic infection.

    2. Blindness.

J. Education.

    1. Continue treatment for at least 7 days or for at least 3 days after symptoms have resolved.

    2. Very contagious; meticulous handwashing and no sharing of linens.

    3. No school or daycare until antibiotic treatment for 24 hours.

    4. Instillation of ophthalmic ointment will blur vision.

III. CHLAMYDIAL CONJUNCTIVITIS

Chlamydial conjunctivitis, 077.99	Pneumonia, 486.
Chlamydial pneumonia, 483.1	Rhinorrhea, 478.1
Cough, 786.2	Tachypnea, 786.06
Hyperemic conjunctiva, 372.71	

A. Etiology.

    1. Chlamydia trachomatis.

B. Occurrence.

    1. Neonatal occurrence, acquired from infected cervix during birth.

    2. Adult occurrence, acquired through sexual contact.

C. Clinical manifestations.

    1. Purulent discharge.

      2.   May occur in one or both eyes.

      3.   Neonatal infection appears from day 2 to week 8.

D. Physical findings.

      1.   Mucopurulent discharge.

      2.   Hyperemic conjunctiva.

      3.   May see Chlamydia pneumonia in infants.

E. Diagnostic tests.

      1.   Giemsa-stained epithelial cells from conjunctival scraping.

      2.   Conjunctival culture from swab (requires special tissue culture techniques).

      3.   Immunofluorescent staining of conjunctival scraping.

      4.   Chlamydial antigen test.

F. Differential diagnosis.

Congenital glaucoma, 743.2	Conjunctivitis, viral, 077.99
Conjunctivitis, bacterial, 372.3	Neisseria gonorrhoeae conjunctivitis, 098.4

      1.   Neisseria gonorrhoeae conjunctivitis (refer to ophthalmologist).

      2.   Bacterial conjunctivitis.

      3.   Viral conjunctivitis.

      4.   Congenital glaucoma (refer to ophthalmologist).

G. Treatment.

      1.   Refer all neonates for evaluation and treatment (systemic oral erythromycin).

      2.   Refer mother and mother's sexual partner for evaluation and treatment.

      3.   Report to appropriate authority (sexually transmitted infection).

H. Follow up.

      1.   Return in 3 days to monitor eye infection.

      2.   Return sooner if infant has signs of pneumonia or parental concerns.

I. Complications.

      1.   Other sexually transmitted infections.

J. Education.

      1.   Review good handwashing with family.

      2.   Mother and partner need treatment because disease is usually transmitted vaginally during birth.

      3.   Eye infection can be associated with pneumonia that started during first 6 weeks with cough, rhinorrhea, tachypnea.

      4.   Infant may need second round of erythromycin; efficacy is 80%.

IV. VIRAL CONJUNCTIVITIS

Conjunctivitis, viral, 077.99	Pharyngitis, 462
Diffuse conjunctival hyperemia, 372.71	Upper respiratory infection, 465.9

A. Etiology.
  1. Adenovirus (most).
  2. Herpes simplex.
  3. Varicella zoster.
  4. Coxsackie.
B. Occurrence.
  1. Common in all age groups.
  2. Very contagious; 8-day incubation period.
C. Clinical manifestations.
  1. Pinkish-red eyes.
  2. Watery or serous discharge, with crusty eyelids on awakening.
  3. May complain of gritty sensation in eye.
  4. May complain of sore throat, upper respiratory infection, flulike symptoms.
  5. One or both eyes involved.
  6. Vesicles on skin around eye (herpes).
D. Physical findings.
  1. Diffuse conjunctival hyperemia with follicles.
  2. Watery or serous discharge.
  3. Discomfort, not acute pain.
  4. Preauricular and submandibular adenopathy.
  5. May see concurrent pharyngitis and/or upper respiratory infection.
  6. Vesicular lesions on skin around eyes (herpes).
  7. Normal vision.
E. Diagnostic tests.
  1. None.
  2. Culture if conjunctivitis is persistent or does not respond to treatment.
F. Differential diagnosis.

Blepharitis, 373	Corneal abrasion, 918.1
Conjunctivitis, allergic, 372.14	Corneal ulcer, 370
Conjunctivitis, bacterial, 372.3	Nasolacrimal duct obstruction, 375.56

  1. Bacterial conjunctivitis.
  2. Allergic conjunctivitis.

     3. Nasolacrimal duct obstruction.

     4. Blepharitis.

     5. Corneal abrasion or ulcer (refer to ophthalmologist).

G. Treatment.

     1. Antibiotics not indicated.

     2. Cool, wet compresses.

     3. Artificial tears.

     4. Refer if suspect conjunctivitis due to herpes.

H. Follow up.

     1. No routine follow up necessary.

     2. Recheck if fails to improve in 10–14 days; sooner if worsens.

I. Complications.

Secondary bacterial infection, 041.9

     1. Secondary bacterial infection.

J. Education.

     1. Very contagious; meticulous handwashing and no sharing of linens.

     2. Avoid touching eyes.

     3. Will last about 12–14 days.

     4. No school or daycare until discharge is resolved.

V. CONGENITAL NASOLACRIMAL DUCT OBSTRUCTION (DACRYOSTENOSIS)

A. Definition. Congenital nasolacrimal duct obstruction (dacryostenosis), 375.56 Defect of lacrimal drainage system resulting in blockage.

B. Etiology.

     1. Imperforate membrane at distal end of nasolacrimal duct.

C. Occurrence.

     1. Occurs in up to 6% of all newborn infants.

     2. Both eyes involved, 33%; one eye involved, 66%.

D. Clinical manifestations.

     1. Persistent, excessively watery eyes.

     2. Mucopurulent discharge.

     3. Matted eyes on awakening.

E. Physical findings.

     1. Watery eyes, often overflowing onto cheek.

     2. Sclera clear.

     3. Reflux of mucopurulent discharge from punctum easily obtained with gentle pressure over nasolacrimal sac.

     4. May see concurrent erythema or irritation of skin around eyes.

F. Diagnostic tests.
   1. Gentle pressure over nasolacrimal sac produces mucopurulent discharge from punctum.
G. Differential diagnosis.

Blepharitis, 373	Conjunctivitis, viral, 077.99
Conjunctivitis, bacterial, 372.3	Dacryocystitis, 375.3

   1. Viral conjunctivitis.
   2. Bacterial conjunctivitis.
   3. Blepharitis.
   4. Dacryocystitis.
H. Treatment.
   1. Massage lacrimal sac several times a day.
   2. If secondarily infected, treat with anti-infective (see Bacterial Conjunctivitis).
   3. Refer to ophthalmologist if not resolved by 12 months of age.
I. Follow up.
   1. Recheck at all well-baby exams and as needed.
J. Complications.

Conjunctivitis, bacterial, 372.3
Dacryocystitis, 375.3
Periorbital or orbital cellulites, 376.01

   1. Bacterial conjunctivitis.
   2. Dacryocystitis.
   3. Periorbital or orbital cellulites.
K. Education.
   1. Wash hands before touching infant's eyes.
   2. Teach massage technique: place index finger over lacrimal sac, exert gentle downward pressure, and slide finger downward toward mouth.

VI. BLEPHARITIS

A. Definition.

Blepharitis, 373
Conjunctivitis, 372.3
Inflammation or infection of margins of eyelid.

B. Etiology.
   1. Seborrhea.
   2. Staphylococcal.
   3. Pediculus pubis or P. capitis.
C. Occurrence.
   1. Can occur in all age groups.
D. Clinical manifestations.
   1. Red eyelid margin.
   2. Itching or burning of eyelid margin.
   3. Crusting or scaling of eyelid margin.
   4. Commonly bilateral and chronic or recurrent.
E. Physical findings.
   1. Seborrhea.
      a. Easy-to-remove yellow, greasy scales along base of eyelashes.
      b. May see concurrent and similar scales on eyebrows, scalp, external ears.
   2. Staphylococcal.
      a. Fibrinous, difficult-to-remove scales along base of eyelashes.
      b. Inflammation or ulceration of lid margins.
      c. Loss of eyelashes.
      d. May see concurrent conjunctivitis.
   3. Pediculosis.
      a. Lice along lid margins.
      b. May see concurrent pubic or head lice.
F. Diagnostic tests.
   1. Culture of lid margin indicated only if fails to respond to treatment.
G. Differential diagnosis.

Conjunctivitis, allergic, 372.14	Dermatitis, contact, 692.9
Conjunctivitis, bacterial, 372.3	Nasolacrimal duct obstruction, 375.56
Conjunctivitis, viral, 077.99	Seborrheic dermatitis, 690.1
Dermatitis, atopic, 691.8	

   1. Conjunctivitis (allergic, bacterial, or viral).
   2. Nasolacrimal duct obstruction.
   3. Atopic or contact dermatitis.
   4. Seborrheic dermatitis.

H. Treatment.
   1. Clean eyelid margins twice a day with diluted baby shampoo.
   2. Seborrhea blepharitis: treat eyebrows, scalp, ears with selenium sulfide shampoo.
   3. Staphylococcal blepharitis: apply topical anti-infective ointment (erythromycin ophthalmic ointment or bacitracin/polymyxin B ophthalmic ointment).
   4. Pediculosis blepharitis: remove parasite by smothering with ophthalmic petrolatum along lid margins.
I. Follow up.
   1. No routine follow up necessary.
   2. Recheck if fails to improve; sooner if worsens.
J. Complications.

Conjunctivitis, 372.3

Hordeolum, external, 373.11

Hordeolum, internal, 373.12

---

   1. Loss of eyelashes.
   2. Conjunctivitis.
   3. Hordeolum or chalazion.
K. Education.
   1. Frequent handwashing.
   2. Discourage rubbing of eyes.

VII. HORDEOLUM

Hordeolum, external, 373.11

Hordeolum, internal, 373.12

A. Definition. Infection of meibomian glands (internal hordeolum) or glands of Zeis or Moll (external hordeolum or stye) of eyelid.
B. Etiology.
   1. Usually Staphylococcal aureus.
C. Occurrence.
   1. Can occur at any age.
D. Clinical manifestations.
   1. Internal: painful and tender eyelid, red eye, usually without pustule.
   2. External: painful and tender eyelid, red eye, usually with pustule.

E. Physical findings.
  1. Internal: large, erythematous, tender mound of one eyelid with associated mild conjunctival hyperemia.
  2. External: smaller, more superficial eyelid pustule with associated mild conjunctival hyperemia.
F. Diagnostic tests.
  1. None indicated.
G. Differential diagnosis.

> Chalazion, 373.2
> Eyelid abscess, 373.13

  1. Chalazion.
  2. Eyelid abscess.
H. Treatment.
  1. Frequent, warm compresses.
  2. May use topical antiinfective ointment (erythromycin ophthalmic ointment or bacitracin/polymyxin B ophthalmic ointment).
  3. Refer if mass fails to disappear after several weeks (may need surgical incision and drainage).
I. Follow up.
  1. No routine follow up necessary.
  2. Recheck if fails to resolve or worsens.
J. Complications.

> Orbital or eyelid cellulitis, 376.01

  1. Orbital or eyelid cellulitis.
K. Education.
  1. Frequent handwashing.
  2. Avoid rubbing eyes.

VIII. CHALAZION

A. Definition.

> Chalazion, 373.2
> Inflammation of meibomian glands of eyelid.

  B. Etiology.
     1. Granulomatous inflammation.
  C. Occurrence.
     1. Can occur at any age.
  D. Clinical manifestations.
     1. Hard mass in upper or lower eyelid.
     2. Not red or pustular.
     3. Chronic appearance.
  E. Physical findings.
     1. Firm, nontender nodule in upper or lower eyelid.
     2. Not erythematous or pustular.
     3. No eye discharge.
  F. Diagnostic tests.
     1. None indicated.
  G. Differential diagnosis.

Dacryocystitis, 375.3	Hordeolum, internal, 373.12
Eyelid abscess, 373.13	Orbital cellulitis, 376.01
Hordeolum, external, 373.11	

     1. Hordeolum (internal or external).
     2. Orbital cellulitis.
     3. Dacryocystitis (inflammation of the lacrimal sac).
     4. Eyelid abscess.
  H. Treatment.
     1. Most spontaneously subside without treatment.
     2. Surgical removal if size distorts vision.
  I. Follow up.
     1. No routine follow up necessary.
     2. Recheck if fails to improve or worsens.
  J. Complications.

Distorted vision, 368.15

     1. Distorted vision secondary to size of lesion.
  K. Education.
     1. Frequent handwashing.
     2. Avoid rubbing eyes.

IX. CHEMICAL BURN

A. Definition.

Burn of the eye, 940.9	Opacity of corneal tissue, 371
Eye pain, 379.91	Photophobia, 368.13
Eyelid burn, 940.9	Swollen corneas, 379.92

Instillation of alkali or acid solution or substance to eye. True emergency needs immediate referral to ophthalmologist.

B. Etiology.
1. Installation of alkali or acid solution or substance into eye.

C. Occurrence.
1. Boys > girls.
2. 11- to 15-year olds have highest rate of injury.

D. Clinical manifestations.
1. Eye pain.
2. Unable to open eye(s).

E. Physical findings.
1. Eyelid burn.
2. Opacity of corneal tissue, pale surrounding tissue.
3. Photophobia.
4. Tearing, swollen corneas.

F. Diagnostic tests.
1. None.

G. Differential diagnosis.

Eyelid injury, 921.1
Foreign body, eye, 930

1. Foreign body.
2. Type of chemical burn.
3. Eyelid injury.

H. Treatment.
1. Emergency treatment is immediate irrigation with copious amounts of water or saline.
2. Emergency referral to ophthalmologist.

    I.   Follow up.
        1. Per ophthalmologist.
    J. Complications.

Loss of vision, 369.9

        1. Loss of vision.
    K. Education.
        1. Prevention is most important.
        2. Need to know name of chemical in eye; acid burns affect cornea and anterior chamber of eye.
        3. Alkali burns can continue for days.

X. CORNEAL ABRASION (SUPERFICIAL)

    A. Definition.

Corneal abrasion (superficial), 918.1	Eye pain, 379.91
Decreased vision, 369.9	Photophobia, 368.13
Excessive tearing, 375.2	

        Scratched, abraded, or denuded cornea.
    B. Etiology.
        1. Usually due to accidental contact with object (fingernail, branches, bushes, paper, contact lens overwear).
    C. Occurrence.
        1. Can occur at any age.
    D. Clinical manifestations.
        1. Pain.
        2. Excessive tearing.
        3. Photophobia.
        4. Decreased vision.
    E. Physical findings.
        1. May see uneven light reflection or cloudiness of cornea.
        2. May see foreign body.
        3. After staining with fluorescein and using cobalt-blue light or Wood's lamp, will see area of green staining (persists with blinking).
        4. Decreased visual acuity.

F. Diagnostic tests.
1. Fluorescein staining and cobalt-blue light or Wood's lamp.
G. Differential diagnosis.

Foreign body, eye, 930
---

1. Foreign body.
H. Treatment.
1. Instill topical ophthalmic anti-infective ointment (erythromycin ophthalmic ointment or bacitracin/polymyxin B ophthalmic ointment).
2. Patching not recommended.
I. Follow-up.
1. Recheck in 24–48 hours, or sooner if worsens.
J. Complications.

Impaired vision, 369.9

Eye infection, 360
---

1. Infection.
2. Impaired vision.
K. Education.
1. Frequent handwashing.
2. Avoid use of contact lenses for at least 1 week following healing of abrasion.

XI. FOREIGN BODY (CONJUNCTIVAL, CORNEAL)

A. Definition.

Excessive tearing, 375.2	Photophobia, 368.13
Foreign body, eye, 930	Sensation that something is in eye, 368.9
Presence of abnormal substance or object in eye.	

B. Etiology.
1. Usually object is airborne.
C. Occurrence.
1. Can occur at any age.

    D. Clinical manifestations.
       1. Excessive tearing.
       2. Photophobia.
       3. Sensation that something is in eye.
    E. Physical findings.
       1. Excessive tearing.
       2. Use bright light or magnification to visualize corneal and conjunctival surfaces for foreign body.
       3. May need to evert upper eyelid to find foreign body.
    F. Diagnostic tests.
       1. None.
    G. Differential diagnosis.

Eye infection, 360

Perforation of ocular globe, 370.06

---

       1. Infection.
       2. Perforation of ocular globe.
    H. Treatment.
       1. Test visual acuity.
       2. Remove foreign body if possible with moistened, cotton-tipped applicator.
       3. After removal of foreign body, inspect for corneal abrasion using fluorescein.
       4. Refer to ophthalmologist if large abrasion or unable to find foreign body.
    I. Follow up.
       1. Recheck in 24 hours or sooner if worsens.
    J. Complications.
       1. Infection.
       2. Damage to cornea.
    K. Education.
       1. Avoid rubbing eyes.
       2. Teach prevention of eye injuries (protective eyewear).

XII. HEMORRHAGE (SUBCONJUNCTIVAL)

    A. Definition.

Hemorrhage (subconjunctival), 372.72

Ruptured blood vessel in eye, 459

B. Etiology.
  1. Sudden increase in intrathoracic pressure (coughing, sneezing).
  2. Direct ocular trauma.
C. Occurrence.
  1. Can occur at any age.
D. Clinical manifestations.
  1. Ruptured blood vessel in eye.
E. Physical findings.
  1. Blotchy, bulbar erythema of conjunctiva.
F. Diagnostic tests.
  1. None.
G. Differential diagnosis.
  1. Ocular trauma.
H. Treatment.
  1. None; will spontaneously resolve in 5–7 days.
  2. Refer to ophthalmologist if due to trauma.
I. Follow up.
  1. No routine follow up necessary.
  2. Recheck if fails to disappear in 5–7 days, or worsens.
J. Complications.
  1. Usually none.
K. Education.
  1. Teach measures to avoid increasing intrathoracic pressure.

XIII. HYPHEMA

A. Definition.

Eye pain, 379.91
Hyphema, 364.41
Impaired vision, 369.9

Blood in anterior chamber of eye.
B. Etiology
  1. Usually due to blunt or perforating trauma to eye.
C. Occurrence.
  1. Variable.
D. Clinical manifestations.
  1. Bright or dark red area near iris.
  2. Painful.

E. Physical findings.
 1. Bright or dark red fluid level between cornea and iris.
F. Diagnostic tests.
 1. X-rays, CT scan for other injuries.
G. Differential diagnosis.
 Foreign body, conjunctival, 930.1
 1. Type of foreign body.
H. Treatment.
 1. Immediate referral to ophthalmologist.
I. Follow up.
 1. Per ophthalmologist.
J. Complications.
 Impaired vision, 369.9
 1. More extensive ocular injury.
 2. Rebleeding, which may result in vision impairment.
K. Education.
 1. Children sometimes take weeks for vision to return to normal.
 2. Prevention is best.
 3. Encourage parents to continue follow up as recommended by ophthalmologist.

XIV. OCULAR TRAUMA

A. Definition.

Blurred vision, 368.8	Eye pain, 379.91
Decreased/impaired vision, 369.9	Eye redness, 379.93
Double vision, 368.2	

Indirect or direct serious injury to eye.
B. Etiology.
 1. Fireworks, sticks, stones, BB shots.
 2. Sports related.
C. Occurrence.
 1. One-third of all causes of acquired blindness.
 2. Males > females 4:1.
D. Clinical manifestations.
 1. Double, blurred, or decreased vision.
 2. Eye pain or pain in surrounding area.
 3. Tearing.

E. Physical findings.
   1. Unable to open eye.
   2. Tearing.
   3. Corneal redness.
F. Diagnostic tests.
   1. X-rays if orbital fracture or nasal fracture is suspected.
G. Differential diagnosis.

> Laceration to ocular globe or orbit, 871.4
>
> Orbital wall fracture, 802.8
>
> Perforation to ocular globe or orbit, 370.06

   1. Laceration to ocular globe or orbit.
   2. Perforation to ocular globe or orbit.
   3. Orbital wall fracture.
H. Treatment.
   1. Referral to ophthalmologist.
I. Follow up.
   1. Per ophthalmologist.
J. Complications.

> Blindness, 369
>
> Eye infection, 360

   1. Extensive ocular injury.
   2. Blindness.
   3. Infection.
K. Education.
   1. Prevention: use of goggles or glasses when spraying.
   2. Do not instill any medication.
   3. Immediate referral to ophthalmologist.

XV. PRESEPTAL CELLULITIS (PERIORBITAL CELLULITIS)

A. Definition.

> | | |
> |---|---|
> | Dental abscess, 522.5 | Periorbital cellulitis, 376.01 |
> | Edematous, 782.3 | Sinusitis, 473.9 |
> | Erythema, unspecified, 695.9 | Swelling of the eye, 379.92 |
> | Fever, 780.6 | |

Inflammation and infection of eyelids and periorbital tissue.

B. Etiology.
   1. Staphylococcal aureus.
   2. Streptococcus pneumoniae.
   3. Streptococcus pyogenes.
   4. Haemophilus influenzae type B.
C. Occurrence.
   1. Common in young children secondary to trauma, infected wound or insect bite, severe sinusitis, dental abscess.
D. Clinical manifestations.
   1. Red, painful swelling around eye.
   2. May or may not have fever.
   3. History of local trauma to area, insect bite, sinusitis, dental abscess.
E. Physical findings.
   1. Erythematous, edematous, tender, warm area around eye.
   2. Regional adenopathy.
F. Diagnostic tests.
   1. CBC (will indicate leukocytosis in severe cases).
   2. Blood culture.
   3. Head CT scan (helps delineate extent of disease).
G. Differential diagnosis.

Conjunctivitis, 372.3	Retinoblastoma, 190.5
Contact dermatitis, 692.9	Rhabdomyosarcoma, 171.9
Neuroblastoma, 160	

---

   1. Severe contact dermatitis.
   2. Severe conjunctivitis.
   3. Ophthalmic malignancy or tumor (retinoblastoma, rhabdomyosarcoma, neuroblastoma).
H. Treatment.
   1. Uncomplicated and older than 2 months of age: ceftriaxone then oral antibiotics, oral antiinfective (amoxicillin-clavulanate, cephalexin, or erythromycin).
   2. Complicated/extensive or younger than 2 months of age: requires hospitalization and intravenous antibiotics.
I. Follow up.
   1. Daily follow up is necessary to monitor for rapid improvement.

J. Complications.

Eyelid abscess, 373.13
Loss of vision, 369.9
---

1. Spread of infection with possible abscess formation.
2. Loss of vision.
K. Education.
1. Frequent handwashing.
2. Teach prevention (avoid trauma, use insect repellent, cleanse wounds).

BIBLIOGRAPHY

American Academy of Ophthalmology. *Preferred Practice Patterns*. http://one.aao.org/CE/PracticeGuidelines/ PPP.aspx. Accessed September 8, 2010.

Ehlers JP, Shah CP, eds. *The Willis Eye Manual: Office and Emergency Room Diagnosis and Treatment of Eye Disease*. 5th ed. Baltimore, MD: Lippincott Williams & Wilkins; 2008.

Hunter A. Problems related to the head, eyes, ears, nose, throat or mouth. In: Barnes K, ed. *Paediatrics—A Clinical Guide for Nurse Practitioner*s. Philadelphia, PA: Butterworth-Heinemann; 2003.

Kliegman RM, Behrman RE, Jenson HB, et al. *Nelson Textbook of Pediatrics*. 18th ed. Philadelphia, PA: Saunders; 2007.

Nelson LB, Olitsky SE, eds. *Harley's Pediatric Ophthalmology*. 5th ed. Philadelphia, PA: Lippincott Williams & Wilkins; 2005.

Trobe JD. *The Physician's Guide to Eye Care*. 3rd ed. San Francisco, CA: American Academy of Ophthalmology; 2006.

CHAPTER 22

Ear Disorders

Jane A. Fox

I. FOREIGN BODY

Decreased hearing, 389.9	Otitis externa, 380.1
Discharge from ear, 388.6	Pain or itching, 388.7
Foreign body, ear, 931	

A. Etiology.
  1. Usually results from young children or their companions placing stones, erasers, vegetables (beans, peas, string beans), paper, jellybeans, toy parts, or small alkaline batteries in their ear(s).
  2. Insects may become lodged in ear.
  3. Chronic irritation or inflammation (e.g., otitis externa may result from putting objects in ear).
B. Occurrence.
  1. Most common between 2 and 4 years of age.
C. Clinical manifestations.
  1. Presenting complaints may include:
    a. Pain or itching.
    b. Decreased hearing.
    c. Buzzing if insect is in ear canal.
    d. Feeling of fullness in ear or pressure.
    e. Discharge from ear.
D. Physical findings.
  1. Foreign object or insect visualized on otoscopic exam.
  2. Check all body orifices if foreign body found in one.
  3. Carefully check ear after removal of foreign object for additional ones.
E. Diagnostic tests.
  1. Usually none.

F. Differential diagnosis.

Contact dermatitis and eczema, 692.9	Otitis media, 382.9
Impacted cerumen, 380.4	Psoriasis, 696.1
Otitis externa, 380.1	Trauma, 959.09

  1. Foreign body: object or insect is visualized on otoscopic exam.
  2. Otitis media (OM).
  3. Otitis externa.
  4. Trauma.
  5. Impacted cerumen.
  6. Dermatologic disorders (psoriasis or eczema).
G. Treatment.
  1. Remove foreign body. If bleeding occurs, object must be removed.
  2. Have child lie down, restrain head if needed.
  3. *Do not irrigate* if foreign body is vegetable or wood and/or suspect perforation of tympanic membrane.
  4. Insect in ear: Kill insect by filling ear canal with mineral oil or alcohol before removal. Ticks: Dislodge ticks by filling canal with 70% alcohol and then remove.
  5. Removal of objects.
    a. Best: Remove objects using an otoscope with an opening head for visualization.
    b. Objects that are soft and unwedged.
      • Remove by irrigation with tepid water (body temperature) and water pik on low setting or an 18-gauge butterfly catheter with needle cut off. Pulsating water should help dislodge object.
      • Insert pliable tubing into ear canal behind foreign body.
  6. If object does not completely occlude canal, can use ear loop, curette, forceps for removal.
  7. Refer to otolaryngologist if:
    a. Object is an alkaline battery.
    b. Object cannot be easily removed.
    c. Ear canal is swollen or bleeding.
    d. Object is tightly wedged in canal.
    e. Child is unable to cooperate.
H. Follow up.
  1. Generally none, well-child care.
I. Complications.

Perforation of tympanic membrane, 384.2

      1.   Perforation of tympanic membrane (TM).
J. Education.
      1.   Advise parents not to attempt to remove foreign body.
      2.   Tell parents some bleeding may occur after removal.
      3.   Cleaning ear canal is not necessary.

II. HEARING LOSS: CONDUCTIVE, SENSORINEURAL

Allergies, 477.9	Hearing loss, sensorineural, 389.1
Anomalies of external ear, 744.3	Impacted cerumen, 380.4
Cholesteatoma, 385.3	Middle ear anomalies, 744.03
Decreased hearing, 389.9	Middle ear effusions, 389.03
Delayed language development, 315.39	Neck anomalies, 744.9
Foreign body, ear, 931	Otitis externa, 380.1
Head and ear trauma, 959.09	Otitis media, 382.9
Head anomalies, 756	TM perforation, 384.2
Hearing loss, conductive, 389	

A. Etiology.
      1.   Genetic or hereditary factors, environmental or acquired diseases, malformations.
      2.   Trauma.
      3.   Congenital perinatal infections.
      4.   About 33% of cases of hearing impairment: cause unknown.
B. Occurrence.
      1.   About 15% of school-age children have significant conductive hearing losses.
      2.   OM and its sequelae most common cause of conductive hearing losses during childhood.
      3.   Acquired conductive hearing losses most common types of hearing loss in childhood.
C. Clinical manifestations.
      1.   *Conductive hearing loss* (middle ear hearing loss).
          a. Decreased hearing.
          b. May have history of middle ear effusions.
          c. OM and its sequelae.
          d. Foreign body and/or impacted cerumen.

    e. May report delayed language and speech development or parental
       concern about child's ability to hear.
    f. Allergies.
    g. Head or ear trauma.
    h. Middle ear anomalies.
    i. Cholesteatoma can cause hearing loss.
  2. *Sensorineural hearing loss* (perceptive or nerve deafness) may report dis-
     tortion of sound and problems in discrimination of sounds. Hearing loss
     often involves high-range frequencies, speech difficulties.
D. Physical findings.
  1. Conductive hearing loss (middle ear hearing loss).
    a. Possible:
       • Otitis externa.
       • OM.
       • Foreign body.
       • Impacted cerumen.
       • Growths or tumors, cholesteatomas.
       • TM perforation.
    b. Rinne test on affected side; bone conduction (BC), air conduction
       (AC).
    c. Weber test sounds lateralized to involved side.
    d. Average hearing loss 27–31 dB (mild), may be intermittent, may occur
       in one or both ears.
  2. Sensorineural hearing loss (perceptive or nerve deafness).
    a. Possible dysmorphic facial features suggesting presence of syndrome.
    b. Head and/or neck anomalies.
    c. Anomalies of pinnae and external ear canals.
    d. Weber test sounds louder in unaffected ear.
    e. Rinne test: in normal ear or ear with sensorineural hearing loss,
       AC, BC.
  3. Audiometric testing: soft sounds not well perceived, loud sounds per-
     ceived almost normally. In older children, if normal in high and low
     frequencies but poor in middle frequencies, suspect congenital hearing
     loss.
  4. Acquisition of language skills affected.
E. Diagnostic tests.
  1. Evoked otoacoustic emissions (EOAE) testing (can be performed on chil-
     dren of all ages): newer type of newborn screening, 10 minutes.
  2. Automated auditory brainstem response (AABR): for newborn screening,
     10 minutes.

3. Brainstem auditory evoked response (BAER): newborn screening, 90 minutes; often used in children of all ages who are unable to cooperate for audiometry testing.
4. Behavioral observation audiometry.
5. Pure tone audiometry for children 5 years of age.
6. Tympanometry identifies a middle ear effusion.
7. Impedance audiometry.
8. Language screening: Early Language Milestone Scale.

F. Differential diagnosis.

Hearing loss, conductive, 389

Hearing loss, sensorineural, 389.1

Mixed conductive sensorineural loss, 389.2

---

1. Careful history and thorough physical examination, including screening and laboratory data, essential in identifying those at risk and in early detection of hearing losses.
2. Hearing disorders classified into three categories:
   a. Conductive hearing loss.
   b. Sensorineural hearing loss.
   c. Mixed conductive sensorineural loss.

G. Treatment.
1. Refer for audiologic testing.
2. Surgery for conductive hearing loss (usually bilateral myringotomy with tubes).
3. Refer to multidisciplinary team, hearing center, or ENT specialist if hearing impairment detected.
4. For sensorineural loss:
   a. Amplification (hearing aids; bilateral is best) benefits most children.
   b. Cochlear implants with sensorineural loss, if done within 4 years of hearing loss.
   c. Clarion CII Bionic Ear System for deafness.

H. Follow up.
1. Determined by type and cause of hearing loss.
2. Well-child care.

I. Complications.

Speech and language disorder, 315.39

---

1. Speech and language disorders.

J. Education.
1. Early detection imperative to minimize negative consequences for language, other development.
2. Disease process, type of loss, causes. Conductive loss usually reversible, sensorineural loss often irreversible.
3. To decrease incidence of communication disorder in child with middle ear disease:
   a. When speaking to child, turn off sources of background noise (e.g., dishwasher, television, radio, stereo, computer games, etc.).
   b. Make sure child is looking directly at speaker and that speaker has child's attention.
   c. Speak louder than normal.
   d. Child should sit in front of classroom (may need referral for full evaluation of hearing needs).
4. Effects on child.
   a. Speech and language development.
   b. Social development.
   c. Learning process.
5. Needs of child.
   a. Emotional.
   b. Social.
   c. Educational.
6. Parents' role.
   a. Care and function of hearing aids, if indicated.
   b. Medic alert bracelet.
7. Parent support groups.
8. Support groups for the child.
9. Prevention: Limit exposure to loud noise.

III. OTITIS EXTERNA

Contact dermatitis and eczema, 692.9	Psoriasis, 696.1
Otitis externa, 381.1	Seborrhea, 706.3
Perforation of the tympanic membrane, 384.2	

A. Etiology.
1. Bacteria: *Pseudomonas aeruginosa* (most common); *Streptococcus* species, *Staphylococcus epidermidis, Proteus* species, *Mycoplasma* species.
2. Fungi: *Aspergillus* species, *Candida* organisms.

3. Excess cerumen or loss of protective cerumen from exposure to excess moisture.
4. Trauma to the ear canal caused by overzealous cleaning with a cotton-tipped applicator or a foreign body.
5. Allergic reaction to chemical or physical agents; contact dermatitis.
6. Excessive wetness from swimming, bathing, or high humidity.
7. Excessive dryness; child or family history of eczema, psoriasis, seborrhea.
8. Purulent otitis media with perforation of the tympanic membrane and drainage may masquerade as otitis externa, usually painless with no swelling of the canal.

B. Occurrence.
1. Most common in hot, muggy weather, summer months.
2. Persons who are swimmers or divers are more susceptible.
3. Higher incidence in those with smaller ear canals.
4. Males and females equally affected.
5. Affects all ages.

C. Clinical manifestations.
1. Ear pain and itching (common in fungal infections) in the ear, especially when chewing or pressure on tragus.
2. Feeling of fullness or obstruction of ear.
3. Frequently, a history of exposure to water.
4. Purulent discharge and hearing loss (conductive) possible.

D. Physical findings.
1. Pain on movement of pinna or tragus.
2. Periauricular adenitis may occur, but not necessary for diagnosis.
3. External canal: gross edema and erythema of canal, accumulation of moist debris in canal. Patient may resist insertion of ear speculum.
4. Tympanic membrane often difficult to visualize and may be mildly inflamed but is mobile on insufflation.

E. Diagnostic tests.
1. No tests specific to diagnosing otitis externa.
2. Gram stain and culture of discharge may be helpful, particularly when fungal cause is suspected.

F. Differential diagnosis.

Abscess of otitis externa, 380.1	Furuncle of otitis externa, 680
Contact dermatitis and eczema, 692.9	Mastoiditis, 389.3
Cyst of otitis externa, 382	Otitis externa, malignant, 160.1
Dental infection, 522.4	Otitis media with perforation, 384
Foreign body, ear, 931	Postauricular lymphadenopathy, 289.3

1. Cyst, furuncle, or abscess.
2. Foreign body.
3. Otitis media with perforation.
4. Dental infection.
5. Mastoiditis.
6. Postauricular lymphadenopathy.
7. Eczema or other dermatologic condition.
8. Malignant otitis externa.
G. Treatment.
   1. Clean debris from canal: Insert small gauze wick or absorbent sponge into external canal to carry antibiotic corticosteroid solution into canal if needed (severe swelling).
   2. Ciprofloxacin hydrochloride/hydrocortisone otic suspension (Cipro HC Otic Suspension) has broad spectrum for covering resistant organisms or combination eardrops of antibiotics, hydrocortisone, propylene glycol.
      a. Not recommended for children younger than 1 year of age.
      b. Advise parents to warm bottle in hands for 1–2 minutes before use and then place 3 drops in affected ear(s) 2 times a day for 7 days.
   3. Ofloxacin solution 0.3% otic drops (Floxin) every 12 hours.
      a. Highly effective if *Pseudomonas aeruginosa* and *Staphylococcus aureus* are causes in patients 1 year of age and older.
      b. Age 1–12 years: 5 drops in affected ear(s) 2 times daily for 10 days.
      c. Older than 12 years of age: 10 drops in affected ear(s) twice daily for 10 days.
   4. Analgesics for pain.
   5. Oral antibiotics only if signs of invasive infection.
      a. Cellulitis of auricle.
      b. Fever.
      c. Tender postauricular lymph nodes.
   6. Topical treatment is always needed to treat otitis externa.
   7. Keep ear dry.
   8. Do not use cotton swabs.
H. Follow up.
   1. Mild cases: none.
   2. Immediate recheck: pain worsens or sensitivity to eardrops.
   3. Return visit in 2–3 days if marked cellulitis or tympanic membrane was not visualized.
   4. Return visit if symptoms worsen, do not improve in 48 hours, or recur.
   5. Telephone if severe pain.
   6. Recheck in 10 days and continue treatment, if not completely resolved.

I. Complications.

Cellulitis of surrounding tissue, 380.1	Stenosis of auditory canal, 380.5
Irritated furunculosis, 680	Transient conductive hearing loss, 388.02
Malignant otitis externa, 172.3	

   1. Cellulitis of surrounding tissue.
   2. Irritated furunculosis.
   3. Malignant otitis externa (uncommon) seen in chronically ill or immuno-suppressed children.
   4. Stenosis of auditory canal.
   5. Transient conductive hearing loss.
J. Education.
   1. Explain cause and treatment plan.
     a. Keep ear dry: no swimming during acute phase, can use cotton coated with petroleum jelly or lamb's wool when showering or shampooing to occlude canal; remove immediately when finished.
     b. Side effects of eardrops: local stinging or burning sensation and rash where drops have come in contact with skin.
     c. Avoid earplugs and use of cotton swabs.
     d. Acute pain should subside within 48 hours.
   2. Keep foreign objects out of ears.
   3. Prevention of recurrence (common): Instill 2–3 drops of isopropyl alcohol in ear canals after swimming, showering, or during hot, humid weather; shake excess water out of ears.

IV. ACUTE OTITIS MEDIA (AOM)

Enlarged tonsils (pharyngitis), 462	Otitis media, chronic, 381.01
Fever, 780.6	Perforation of tympanic membrane, 384.2
Influenza virus (types A and B), 487.1	Respiratory syncytial virus (RSV), 079.6
Otitis media, 382.9	Upper respiratory infection, 465.9
Otitis media, acute, 392.9	

A. Etiology.
   1. *Streptococcus pneumoniae* (most common causative organism).
   2. Nontypeable *Haemophilus influenzae* causes about 27% of the bacterial otitis.

3. Less frequent pathogens include *Moraxella (Branhamella) catarrhalis* and Group A beta-hemolytic streptococci.
4. *Staphylococcus aureus* and *Pseudomonas aeruginosa:* common in chronic serous otitis media, especially if perforation of tympanic membrane present.
   a. Group A beta-hemolytic streptococci, *Escherichia coli, S. aureus:* more common in neonates.
5. Viruses, particularly respiratory syncytial virus (RSV), influenza virus (types A and B), and adenovirus, increase the risk, possibly by impairing eustachian tube function. Infants have increased susceptibility to OM, possibly due to short horizontal position of eustachian tube.
6. Viruses may be involved in about 40% of cases of AOM.
7. Bacterial resistance is increasing problem: Certain strains of *H. influenzae* and most strains of *M. catarrhalis* are resistant to amoxicillin because of beta-lactamase production. Another concern is drug-resistant *S. pneumoniae* (DRSP).
8. The groups most at risk for DRSP are:
   a. Children younger than 24 months of age.
   b. Those who have recently received beta-lactam drugs, were recently treated with antibiotics, and/or had a recent ear infection.
   c. Children exposed to large numbers of other children (e.g., daycare attendance in children 2 months to younger than 5 years of age, or household crowding in children older than 2 years of age).
   d. Those with immune deficiencies (e.g., sickle cell disease, HIV, malignancy). The proportion of penicillin-resistant *S. pneumoniae* strains may be 40–50% and half of these may be highly resistant.
B. Occurrence.
   1. After upper respiratory infection (URI), OM most common disease of childhood; peak prevalence from 6 to 36 months of age. Incidence declines at about 6 years of age.
   2. Incidence has dramatically increased since 1985; greatest in children younger than 2 years of age.
   3. By 3 years of age, most have had at least 1 acute infection; 33% have had 3.
   4. Those with first episode early in life have increased risk for developing chronic ear disease.
   5. More common in boys than in girls.
   6. Caucasians, Native Alaskans, Native Americans have higher incidence than African Americans.
   7. More frequent in low-income and large families and those children in group daycare settings.

8. Those immunocompromised, including those with AIDS, have higher incidence.
9. Smoking in household increases incidence.
10. Bottle-fed infants have higher incidence than breastfed infants.
11. Incidence, prevalence of otorrhea: tympanostomy tubes in place longer.

C. Clinical manifestations.
1. Diagnosis of AOM requires:
   a. History of acute onset of signs and symptoms.
   b. Presence of middle ear effusion.
   c. Signs and symptoms of middle ear inflammation.
   d. Distinct erythema of TM or distinct otalgia (discomfort clearly related to the ear[s] that causes sleep disturbances and/or interferes with normal activity).
2. Most common younger than 2 years of age.
3. Acute onset of ear pain and fever; pulling, tugging, rubbing at infected ear.
4. Occasionally asymptomatic.
5. Fever in 50% of cases.
6. Other associated symptoms: irritability, disturbed sleep, restlessness, rhinorrhea or URI, cough, malaise, sore throat, stiff neck, refusal of bottle, change in eating habits, vomiting, diarrhea.
7. May report recent URI, previous ear infections, allergies, taking bottle to bed, infant supine when feeding from bottle, attending daycare, other siblings sick.
8. Hearing loss.

D. Physical findings.
1. Fever is common.
2. Signs of URI or allergies.
3. Possible red, enlarged tonsils (pharyngitis).
4. Cervical nodes often enlarged.
5. Otoscopic findings: Middle ear effusion must be present as evidenced by any of the following: bulging TM, decreased or absent mobility of the TM as noted with pneumatic otoscopy, air fluid level behind the TM, otorrhea reflectometry.

E. Diagnostic tests.
1. Pneumatic otoscopy to assess mobility of TM.
2. Tympanometry: to supplement but not replace pneumatic otoscopy, for children older than 6 months of age.
3. Acoustic reflectometry.
4. Tympanocentesis with culture and sensitivity testing is diagnostic of organism.

Table 22-1 Recommended Antibacterial Agents for Patients Who Are Being Treated Initially with Antibacterial Agents or Have Failed 48 to 72 Hours of Observation or Initial Management with Antibacterial Agents

Temperature ≥ 39 °C and/or severe otalgia	At diagnosis for patients being treated initially with antibacterial agents		Clinically defined treatment failure at 48–72 hours after initial management with observation option		Clinically defined treatment failure at 48–72 hours after initial management with antibacterial agents	
	Recommended	Alternative for penicillin allergy	Recommended	Alternative for penicillin allergy	Recommended	Alternative for penicillin allergy
No	Amoxicillin, 80–90 mg/kg per day	Non-type I: cefdinir, cefuroxime, cefpodoxime; type I: azithromycin, clarithromycin	Amoxicillin, 80–90 mg/kg per day	Non-type I: cefdinir, cefuroxime, cefpodoxime; type I: azithromycin, clarithromycin	Amoxicillin-clavulanate, 90 mg/kg per day of amoxicillin component, with 6.4 mg/kg per day of clavulanate	Non-type I: ceftriaxone, 3 days; type I: clindamycin
Yes	Amoxicillin-clavulanate, 90 mg/kg per day of amoxicillin, with 6.4 mg/kg per day of clavulanate	Ceftriaxone, 1 or 3 days	Amoxicillin, clavulanate, 90 mg/kg per day of amoxicillin, with 6.4 mg/kg per day of clavulanate	Ceftriaxone, 1 or 3 days	Ceftriaxone, 3 days	Tympanocentesis, clindamycin

Source: American Academy of Pediatrics/American Academy of Family Physicians Subcommittee on Management of Acute Otitis Media. Clinical practice guideline: diagnosis and management of acute otitis media. *Pediatrics.* 2004;113(5):1451-1465.

F.   Differential diagnosis.

Dental abscess, 522.5	Mastoiditis, 389.3
Dysfunction 524.6	Otitis externa, 380.1
Eustachian tube dysfunction, 381.81	Otitis media, acute with effusion, 381
Foreign body, ear, 931	Sinusitis, 473.9
Furuncle, 680	Temporomandibular joint (TMJ)
Immune deficiency, 279.3	Tonsillitis, 463
Impacted teeth, 520.6	Lymphadenitis, 289.3

1. Otitis externa, otitis media with effusion (OME), sinusitis.
2. Mastoiditis, furuncle.
3. Foreign body, trauma.
4. Eustachian tube dysfunction.
5. Lymphadenitis.
6. Dental abscess, tonsillitis, impacted teeth.
7. Temporomandibular joint (TMJ) dysfunction.
8. Immune deficiency.

G.   Treatment (**Table 22-1**).

1. Pain management, especially during the first 24 hours, is a priority regardless of whether antimicrobial agents are prescribed. Acetaminophen and ibuprofen are the mainstays. Adequate dosage is important.
2. Observation involves deferring treatment for 48–72 hours in otherwise healthy children 6 months to 2 years of age with nonsevere illness at presentation *and* uncertain diagnosis and in children ages 2 years and older who present without severe symptoms *or* an uncertain diagnosis. There should also be a reliable parent or caregiver able to obtain medication if needed and adequate facilities for follow up and reevaluation.
3. Prescribe antibiotics with caution. More than 80% of cases resolve spontaneously.
4. For children age 2 years and older who appear well, discuss treatment options with parents which include:
   a. Safety-net antibiotic prescription (SNAP) is a prescription for an appropriate antibiotic written to be filled within 5 days of the office visit. Parents are instructed not to fill the SNAP unless symptoms worsen at any time or symptoms do not improve during the waiting period of 48–72 hours. Instruct parents that child's condition may

quickly progress to a more severe case and to call and make a return visit if this occurs.

   b. 5-day course of high-dose amoxicillin (if no history of allergy).

5. Begin antimicrobial therapy (**Box 22-1**) if no improvement or condition has worsened within 24–72 hours.

6. Antibiotic therapy is indicated for symptomatic AOM, particularly in children younger than 2 years of age.

7. Prescribe amoxicillin (drug of choice) or ampicillin if causative organism unknown (most cases).

8. Initially prescribe amoxicillin 40–45 mg/kg per day for 5–7 days in uncomplicated cases in children younger than 2 years of age who do not attend daycare, have not taken antibiotics within the past 3 months, except in areas of high resistance. This dose may fail to eradicate DRSP.

9. If child attends daycare, has taken antibiotics recently, or has history of recent AOM, prescribe amoxicillin 80–90 mg/kg per day in 2 divided doses for 10 days.

10. Prescribe adequate dose for initial treatment of symptomatic children. If allergic to penicillin, treat with azithromycin (for children allergic to beta-lactam).

11. Not recommended in children younger than 6 months of age: 30 mg/kg (max 500 mg) once daily for 3 days; or 10 mg/kg (max 500 mg) once, then 5 mg/kg (max 250 mg) once daily for 4 days. Can also prescribe oral cephalosporins, macrolides, or trimethoprim-sulfamethoxazole (TMP-SMX; rates of resistance to pneumococci are high). Treat for 10 days.

12. Begin second-line therapy in cases of documented amoxicillin failure (e.g., persistent fever, ear pain, irritability, TM findings after 3 days of treatment of redness, bulging, or otorrhea). Drug must be active against beta-lactamase-producing strains of *H. influenzae* or *M. catarrhalis,* DRSP (e.g., oral amoxicillin-clavulanate [Augmentin]); give in higher doses of 80–90 mg/kg per day of amoxicillin component, clavulanate dose remains at 10 mg/kg per day or ceftriaxone (Rocephin) 50 mg/kg (max 1 g) IM once for severe infections and/or if compliance is concern.

13. If recurrence of acute symptoms after full course of amoxicillin, retreat with second-line antibiotic. First drug of choice is amoxicillin-clavulanate. Oral cephalosporins (except cefuroxime axetil) and macrolides do not provide adequate coverage against resistant strains of *S. pneumoniae.*

14. Pain control (see beginning of section): warm compresses, an analgesic with antipyretic effects (e.g., acetaminophen or ibuprofen), and eardrops

Box 22-1 Antibiotics Labeled for the Treatment of Acute Otitis Media

Penicillins

Amoxicillin (first-line therapy)
Amoxicillin-clavulanate (Augmentin) (second-line therapy)

Sulfa-based combinations

Erythromycin-sulfisoxazole (Pediazole)
Trimethoprim-sulfamethoxazole (Bactrim, Septra)

Macrolide/azalide (second-line therapy)

Azithromycin (Zithromax)
Clarithromycin (Biaxin)

Second-generation cephalosporins

Cefaclor (Ceclor)
Cefprozil (Cefzil)
Cefuroxime axetil (Ceftin)
Loracarbef (Lorabid)

Third-generation cephalosporins

Cefdinir (Omnicef)
Cefixime (Suprax)
Cefpodoxime proxetil (Vantin)
Ceftibuten (Cedax)
Ceftriaxone (Rocephin)

Topical antimicrobial agents (approved for use with tympanostomy tubes or nonintact tympanic membrane

Ciprofloxacin/dexamethasone (Ciprodex Otic Suspension)
Ofloxacin (Floxin Otic Solution)

Source: Pichichero ME. Acute otitis media. Part II. Treatment in an era of increasing antibiotic resistance. *Am Fam Phys.* 2000;61:2410-6,. American Academy of Family Physicians website: www.aafp.org/afp/20000415/2410.html. Accessed June 16, 2011.

with benzocaine and antipyrine (Auralgan). Immediate treatment for pain is very important.

15. Children with frequent AOM: evaluate for anemia. If iron deficiency is diagnosed (hemoglobin 10 g/dL), begin iron supplementation to achieve at least a hemoglobin level of 11 g/dL.

16. Persistent AOM likely caused by different pathogen than initial infection: treat with antibiotic (e.g., cefaclor, TMP-SMX, erythromycin-sulfisoxazole, amoxicillin-clavulanate potassium, cefixime).

17. Recurrent AOM: American Academy of Pediatrics and the CDC suggest placement of tympanostomy tubes rather than antibiotic prophylaxis. If must prescribe antibiotics: sulfisoxazole most effective at preventing recurrences.

18. Pneumococcal vaccine (PCV 13, Prevnar) in children during first year of life, as well as high-risk children younger than 1 year of age.

19. Influenza vaccine in high-risk children.

20. Surgical intervention: tympanostomy tubes (performed by an ENT surgeon) possible in children with chronic middle ear fluid (3 months or 4 persistent episodes) who fail to respond to antimicrobial therapy; children with recurrent AOM; suppurative complications; those with eustachian tube dysfunction.

21. Adenoidectomy in children younger than 4 years of age with recurrent AOM may be performed as substitute for, or in conjunction with, insertion of tympanostomy tubes.

22. Tympanocentesis (performed by an ENT specialist) and culture of exudate: if diagnosis is uncertain, child is seriously ill or toxic, response to antibiotic therapy is unsatisfactory, suppurative complications develop, otitis media in newborn or in immunologically deficient patients, or AOM develops despite receiving antibiotic therapy.

23. Refer for audiologic testing if fail hearing screen.

24. Consult/refer to physician: infant younger than 2 months of age, signs of meningitis.

25. ENT referral: hearing loss or delayed speech, 3 infections in 6 months or 4 in 12 months.

H. Follow up.

1. Younger than 3 months of age: revisit 1 to 2 days (higher incidence of treatment failure).

2. Children 3 months of age and older: revisit in 48–72 hours if no improvement or condition worsens (need to change antibiotics).

3. Return visit 4–8 weeks to evaluate for OME and reinforce teaching.
4. Persistent AOM: prescribe second-line antibiotic (e.g., amoxicillin-clavulanate, cefuroxime, or ceftriaxone IM); recheck every 2–4 weeks until resolved.
5. Return visit if signs or symptoms of ear infection, trouble hearing, fever with/without ear pain.
  I. Complications.

Cerebral thrombophlebitis, 325	Meningitis, 322.9
Cholesteatoma, 385.3	Ossicle necrosis, 385.24
Facial nerve paralysis, 767.5	Otitis media, acute, 382.9
Hearing loss, 389.9	Otitis media, acute with effusion, 381
Labyrinthitis, 386.3	Perforation of tympanic membrane, 384.2
Language delay, 315.39	Pseudotumor cerebri, 348.2
Mastoiditis, 389.3	Tympanosclerosis, 385.09

1. Perforation of TM.
2. Hearing loss, language delay.
3. Persistent AOM, persistent OME.
4. Mastoiditis, cholesteatoma.
5. Meningitis.
6. Facial nerve paralysis.
7. Labyrinthitis.
8. Tympanosclerosis.
9. Ossicle necrosis.
10. Pseudotumor cerebri.
11. Cerebral thrombophlebitis.
  J. Education.
1. Causes of ear infections.
2. Risk factors/modification: passive smoke, bottle propping, allergies, sinusitis, use of pacifier after age 6 months, breastfeeding (may protect), immunizations.
3. Treatment plan: If antibiotics prescribed, call if symptoms worsen or do not improve in 48 hours; give exactly as prescribed.
4. Pain relief measures.
5. Importance of follow-up.

V. OTITIS MEDIA WITH EFFUSION (OME)

Allergies, 477.9	Otitis media, 382.9
Cervical lymphadenopathy, 785.6	Otitis media, acute, 382.9
Enlarged tonsils, 474.11	Otitis media with effusion, chronic, 380.23
Eustachian tube dysfunction (ETD), 381.81	Perforated tympanitic membrane, 384.2
Hearing loss, 389.9	Sleep disturbances, 780.5
Irritability, 799.2	Speech and language disorder, 315.39

A. Etiology.
   1. Multifactorial: eustachian tube dysfunction (ETD), infection, allergies.
   2. Bacteria are same as for AOM, except frequency of *H. influenzae* is greater in OME.
   3. If TM perforated in chronic OME: *S. aureus* and *P. aeruginosa* most likely causative organisms.
B. Occurrence.
   1. See AOM section earlier in this chapter.
   2. Usually follows episode of AOM.
   3. Children who are diagnosed with AOM during the first year of life are much more likely to develop chronic OME.
   4. Sixty-six percent of children with AOM have middle ear effusion or high negative middle ear pressure 2 weeks after diagnosis; 33% have middle ear effusion 1 month after diagnosis, regardless of antibiotic therapy.
   5. OME most common cause of hearing loss in children.
C. Clinical manifestations.
   1. May be asymptomatic.
   2. Complaint of hearing loss (older children).
   3. Possible language delay.
   4. Feeling of fullness in affected ear, clogged/crackling sensation in ear, "talking in tunnel."
   5. Irritability.
   6. Sleep disturbances.
   7. Poor school performance.
   8. Allergies.
   9. Frequent episodes of otitis media.
D. Physical findings.
   1. Possible indicators of allergies.
   2. Possible enlarged tonsils.

3. Possible cervical lymphadenopathy.
4. External canal may have discharge.
5. TM: often retracted or convex, opaque; diffuse light reflex; may be translucent with air-fluid level or air bubbles present or amber with blue-gray fluid noted, no visible landmarks.
6. Pneumatic otoscopy: decreased or irregular mobility to both negative and positive pressure.
7. Weber test: lateralization to involved ear.
8. Rinne test: BC AC (abnormal).
9. Hearing impairment.
10. Tympanometry: fluid present.
E. Diagnostic tests.
   1. Pneumatic otoscope for primary diagnosis, confirmed by tympanometry.
   2. Tympanometry: tympanogram is flat with an effusion.
   3. Audiometry.
   4. Acoustic reflectometry.
   5. Otoacoustic emissions.
   6. Tympanocentesis.
F. Differential diagnosis.

Anatomic abnormalities, 759.9	Nasopharyngeal carcinoma, 147.9
Hearing loss, 389.9	Otitis media, acute, 382.9

   1. All possible causes of hearing loss.
   2. Anatomic abnormalities.
   3. AOM.
   4. Nasopharyngeal carcinoma (if unilateral OME).
G. Treatment.
   1. Most cases of OME resolve spontaneously within 3 months.
   2. Document at each visit: laterality, duration of effusion, and presence and severity of associated symptoms.
   3. Distinguish the child who is at risk for speech, language, or learning problems from other children with OME and more quickly evaluate hearing, speech, and language and need for intervention in children at risk.
   4. Refer for hearing evaluation when OME persists for 3 months or longer or at any time there is a language delay, learning problems, or a significant hearing loss is suspected in a child with OME.
   5. Not recommended for treatment of OME in an otherwise healthy child 2 months through 12 years: Antihistamines and decongestants are ineffective for OME and should not be used for treatment. Antimicrobials and

corticosteroids do not have long-term efficacy and should not be used for routine management.

6. Observation or antibiotic therapy treatment options for children with effusion less than 4–6 months and any time in children without a 20-dB hearing threshold level or worse in the better hearing ear.

7. Antibiotics: consider beginning with a beta-lactamase-resistant antibiotic (e.g., amoxicillin-clavulanate potassium) for 2–3 weeks.

8. Myringotomy and tympanostomy tubes: *consider* if bilateral effusion for a total of 3 months and bilateral hearing deficiency (defined as a 20-dB hearing threshold level or worse in the better hearing ear). *Recommended* after a total of 4–6 months of bilateral effusion with a bilateral hearing deficit.

H. Follow up.
  1. Return visit in 1 month, sooner if acute symptoms develop.
I. Complications.

Hearing loss, 389.9

Otitis media, acute, 382.9

Speech delay, 315.39

---

  1. Hearing loss, speech delay.
  2. Recurrent AOM.
J. Education.
  1. Diagnosis; OME usually resolves spontaneously without treatment in 3 months.
  2. Treatment plan.
  3. Signs of hearing loss.
  4. Modify risk factors.
  5. Relationship between speech and language development and hearing.
  6. Importance of follow up.

VI. EUSTACHIAN TUBE DYSFUNCTION (ETD)

A. Etiology.
  1. Eustachian tube (ET) is narrower and oriented horizontally in children which predisposes them to ventilation and drainage problems.
  2. Upper respiratory infections.
  3. Pressure changes that occur, such as with plane travel, may lead to acute ETD.
  4. Otitis media, serous effusions, cholesteatoma may cause chronic ETD from negative middle ear pressure.

5. Gastroesophageal reflux (GERD).
6. Enlarged adenoids.
7. Allergies.
8. Down syndrome (associated with small ETs).
9. Smoking.

B. Occurrence.
   1. Most common in children younger than 5 years.
   2. Usually decreases with age but may persist to adulthood.

C. Clinical manifestations.
   1. Presenting complaints may include:
      a. Fullness, clogged feeling in ear.
      b. Ear discomfort (may be relieved by "popping ears").
      c. Hearing loss.
      d. Symptoms can be unilateral or bilateral.
      e. Allergic symptoms.
      f. Dizziness or lightheadedness.

D. Physical findings.
   1. Retracted TM, effusion, decreased movement on pneumoscopy.
   2. Nasal obstruction.
   3. Tuning fork test lateralizes to the affected ear if conductive hearing loss present.

E. Diagnostic tests.
   1. Usually none.
   2. Tympanography will confirm diagnosis.
   3. Audiometry may be needed to determine hearing loss.

F. Differential diagnosis.
   1. Otitis media.
   2. Otitis media with effusion (OME).
   3. Otitis externa.
   4. Sinus infection.
   5. Perforation of the TM.
   6. Bullous myringitis.
   7. Patulous eustachian tube (ET remains open for a prolonged period of time).

G. Treatment.
   1. Decongestants.
      a. Pseudoephedrine (Sudafed, Actifed), OR:
      b. Topical nasal sprays (avoid use longer than 3 days)—phenylephrine (Neo-Synephrine topical), oxymetazoline (Afrin).
   2. Nasal steroids (especially helpful to those with allergic rhinitis, most approved for children 6 years and older).

a. Beclomethasone (Beconase).
b. Budesonide (Rhinocort).
c. Fluticasone (Flonase) approved for those 4 years of age and older.
d. Fluticasone furoate (Veramyst) approved for those 2 years of age and older.
e. Mometasone (Nasonex) approved for those 2 years of age and older.
3. Second generation H1 antihistamines (may be beneficial for those with allergic rhinitis).
a. Loratadine (Claritin).
b. Desloratadine (Clarinex).
c. Fexofenadine (Allegra).
d. Cetirizine (Zyrtec).
4. Antibiotics: not usually indicated unless AOM present.
a. Amoxicillin for 10 days—most effective.
5. Tympanic perforation or ventilation tubes present.
a. Topical antibiotic drops with topical steroid if discharge present.
b. Neomycin-polymyxin-hydrocortisone (Cortisporin) otic drops.
c. Ciprofloxacin-hydrocortisone (Cipro HC).
6. Pain management.
a. Anti-inflammatories such as acetaminophen or ibuprofen, others.
7. GERD—omeprazole (Prilosec).
8. Patulous (abnormally open) ET—Premarin nose drops or nasal spray.
H. Follow up.
1. Check tubes every 3 months, if present.
2. If OME present, check for resolution in 3 months.
3. Return visit if symptoms worsen or change.
I. Complications.
1. TM perforation.
2. Hearing loss.
3. Cholesteatoma.
4. Meningitis.
5. Brain abscess.
6. Labyrinthitis.
7. Subdural empyema.
8. Subperiosteal abscess.
9. Facial paralysis.
10. Death.
J. Education.
1. Diagnosis: importance of treating cause.
2. Treatment plan.

3. Modification of risk factors.
4. Importance of follow up.
5. Relationship between speech, language and hearing.

BIBLIOGRAPHY

American Academy of Family Physicians, American Academy of Otolaryngology-Head and Neck Surgery, and American Academy of Pediatrics Subcommittee on Otitis Media with Effusion. *Clinical practice guideline: Otitis media with effusion.* Published May 3, 2004: http://www.aafp.org/online/etc/medialib/ aafp_org/documents/clinical/clin_recs/ome.Par.0001.File.dat/OMEFinal.pdf. Accessed June 6, 2011.

American Academy of Pediatrics and American Academy of Family Physicians Subcommittee on Management of Acute Otitis Media. Diagnosis and management of acute otitis media. *Pediatrics* 2004;113(5):1451-1465.

Corbeel L. What is new in otitis media? *European J Pediatrics.* 2007;166:511-519.

Daly KA, et. al. Epidemiology, natural history, and risk factors: Panel report from the ninth International Research Conference on otitis media. *Int J Pediatr Otorhinolaryngol.* 2010;74(3):231-240.

Gunasekera H, Morris P, McIntyre P, et al. Management of children with otitis media: A summary of evidence from recent systemic reviews. *J Pediatr Child Health.* 2009;45(10):554-563.

Leo G, Piacentini E, Incorvaia C, et al. Sinusitis and eustachian tube dysfunction in children. *Pediatric Allergy Immunol.* 2007;18(Suppl. 18):35-39.

Meropol S. Valuing reduced antibiotic use for pediatric acute otitis media. *Pediatrics.* 2008;12:669-673.

Rosenfeld RM. Antibiotic use for otitis media: Oral, topical, or none? *Pediatr Ann.* 2004;33:833-842.

Stool SE, et al. Managing otitis media with effusion in young children. In: *Quick Reference Guide for Clinicians.* AHCPR Publication 94-0623. Rockville, MD: Agency for Health Care Policy and Research, Public Health Service, U.S. Department of Health and Human Services; 1994.

Takata G, et al. Evidence assessment of the accuracy of methods of diagnosing middle ear effusion in children with otitis media with effusion. *Pediatrics.* 2003;112:1379.

Vernacchio L, Vezina R, Mitchell A. Management of acute otitis media by primary care physicians: Trends since the release of the 2004 American Academy of Pediatrics/American Academy of Family Physicians Clinical Practice Guideline. *Pediatrics.* 2007;120:281-287.

CHAPTER 23

Sinus, Mouth, Throat, and Neck Disorders

Susan G. Rains

I. ALLERGIC RHINITIS

Allergic conjunctivitis, 372.14	Noisy breathing/snoring, 786.09
Allergic rhinitis due to other allergens, 477.8	Rhinorrhea, 478.1
	Sneezing, 784.9
Allergic rhinitis due to pollen (seasonal rhinitis), 477.9	Stuffy nose, 478.1
	Wheezing, 786.07
Cough, 786.2	
Halitosis, 784.9	
Nasal obstruction, 478.1	

A. Etiology.
  1. Atopic predilection.
     a. Very common atopic disease of childhood, second only to asthma.
     b. Often same mediators that produce asthma.
     c. Genetic factors: increased IgE production in response to allergens.
  2. Environmental factors.
     a. Common allergens.
        • Seasonal (rare in children younger than 3 years of age).
          i. Nonflowering, wind-pollinated plants.
          ii. Tree pollens: early spring.
          iii. Grasses: late spring and early summer.
          iv. Weeds: fall.
        • Perennial: animal dander, dust (mites), molds (spores), mildew, feathers, cockroaches.

B. Occurrence.
1. Affects about 40% of children and 30% of adolescents.
2. If one parent affected, child has 30% chance of developing allergies; both parents, 70% chance.
3. The incidence in males is slightly higher.
C. Clinical manifestations.
1. Stuffy nose, sneezing, itching, runny nose, noisy breathing/snoring, cough, halitosis, frequent clearing of throat, plugged ears, wheezing.
2. Possibly associated signs of allergic conjunctivitis: itchy, injected conjunctiva, puffy lids, tearing or clear mucous drainage in eye.
3. Has significant decrement on measurements of vigilance and a broad range of cognitive functioning.
D. Physical findings.
1. Nasal mucosa is usually pale, edematous, boggy.
2. Thin, watery rhinorrhea.
3. Allergic salute may cause external, transverse crease near end of nose.
4. Nasal obstruction may cause mouth breathing.
5. Allergic shiners (dark circles under eyes), due to venous pooling.
E. Diagnostic tests.
1. Nasal smear for presence of eosinophils: 10% is positive (intranasal steroids may decrease percentage).
2. Skin testing.
F. Differential diagnosis.

Choanal atresia, 748	Rhinitis, drug or food induced, 477.1
Cystic fibrosis, 277	Rhinitis medicamentosus, 372.05
Dermatoid cyst, 706.2	Rhinorrhea, 478.1
Deviated septum, 470	Sinusitis, 473.9
Headache, 784	Sinusitis, chronic, 473.9
Nasal foreign body, 932	Upper respiratory infection, 465.9
Nasal glioma, 748.1	Vasomotor rhinitis, 477.9
Nasal polyp, 471.9	Viral URI, 465.9

1. Infection.
a. Viral upper respiratory infection (URI): red and swollen turbinates, thicker, more purulent rhinorrhea; duration 10–14 days, clustered fall–spring.

      b. Sinusitis: possibly symptoms of URI, also headache, facial pressure; duration longer than viral URI but more limited than solely allergic rhinitis.

  2. Nasal foreign body: unilateral purulent nasal discharge, foul odor.

  3. Nasal polyp, dermatoid cyst, nasal glioma.

  4. Cystic fibrosis (patients often have nasal polyps and chronic sinusitis).

  5. Choanal atresia, deviated septum.

  6. Vasomotor rhinitis: sudden appearance and disappearance of symptoms in response to irritants.

  7. Rhinitis medicamentosus: abuse of nasal spray/drops.

  8. Drug- or food-induced rhinitis.

G. Classification.

  1. Mild, moderate, severe.

  2. Intermittent or persistent.

H. Treatment.

  1. Avoidance.

      a. Minimize exposure to dust mites, especially in child's bedroom: remove wall-to-wall carpets, curtains, bed ruffles, stuffed animals; wash cotton bedding in hot water frequently, use nonallergenic bedding covers.

      b. Minimize exposure to animal dander.

      c. Minimize exposure to pollens: close windows, use air conditioning, filters on air systems, keep humidity low in home, remove house plants.

      d. Avoid activities such as leaf raking, lawn mowing, furniture dusting.

      e. Avoid talcs, perfumes, cigarettes, wood smoke.

  2. Pharmacotherapy.

      a. Antihistamines.

        • First generation (sedating unless child has adverse hyperactive response). Diphenhydramine (Benadryl), chlorpheniramine, combined products: 5 mg/kg/day, divided qid.

        • Second generation. Loratadine (Claritin, generic and brand preparations now available OTC), age 2–5 years: 5 mg PO daily; older than 6 years: 10 mg. Cetirizine (Zyrtec, generic and brand preparations now available OTC), age 2–5 years: 2.5–5 mg PO daily; older than 6 years: 10 mg. Fexofenadine (Allegra); age 2–11 years: 30 mg bid; older than 12 years: 60 mg tab bid or 180 mg daily. Desloratidine (Clarinex): age 6–11 months: 1 mg/day, 12 months to 5 years: 1.25 mg/day, 6–11 years: 2.5 mg/day, 12 years and older 5 mg/day. Levoceterizine (Xyzal): 6–11 years: 2.5 mg HS, 12 years and older 5 mg HS.

   b. Intranasal steroids, e.g., fluticasone propionate (Flonase 0.05%—only one available generically); mometasone furoate (Nasonex); triamcinolone acetonide (Nasocort AQ); budesonide (Rhinocort Aqua).
- 4–12 years of age: 1 spray each nostril daily.
- Older than 12 years of age: 2 sprays/nostril.

   c. Topical cromolyn (NasalCrom): 1 spray tid–qid, 2–4 weeks for effect (available OTC).

   d. Nonsedating nasal anti-histamine: Patanse (Olopatadine), ages 6–11 years: 1 spray/nostril q day; 12 years 2 sprays/nostril q day.

   e. Nasal decongestants (not recommended due to rebound effect secondary to abuse).
- Oral often combined with antihistamines.
- Topical not recommended due to rebound and abuse potential.

  3. Immunotherapy (hyposensitization): "allergy shots," especially recommended for children who suffer perennially and do not respond to medications.

I. Follow up.

  1. 2–4 weeks after initial treatment, sooner if needed, then 3–6 months.

J. Complications.

Dental malocclusion, 524.5	Loss of smell, 781.1
Hearing loss, 389.9	Otitis media, 382.9
Hoarseness, 784.49	Sinusitis, chronic, 473.9

  1. Chronic sinusitis.
  2. Recurrent otitis media.
  3. Hoarseness.
  4. Loss of smell or hearing.
  5. High-arched palate, dental malocclusion from chronic mouth breathing.

K. Education.

  1. Chronicity of problem.
  2. Avoidance of allergens (recent evidence that exposure to cats, dogs in first year of life decreases development of allergies later in childhood).
  3. Medication administration and side effects.

II. APHTHOUS STOMATITIS

Aphthous stomatitis, 528.2	Fever, 780.6
Cheilitis	Lymphadenopathy, 785.6
Deficiencies of B12, 266.2	Malabsorption syndromes, 579.9
Deficiencies of folic acid, 266.2	Painful sores in mouth, 528.9
Deficiencies of iron, 280.9	

A. Etiology.
  1. Commonly known as canker sores, aphthous stomatitis is recurrence of painful, discrete, shallow ulcers on unattached mucous membranes of mouth.
  2. Considered to be immune-mediated destruction of epithelium, cause is multifactorial, including infection, autoimmune disease, allergies, nutritional deficiencies, and trauma.
  3. Associated risk factors.
     a. Genetic: positive family history.
     b. Deficiencies of iron, vitamin B12, folic acid.
     c. Chronic illness such as IBD, celiac disease, immune suppression, lupus, JRA.
     d. NSAID or ACE inhibitor usage.
     e. Childhood: higher incidence (peak 10–19 years).
B. Occurrence.
  1. Incidence: up to 20% of population.
  2. Precipitating factors.
     a. Stress/trauma: emotional, physical, hormonal.
     b. Foods: chocolate, nuts, tomatoes.
     c. Malabsorption syndromes.
C. Clinical manifestations.
  1. Aphthous minor: 80% of cases: 1–5 mm lesions; heal in 5–12 days; no scarring.
  2. Aphthous major: 15% of cases > 1 cm lesions; last 4 weeks; may scar.
  3. Patient complains of single or multiple painful sores in mouth.
  4. Tingling or burning may precede appearance of lesions.
D. Physical findings.
  1. Painful, yellow, gray, ulcerative lesions with erythematous halo on mucosa.

    2. 1–5 ulcerative oval or circular ulcers with an erythematous periphery and pale white/gray or yellow center.

    3. Size: 2–10 mm.

    4. Absence of systemic symptoms (i.e., fever, lymphadenopathy).

E. Diagnostic tests.

    1. None.

F. Differential diagnosis.

Fever, 780.6	Herpes simplex, 054.9
Herpangina-ulcerative pharyngitis, 074	Lymphadenopathy, 785.6

    1. Infections:

      a. Herpes simplex (rare).
- Small, irregular vesicles that rupture and leave ulcers.
- Red at periphery with gray center.
- Patient often febrile with significant lymphadenopathy.
- Recurrent herpes infections remain localized to lips, rarely cross mucocutaneous junction.
- Primary infections sometimes involve oral mucosa.

      b. Coxsackie—hand, foot and mouth disease.
- Sometimes ulcers in the mouth (and will have papules on hands and feet, perhaps buttocks).

    2. Traumatic (injury).

    3. Herpangina—ulcerative pharyngitis (not stomatitis); fever, lymphadenopathy.

    4. Angular cheilitis—erythematous, painful fissures at corners of the mouth. May be caused by lipsucking, sensitivity to agent with which in contact. Treatment is topical with an antibiotic, anti-yeast or low-dose steroid ointment.

G. Treatment.

    1. Supportive.

      a. Oral analgesics such as acetaminophen or ibuprofen.

      b. Topical anesthetics: especially prior to eating/drinking.
- Viscous Xylocaine dabbed on lesions with cotton swab.
- Mouthwashes.
  - i. Diphenhydramine elixir: antacid suspension (aluminum and magnesium hydroxide combination): mix 1:1 (parent can do this).

        ii. Pharmacist may add lidocaine 1% for older child to swish and spit.
- 0.1% Triamcinolone (Kenalog) in Orabase: dab on lesions qid.

    c. Avoid acidic, salty foods and drinks.

    d. Good oral hygiene.
- Rinse mouth frequently with clear water.
- Offer water to young children frequently, especially after eating or drinking other fluids.

H. Follow up.
1. None if healed.

I. Complications.
1. Generally none. Young child may refuse to drink.
2. Referral if persists 3 weeks or no urine output for 12 hours.

J. Education.
1. Avoidance of triggers/precipitating factors.

III. CAT-SCRATCH DISEASE

Cat-scratch disease, 078.3	Nonpruritic vesicle or papule(s), 216.3
Conjunctivitis, nonsuppurative, 372.3	Ocular granuloma, 376.11
Fever, 780.6	Skin lesion, 709.9
Lymphadenopathy, 785.6	

A. Etiology.
1. Bacteria *Bartonella henselae* infects humans via cat saliva entering the body through a scratch or bite.
2. 87–99% of patients have had contact with kitten within the last 6 months; 50% have history of scratch.

B. Occurrence.
1. More common in children, (younger than 18 years), especially boys.
2. 20,000 cases/year in United States, primarily July–January.

C. Clinical manifestations.
1. Typical cat-scratch disease.
   a. Primary skin lesion (papule) appears 3–10 days following inoculation.
   b. Regional lymphadenopathy develops in about 2 weeks, persists sometimes for months. 85% have a single node.
   c. Fever, which may be prolonged (up to 2 weeks) in two-thirds of patients.

        d. 10% of nodes may suppurate spontaneously.

        e. Hepatosplenic disease.

  2. Less common clinical manifestations:

        a. Parinaud oculoglandular syndrome.

        b. Neuroretinitis-posterior segment ocular disease.

        c. Encephalopathy.

        d. Radiculopathy.

        e. Facial nerve palsy.

        f. Guillain-Barré syndrome.

        g. Cerebral arteritis.

        h. Transverse myelitis.

        i. Glomerulonephritis.

        j. Thrombocytopenia purpura.

        k. Osteomyelitis.

        l. Arthritis/arthralgia.

        m. Endocarditis.

D. Physical findings (in typical CSD).

  1. Nonpruritic vesicle or papule(s) over site of inoculation.

  2. Lymphadenopathy of area that drains site of inoculation. Most commonly axillary and epitrochlear nodes, then head, neck, and groin in descending order of frequency.

  3. Skin over affected nodes is warm, taut, tender, indurated.

E. Diagnostic criteria: (3 of the following 4):

  1. Cat or flea contact regardless of presence of inoculation site.

  2. Negative serology for other causes of adenopathy, sterile pus aspirated from a node, a positive PCR assay, and/or liver/spleen lesions seen on CT scan.

  3. Positive enzyme immunoassay or IFA with a titer ratio of $\geq$ 1:64.

  4. Biopsy showing granulomatous inflammation consistent with CSD or positive Warthin-Starry silver stain.

F. Differential diagnosis.

Cytomegalovirus, 078.5	Lymphadenopathy, 785.6
Epstein-Barr virus, 075	Mycobacterium, 031.9
Group A streptococcus, 041.01	Neck masses, 784.2
Group B streptococcus, 041.02	Staphylococci, 041.1
HIV, V08	Toxoplasmosis, 130.9
Infectious mononucleosis, 075	

1. Other causes of lymphadenopathy.
   a. Common viral and bacterial infections such as Group A beta-hemolytic streptococci (GABHS), staphylococci, cytomegalovirus (CMV), Epstein-Barr virus (EBV; infectious mono), HIV.
2. Subacute and chronic lymphadenopathy more likely associated with mycobacterium and toxoplasmosis.
3. Neck masses from other sources.

G. Treatment.
   1. Symptomatic.
      a. Antipyretics and analgesics.
      b. Moist wraps/compresses.
      c. Aspiration of painful nodes (avoid I&D).
      d. Antimicrobial treatment for severely ill patients or those with other chronic condition. Not suggested for regional CSD.
      e. For patients with significant lymphadenopathy: Azithromycin (Zithromax): 500 mg day 1, 250 mg days 2–5; younger children 10 mg/kg day 1, 5 mg/kg days 2–5.
      f. Other antibiotics with anecdotal evidence of efficacy: ciprofloxacin, rifampin, trimethoprim-sulfamethoxazole.

H. Follow up.
   1. Every week until resolution of symptoms, dependent on severity of symptoms.

I. Complications.

Aseptic meningitis, 047.9	Osteomyelitis, 730.28
Encephalitis, 323.9	Parinaud oculoglandular syndrome, 378.81
Erythema nodosum, 695.2	Pneumonia, 486
Hepatosplenomegaly, 571.8	Submandibular lymphadenopathy, 785.6
Neuroretinitis, 363.05	Thrombocytopenia purpura, 287.3

1. Parinaud oculoglandular syndrome: inoculation of conjunctiva results in ipsilateral preauricular or submandibular lymphadenopathy.
2. Less commonly: encephalitis, aseptic meningitis, neuroretinitis, thrombocytopenia purpura, erythema nodosum, pneumonia, hepatosplenomegaly, osteomyelitis, endocarditis.

J. Education.
   1. Avoid scratches by decreasing rough play with kittens.
   2. Immediately cleanse wounds from cats.

IV. CERVICAL LYMPHADENITIS

Adenopathy, 785.6	Hepatosplenomegaly, 571.8
Arthralgias, 719.4	Infectious mononucleosis, 075
Kawasaki disease 446.1	Lymphoma, 202.8
Cat-scratch disease, 078.3	Malnutrition, 263.9
Cervical lymphadenitis, 289.3	Mycobacterial infections, 031.9
Cervical lymphadenitis, acute, 683	Night sweats, 780.8
Cervical lymphadenopathy, 785.6	Pharyngitis, 462
Collagen vascular disease, 459.9	Rubella, 056.9
Cough, 786.2	Sore throat, 462
Enlargement of lymph glands, 785.6	Staphylococci, 041.1
Epstein-Barr virus, 075	Staphylococcus aureus, 041.11
Fatigue, 780.79	Toxoplasmosis, 130.9
Fever, 780.6	Upper respiratory infections, 465.9
Group A streptococcus, 041.01	Weight loss, 783.21
Group B streptococcus, 041.02	

A. Etiology.
1. Enlargement of lymph glands of neck generally due to:
    a. Infection, which causes proliferation and invasion of inflammatory cells.
        - Viruses:
            i.   Upper respiratory: respiratory syncytial virus (RSV), adenoviruses, influenza, parainfluenza, rhinoviruses—which usually resolve more quickly than other etiologies.
            ii. EBV.
            iii. CMV—rare.
            iv. Rubella, rubeola, roseola—rare.
            v.   Varicella zoster—rare.
            vi. HSV.
            vii. Coxsackie.
            viii. HIV—rare.
        - Bacteria:
            i.   *Staphylococcus aureus* and GABS: 40–80% of cases.
            ii. Anaerobes—rare.
            iii. *Corynebacterium diphtheriae.*

        iv. *Bartonella henselae* (cat-scratch disease).

        v. Gram-negative rods: *Haemophilus influenzae*, pseudomonas, salmonellae, shigellae, *Francisella tularensis* (tularemia).

- Mycobacterium.
  - i. Mycobacterium tuberculosis.
  - ii. Nontuberculous mycobacteria (NTM).
- Spirochetes.
- Rickettsiae.
- Fungi, including *Histoplasma capsulatum* (histoplasmosis)—rare.
- Protozoa, including *Toxoplasma gondii* (toxoplasmosis)—rare.

  b. Other causes.

- Neoplasms that cause infiltration of neoplastic cells—rare.
- Histiocytosis.
- Collagen vascular diseases: juvenile rheumatoid arthritis (JRA), lupus.
- Sarcoidosis.
- Kawasaki disease.
- Postvaccination: DTaP, polio, typhoid.
- Drugs-phenytoin, INH.

B. Occurrence.
1. About 40% of all children have palpable cervical lymph nodes.
2. Most cases of cervical lymphadenitis resulting from common bacterial and viral infections occur in toddler and preschool age groups.
3. Etiologic and age-related occurrence.
   a. Neonate.
      - Acute unilateral cervical lymphadenitis: *S. aureus*.
      - "Cellulitis-adenitis" syndrome: late-onset Group B streptococcus.
   b. Younger than 5 years of age.
      - Acute pyogenic cervical lymphadenitis: *S. aureus* and GABHS.
      - NTM lymph node infection.
      - Kawasaki disease (also usually unilateral).
   c. School-aged and adolescents: more likely chronic cervical lymphadenitis than acute pyogenic disease.

C. Clinical manifestations.
1. Acute bilateral cervical lymphadenopathy generally caused by URI or strep pharyngitis. Generally associated with EBV (infectious mononucleosis).
2. Acute unilateral cervical lymphadenitis variably associated with fever and suppuration, most often caused by staph and Group A streptococcus.

3. Subacute and chronic lymphadenitis are found in cat-scratch disease, toxoplasmosis, and mycobacterial infections. Nodes become fluctuant and are generally nontender.

4. Painless, possibly matted nodes and especially those in supraclavicular area are more likely malignant.

5. Associated symptoms.
   a. With URI: fever, sore throat, cough.
   b. Lymphoma, TB: fever, night sweats, weight loss.
   c. Collagen vascular disease or serum sickness: fever, fatigue, arthralgias.

D. Physical findings.
   1. General.
      a. Signs of malnutrition, including poor growth: suggestive of chronic disease.
      b. Generalized adenopathy and hepatosplenomegaly: suggestive of malignancy or other noninfectious illnesses and some infectious diseases such as EBV, HIV, TB, histoplasmosis.
   2. Enlargement of the lymph nodes: > 1 cm.
      a. Node-bearing areas: occipital, cervicofacial, axillary, epitrochlear, inguinal, popliteal.
      b. Nodes may be warm, mobile, fixed, fluctuant, solid, smooth.
   3. Presentation, distribution, associated diseases.
      a. Acute posterior cervical lymphadenopathy: rubella, infectious mononucleosis.
      b. Supraclavicular or posterior cervical lymphadenopathy: risk for malignancy.
      c. Cervical lymphadenopathy, associated generalized lymphadenopathy: viral infection.
      d. Generalized lymphadenopathy: associated with leukemia, lymphoma, collagen vascular disease.
      e. Nodes bilateral and soft (not fixed): viral infection.
      f. Tender nodes, possibly fluctuant, not fixed: bacteria.
      g. Redness and warmth: acute pyogenic process.
      h. With fluctuance: abscess formation.
      i. Matted or fluctuant nodes, skin overlying red but not warm: TB.
      j. Nodes hard and fixed, without signs of acute inflammation: associated malignancy.
   4. Associated physical signs.
      a. Markedly red pharynx, possibly exudates, soft palate petechiae: GABHS.
      b. Swelling, redness, tenderness of gums: periodontal disease.

      c. Edema of the soft tissues of the neck: diphtheria.

      d. Sinus tract formation: TB.

      e. Gingivostomatitis: HSV.

      f. Herpangina: coxsackievirus.

      g. Rash: infectious mono, scarlet fever.

      h. Pallor, petechiae, bruises, sternal tenderness.

      i. Hepatosplenomegaly: leukemia.

E. Diagnostic tests.

    1. Appropriate for suspicion of specific entity.

    2. Throat culture.

    3. PPD.

    4. CBC.

    5. Erythrocyte sedimentation rate (ESR) or (CRP) C-reactive protein

    6. Blood cultures.

    7. Liver enzymes.

    8. Serology for specific microorganisms.

    9. Chest X-ray.

  10. Ultrasound of nodes.

  11. Echocardiogram, ECG.

  12. Fine-needle aspiration for Gram stain and culture.

  13. Biopsy: if malignancy suspected.

F. Differential diagnosis.

Neck masses, 784.2
---

    1. Neck masses.

      a. Congenital lesions are generally painless and most likely identified in infancy.

        • Thyroglossal duct cyst: midline between thyroid bone and suprasternal notch, moves upward.

        • Branchial cleft cyst: smooth, fluctuant, proximal, anterior border of sternocleidomastoid muscle.

        • Sternocleidomastoid tumor: mass in belly of the muscle caused by perinatal injury; associated torticollis.

        • Cervical ribs: bony anomaly.

        • Cystic hygroma: fluid filled, easily transilluminated.

        • Hemangioma.

        • Laryngocele: cystic mass extending through the thyrohyoid membrane.

        • Dermoid cyst: midline cyst, also contains solid components.

        • Parotitis: swelling crosses angle of jaw; mumps.

2. To summarize: It is reasonable to safely observe nodes that are bilateral, < 3 cm in size, nonerythematous nor exquisitely tender. Treat empirically if: no accompanying systemic symptoms, node > 2–3 cm, unilateral, or erythematous and tender.

G. Treatment.
   1. Acute cervical lymphadenitis.
      a. Staphylococcus or Group B streptococcus.
         • Patient nontoxic, no abscesses or cellulitis.
            i. Cephalexin—for 10 days; child: 40 mg/kg/day divided bid or qid; adult: 250–500 mg bid or qid.
            ii. Amoxicillin-clavulanate (based on amoxicillin component): 40 mg/kg/day divided bid for 10 days; adult 500–875 mg bid.
            iii. Clindamycin: child older than 1 month of age: 8–25 mg/kg/day in divided doses q6–8h; adult: 150–450 mg q6h, max: 1.8 g/day.
         • Patient toxic or immunocompromised.
            i. IV cefazolin, nafcillin, or clindamycin.
      b. Anaerobes: seen with periodontal/dental disease.
         • Penicillin or clindamycin.
      c. Oral analgesia, warm compresses.
      d. Incision and drainage for suppurative, fluctuant nodes.
   2. Consider referral for biopsy if significant lymphadenopathy (> 2 cm in diameter) persists 2 weeks, or no decrease in size after 4–6 weeks or node(s) are supraclavicular, lack inflammation, are firm or rubbery, develop ulceration, fail to respond to antibiotic treatment or there are systemic symptoms (e.g., fever, weight loss, hepatosplenomegaly).
   3. Cervical lymphadenitis abscess: refer for fine-needle aspiration or excision (I&D).

H. Follow up.
   1. Call if node enlarges, becomes markedly tender, erythematous, indurated.
   2. Call if child appears toxic, has difficulty breathing or swallowing.
   3. If being treated for bacterial infection, call if not better in 48 hours (fever down, tenderness decreased, size of node stable).
   4. Recheck at end of treatment.
   5. Recheck if node(s) persist longer than several weeks.

I. Complications.
   1. Bacterial: suppuration, bacteremia.
   2. Undiagnosed infectious process or malignancy.

J. Education.
1. Address family's fears: primarily those of malignancy.
2. Compliance with medications.
3. Observation: when to call, return to clinic.
4. Hydration.

V. EPISTAXIS

Allergies, unspecified, 477.9	Lymphadenopathy, 785.6
Epistaxis, 784.7	Nosebleeds, 784.7
Hepatomegaly, 789.1	Pale skin, 709.9
Hypertension, 401.9	Petechial rashes, 782.1
Hypovolemia, 276.5	Upper respiratory infections, 465.9

A. Etiology.
1. Bleeding from the nose can be anteriorly from nares (commonly Kiesselbach plexus) or posteriorly into nasopharynx. The nasal mucosa has rich, yet relatively unprotected blood supply. The mucosa is thin, especially in children.
2. Causative factors.
    a. Inflammation.
        •   Infectious processes.
        •   Allergies.
    b. Neoplasms, polyps.
    c. Trauma.
        •   External injury.
        •   Nose picking.
        •   Foreign bodies.
        •   Chemical or caustic agents (including drugs).
3. Rarely.
    a. Systemic illnesses.
        •   Hematologic diseases.
        •   Hypertension.
B. Occurrence.
1. Very common in children.
2. Highest incidence 2–10 years of age.
3. Often familial history.

C. Clinical manifestations.
   1. Complaints of persistent, recurrent nosebleeds.
   2. May have history of:
      a. Recent or current URI.
      b. Allergies (especially nasal).
      c. Tarry stools.
      d. Medication or drug use.
      e. Persistent bleeding or bruising.
      f. Family history of epistaxis or bleeding disorders.
      g. Trauma: nose picking or foreign body insertion.
D. Physical findings.
   1. Vital signs may reflect hypovolemia or underlying cause such as hypertension.
   2. Inspection of nose, nasopharynx, and oropharynx may reveal:
      a. Bleeding most commonly from medial anterior nares.
      b. Dry, crusted mucosa.
      c. Excoriation of mucosa, site of bleeding.
   3. General exam may find lymphadenopathy, hepatomegaly, petechial rashes, or pale skin, mucosa, nail beds.
E. Diagnostic tests.
   1. Vital signs, including blood pressure.
   2. Hematocrit or CBC with platelets.
   3. If severe and persistent:
      a. CBC with platelets.
      b. Prothrombin and partial thromboplastic bleeding time.
F. Differential diagnosis.

Bleeding disorders, 289.9	Polyps, 471.9
Foreign body, nose, 932	Renal disease, 593.9
Hypertension, 401.9	Vascular abnormalities, 785.9

   1. Bleeding disorder: if severe and recurrent, child younger than 2 years, positive family history.
   2. Polyps, vascular abnormalities.
   3. Foreign body.
   4. Hypertension, renal disease.
G. Treatment.
   1. Elevate head and lean forward.
   2. Pinch nares together for at least 10 minutes.

3. Ice to nasal dorsum may be added.
4. Packing (preferably absorbable), topical vasoconstrictive drugs may be needed.
5. Referral to ENT if unmanageable or prolonged or abnormalities of nose.

H. Follow up.
 1. Hct, 6–12 hours after bleed if concern for anemia.
 2. Return if unmanageable and/or persistent.

I. Complications.
 1. Possibly mild anemia.
 2. Rare: airway obstruction, aspiration, vomiting.

J. Education.
 1. Prevention.
  a. Humidification of air in home, especially bedroom.
  b. Nasal saline sprays, drops.
  c. Petroleum jelly applied sparingly to anterior nares.
  d. Protective athletic gear.
  e. Discouragement of nose-picking behaviors and vigorous blowing.
 2. Reassurance: amount of blood always looks greater than it is.

VI. FOREIGN BODY, NASAL

Choking, 784.9	Foreign body, nose, 932
Cough, 786.2	Vomiting, 787.03
Dysphagia, 787.2	

A. Etiology.
 1. Small objects are often inserted into nose by children, causing full or partial obstruction of nares.

B. Occurrence.
 1. Frequent, especially in young children age 3–6 years.

C. Clinical manifestations.
 1. Child may have been observed.
 2. Initially, local symptoms of obstruction: swelling, sneezing, mild discomfort.
 3. Subsequently, persistent, purulent, unilateral discharge; may be bloody or foul smelling.

D. Physical findings.
 1. Dependent on length of time obstruction has been present: see above symptoms. Obstruction is almost always unilateral.

2. Examiner may be able to visualize object with nasal speculum or oto-scope.
3. Common objects include beads, buttons, toy parts, pebbles, candle wax, food, paper, cloth, button batteries.
4. Tend to locate in floor of nasal passage or in the upper nasal fossa.

E. Diagnostic tests.
   1. None.

F. Differential diagnosis.

Adenoiditis, 474.01

Nasal tumors, 471.9

Rhinosinusitis, 473.9

---

   1. Infection.
      a. Rhinosinusitis.
      b. Adenoiditis.
   2. Polyps.
   3. Nasal tumors.

G. Treatment.
   1. Purulent discharge may need to be suctioned in order to visualize object.
   2. An older child may be told to occlude one side of nares and blow vigorously.
   3. A parent may blow gently through the child's mouth while occluding one side of the nose or an Ambu bag may be used.
   4. Removal requires:
      a. Good lighting.
      b. Topical anesthesia (generally lidocaine).
      c. Vasoconstrictor drugs (0.5% epinephrine to reduce mucosa edema).
      d. Alligator forceps, cerumen spoon (curved, wire ones best).
      e. Narrow tip suction.
      f. Passing a thin, lubricated, 5–6 Fr, balloon-tipped catheter past the foreign body, inflating balloon and pulling forward.

H. Follow up.
   1. None, if successful removal and signs of infection clear within 1–2 days.
   2. Referral to ENT if unable or unlikely to remove easily.
   3. Consider behavioral/emotional assessment if is recurrent problem or developmentally inappropriate behavior.

I. Complications.
   1. Chronic infection if undetected and/or not removed.
   2. Trauma to nares from removal procedure.

J. Education.
1. Close observation of children by caregivers.
2. Limit access by small children to small objects.
3. *Note*: If child swallows foreign body, especially coin, radiographic survey must be done to ensure object is in stomach. Child must be observed closely for hoarseness, dysphagia, drooling, gagging, vomiting, coughing, choking, and airway compromise including inspiratory stridor.

VII. INFECTIOUS MONONUCLEOSIS

Abdominal pain, 789	Mild hepatitis, 573.3
Fatigue, 780.79	Myalgia, 729.1
Fever, 780.6	Myocarditis, 429.01
Group A streptococcus, 041.01	Palatal petechiae, 782.7
Group B streptococcus, 041.02	Pharyngitis, 462
Hemolytic anemia, 283.9	Rash, 782.1
Infectious mononucleosis, 075	Splenomegaly, 789.2
Lymphadenopathy, 785.6	Thrombocytopenia, 287.5
Lymphocytosis, 288.8	Tonsillitis, 463
Malaise, 780.79	

A. Etiology.
1. Epstein-Barr (which is a herpesvirus) virus: 90% of cases.
2. Clinical symptoms result from proliferation of b-lymphocytes in the epithelial cells of the pharynx, parotid duct, lymph nodes, spleen.
3. Spread primarily in saliva.
4. Latent, lifelong infection occurs and may be reactivated during immuno-suppression.
B. Occurrence.
1. Humans.
    a. Endemic worldwide in younger children, especially third world countries.
    b. One-third of cases in adolescents in more affluent populations of developed countries.
    c. Almost all adults in United States are seropositive for EBV.
C. Clinical manifestations.
1. Primary EBV infection.
    a. Incubation is 30–50 days.

    b. Primary EBV infection in adolescents presents in > 50% of cases with:
- Fatigue, malaise, myalgia.
- Generalized lymphadenopathy.
- Pharyngitis.
- Possibly fever or prodrome of malaise and fever.

    c. Younger children may experience mild febrile episode, rash, abdominal pain.

D. Physical findings.
1. Tonsillitis, pharyngitis: possibly exudative.
2. Palatal petechiae (transient).
3. Lymphadenopathy.
   a. Anterior and posterior cervical nodes, also axillary or inguinal nodes.
   b. Large, mildly tender.
   c. Epitrochlear nodes highly indicative.
4. Splenomegaly.
   a. Frequent false negatives, if done too early in 50% of cases.
   b. 2–3 cm below costal margin.
   c. Persists for 2–4 weeks past resolution of other symptoms.

E. Diagnostic tests.
1. "Monospot" (mononucleosis rapid slide agglutination test for heterophile antibodies disease process) 25% false negative in the first week of the disease. In children younger than 12 years of age monospot detects 25–50% of cases.
2. CBC with differential.
   a. Lymphocytosis with up to 20,000 WBCs.
   b. Up to 40% atypical lymphocytes. *Note:* 50% lymphocytes with 10–20% atypical lymphocytes diagnostic.
   c. Mild thrombocytopenia 50% of cases.
   d. Positive monocytes on differential.
3. Liver enzymes.
   a. Mild hepatitis common.
   b. Usually asymptomatic.
4. EBV serology: indicated in acutely ill patient.
   a. If monospot negative and strong suspicion.
   b. VCA-IgM test if monospot negative and urgent diagnosis needed such as in a competitive athlete.
5. Throat culture.
   a. Rule out other causes.
   b. 5–25% cases have concurrent GABHS infection.

F. Differential diagnosis.

Adenovirus, 079	Leukemias, 208.9
Cytomegalovirus, 078.5	Pharyngitis, 462
Group A streptococcus, 041.01	Rubella, 056.9
Group B streptococcus, 041.02	Tonsillitis, 463
HIV, V08	Toxoplasmosis gondii, 130.9
Human herpes virus, 054.9	

1. Other causes of infectious mononucleosis-like syndrome (in descending order of incidence):
    a. Cytomegalovirus.
    b. Toxoplasmosis gondii.
    c. HIV-mucocutaneous lesions, diarrhea, nausea and vomiting, weight loss.
    d. Human herpesvirus.
    e. Rubella.
2. Pharyngitis/tonsillitis.
    a. GABHS—absence of hepatosplenomegaly; fatigue less prominent.
    b. Other bacterial causes.
    c. Viruses other than EBV.
3. Leukemias.
4. Infectious mononucleosis should be suspected in any febrile patient with sore throat plus palatal petechiae, splenomegaly, posterior cervical, and possibly axillary or inguinal adenopathy.
G. Treatment.
    1. Supportive.
        a. Analgesics and antipyretics.
        b. Hydration support if needed.
        c. Corticosteroids may be indicated if:
            • Impending airway obstruction or dehydration secondary to severe tonsillopharyngitis.
            • Massive splenomegaly.
            • Myocarditis.
            • Hemolytic anemia.
            • Hemophagocytic syndrome.
H. Follow up.
    1. Fatigue may persist months after recovery. Patient should be allowed to resume school and activities as energy level permits.

      2. Splenomegaly.
        a. Risk of rupture is estimated at 0.1% (50% are spontaneous).
        b. Recheck at weekly intervals.
        c. Avoid contact sports at least 3–4 weeks until fully recovered and spleen no longer palpable.
        d. Consider selective ultrasonography such as when an athlete would like to return to competitive sports in < 4 weeks.

I. Complications.

Airway obstruction, 519.8	Dehydration, 276.5
Antibiotic-induced rash, 693	Splenic rupture, 289.59

    1. Additional complications are rare, but include:
      a. Dehydration.
      b. Antibiotic-induced rash (most commonly when ampicillin or amoxicillin antibiotic used for concurrent bacterial infection).
      c. Thrombocytopenia.
      d. Airway obstruction.
      e. Acute interstitial nephritis.
      f. Hemolytic anemia.
      g. Myocarditis.
      h. Neurologic abnormalities.
      i. Cranial nerve palsies.
      j. Encephalitis.
      k. Retrobulbar neuritis.

J. Education.
    1. Close personal contact is required for transmission.
    2. Recovery often biphasic, with worsening of symptoms after period of improvement.
    3. Full recovery may take months.
    4. Patient should not donate blood.

VIII. PHARYNGITIS

Adenovirus, 079	Neisseria gonorrhoeae, 032.9
Coxsackievirus, 079.2	Peritonsillar abscess, 475
Epstein-Barr virus, 075	Pharyngitis, 462
Group A streptococcus, 041.01	Rheumatic fever, 390
Group B streptococcus, 041.02	Rhinovirus, 079.3

A. Etiology.
   1. Inflammation of mucous membranes and underlying structures of pharynx and tonsils, usually caused by infection.
   2. Causative agents.
      a. Respiratory viruses, including rhinovirus, adenovirus, coxsackievirus, Epstein-Barr virus.
      b. GABHS.
      c. Group C beta-hemolytic strep (not a cause of rheumatic fever), Neisseria gonorrhoeae rarely.
      d. Mycoplasma pneumoniae: possibly 10% occurence in adolescents.
      e. Corynebacterium diphtheriae.
B. Occurrence.
   1. Peak incidence late fall through early spring.
   2. Younger children more commonly present in winter months and with viral pharyngitis.
   3. GABHS has proclivity for 5- to 15-year age group, also peaking in winter.
C. Clinical manifestations.
   1. Viral pharyngitis.
      a. Gradual onset.
      b. Cough, coryza, diarrhea more common.
   2. Coxsackievirus (see "Physical findings"—next section)
   3. Streptococcal.
      a. Rapid onset.
      b. See "Physical findings"—next section.
D. Physical findings.
   1. Viral pharyngitis.
      a. Sore throat, dysphagia.
      b. Low-grade fever.
      c. Possibly diarrhea.
   2. Coxsackievirus.
      a. Fever, headache.
      b. GI complaints.
      c. Possibly papular rash of hand, foot, mouth disease.
      d. Possibly ulcerative lesions in mucosa of mouth.
   3. Streptococcal GABHS.
      a. Moderate to high fever, headache.
      b. Red pharynx: beefy red, swollen uvula and tonsils.
      c. Yellow, blood: tinged exudates.
      d. Petechiae on soft palate, strawberry (coated) tongue.
      e. Tender cervical lymphadenopathy.

    f. Multiple GI complaints.

    g. Accompanying scarlatiniform rash: red, sandpaper-like, clustered in body's "hot spots" (axillae, neck, inguinal, anticubital, popliteal areas).

E. Diagnostic tests.

    1. Throat swab for rapid antigen detection test for GABHS. Negative should also have follow-up throat culture (can also identify carrier state).

    2. Heterophile antibody test for EBV.

    3. CBC.

F. Differential diagnosis.

Allergic rhinitis, generalized, 477.9	Group G streptococcus, 041.05
Group C streptococcus, 041.03	Infectious mononucleosis, 075

    1. Viral vs. bacterial entity.

        a. Infectious mononucleosis.

        b. Group C or G streptococcus.

    2. Allergic rhinitis.

G. Treatment.

    1. Nonpharmacologic.

        a. Encourage fluids: may prefer hot or cold for pain relief.

    2. Pharmacologic.

        a. Topical and oral analgesics and antipyretics.

        b. Antimicrobials: penicillin V recommended.

          • Children < 27 kg: 250 mg bid or tid for 10 days.

          • Children > 27 kg: 500 mg bid or tid for 10 days.

          • IM benzathine penicillin G: if compliance, vomiting issues.

            i. Children < 27 kg: 600,000 units.

           ii. Children > 27 kg: 1.2 million units.

          • Amoxicillin: substituted for taste issues (may benefit 40% of children with adenotonsillar disease, who yield beta-lactamase-producing bacteria).

            i. Once daily dosing of amoxicillin at 50 mg/kg for 10 days is as effective as penicillin V or amoxicillin given in multiple doses for 10 days.

          • Penicillin (PCN) allergic options:

            i. Clindamycin (20 mg/kg/day in 3 divided doses, max 1.8 g/day). In the United States, macrolide resistant rates to group A streptococci (GAS) have been 5–8%.

           ii. Erythromycin estolate or ethylsuccinate: 40 mg/kg/day in 2–4 divided doses.

iii. Clarithromycin: Child: 15 mg/kg/day, max: 1000 mg divided q12h for 10 days. Adult: 500 mg q12h for 10 days.

iv. Azithromycin: 12 mg/kg/day for 5 days.

- First-generation cephalosporin such as cephalexin: also appropriate if retreatment necessary.
- *Note*: As many as 5% of penicillin-allergic people are also allergic to cephalosporins. People with type 1 allergy to PCN should not be treated with a cephalosporin.
- Due to increased treatment failure with PCN, some clinicians are using a first generation cephalosporin in all nonallergic patients.
  i. Cephalexin (25–40 mg/kg/day in 2 divided doses for 10 days).
- Other cephalosporins also have indication for GAS treatment:
  i. Cefprozil (second generation).
  ii. Cefpodoxime, cefdinir (third generation).
- If illness recurs shortly after treatment:
  i. May be retreated with same drug.
  ii. IM penicillin if compliance an issue.
  iii. Narrow spectrum cephalosporin (cephalexin).
  iv. Amoxicillin-clavulanate potassium.

H. Follow up.
  1. Routine reculturing is not necessary.
  2. Encourage patients to call if:
    a. Unable to complete course of medication or retain medication.
    b. Siblings complain of sore throat within 2–5 days: amoxicillin-clavulanate 90 mg/6.4 mg per kg/day. If allergic: 6 months to 12 years of age, cefdinir 7 mg/kg bid or 14 mg/kg daily; 13 years, 300 mg bid 10 days.
    c. No improvement in patient in 48 hours.
    d. Signs and symptoms of renal complications.
    e. Drug reaction.
  3. Possible assessment of carrier state which is common and patients are low risk to transmit and develop invasive disease. Most common scenario is a carrier who is experiencing repeated intercurrent episodes of viral pharyngitis. (In true GAS pharyngitis response to antimicrobial therapy is rapid.) Treatment of carriers is indicated only in very specific cases such as those involving rheumatic fever or glomerulonephritis outbreaks or recurrent, symptomatic GAS pharyngitis in a family after appropriate therapy.
    a. Clindamycin most effective treatment (20 mg/kg/day in 3 divided doses; max 1.8 g/day).

   b. ENT referral for possible tonsillectomy and adenoidectomy, though currently poorly understood and risks of surgery often do not outweigh possible benefits.
   - Multiple bouts of tonsillitis in 1 year despite adequate treatment.
   - Significant upper airway obstruction.
   - Peritonsillar abscess.
I. Complications.

Cervical lymphadenitis, 683	Poststreptococcal glomerulonephritis, 580
Mastoiditis, 383	Rheumatic heart disease, acute, 391.9
Peritonsillar abscess, 475	Streptococcal pharyngitis, 034

   1. Streptococcal pharyngitis.
      a. Suppurative.
         - Peritonsillar abscess.
         - Cervical lymphadenitis.
         - Mastoiditis.
      b. Acute rheumatic fever.
      c. Post-strep glomerulonephritis.
J. Education.
   1. Transmission is person to person via respiratory tract secretions.
   2. Medication compliance is essential.
   3. May return to school/daycare 24 hours after beginning antibiotic therapy.

IX. RHINOSINUSITIS

Allergic rhinitis, 477.9	Immunodeficiency, 279.2
Ciliary dyskinesia, 781.3	Nasal obstruction, 478.1·
Cough, 786.2	Nasal speech, 784.5
Cystic fibrosis, 277	Postnasal secretions, 473.9
Dental pain, 529.6	Proptosis, 376.3
Ear pressure, 388.7	Rhinorrhea, 478.1
Fatigue, 780.79	Rhinosinusitis, bacterial, 473.9
Frontal sinusitis, 473.1	Rhinosinusitis, viral, 472
Gastroesophageal reflux, 530.81	Smoke exposure, 987.9
Halitosis, 784.9	Snoring, 786.09
Headache, 784	Upper respiratory infection, 465.9

A. Etiology.
1. Each case of viral rhinitis is also rhinosinusitis, because mucous membranes of nasal passages, sinus cavities are identical.
2. Sinusitis is inflammation of mucous membranes lining paranasal sinuses, commonly used to describe bacterial rhinosinusitis.
3. Factors that increase risk of sinusitis are:
   a. Smoke exposure.
   b. Cold and dry inspired air.
   c. Preceding or concurrent URI.
   d. Allergic rhinitis.
   e. Swimming.
   f. Gastroesophageal reflux.
   g. Cystic fibrosis.
   h. Immunodeficiency.
   i. Ciliary dyskinesia.
   j. Factors associated with nasal obstruction.
4. Stagnation of secretions occurs within sinus cavities, becoming culture medium for bacteria.
5. Common pathogens.
   a. Streptococcus pneumoniae.
   b. *Haemophilus influenzae.*
   c. Moraxella catarrhalis (becoming most common in children).
B. Occurrence.
1. Complication of 5–10% of viral upper respiratory illnesses in children.
2. In young children, occurs primarily in maxillary sinuses, ethmoids secondly.
3. Frontal sinusitis is rare prior to age 10 years.
C. Clinical manifestations.
1. Acute and persistent nasal and sinus symptoms for 10–30 days.
   a. Subacute: clinical symptoms for 4–12 weeks.
   b. Chronic: symptoms lasting at least 12 weeks.
   c. Recurrent: 4+ incidents/year with complete resolution in interim.
   d. Mild: 10–14 days of persistent anterior or posterior rhinorrhea (discharge)—of any quality, without improvement and fatigue.
   e. Moderate: 10 days of nasal congestion, fever, increased maxillary or frontal tenderness/pressure.
   f. Severe–high fever > 102°F and purulent nasal discharge for at least 3 days in a child who seems ill.
2. May complain of cough (daytime, often worsening at night), rhinorrhea, postnasal secretions, halitosis, dental pain, headache, fatigue, ear pressure, snoring, nasal speech.

    D. Physical findings.
1. Fever.
2. Nasal speech.
3. Halitosis.
4. Purulent drainage in posterior pharynx and/or nose.
5. Nasal mucosa may be erythematous and swollen.
6. Face over paranasal sinuses may be tender to palpation.
7. Headache, especially when bending over.
8. Sinuses opaque, especially in older children.
9. Puffiness around eyes.
10. Proptosis, impaired extraocular movements: associated with orbital infection.

    E. Diagnostic tests.
1. X-rays—findings on plain radiographs correlate poorly with disease and should not be used.
2. CT scan of paranasal sinuses: indicated in complicated, severe, or recalcitrant cases.

    F. Differential diagnosis.

Adenoidal hypertrophy, 474.12	Foreign body, nose, 932
Allergic rhinitis, 477.9	Septal deviation, 470
Choanal atresia, 748	Viral URI, 465.9

1. Viral URI.
2. Allergic rhinitis.
3. Drug induced (rhinitis medicamentosa).
4. Tumors: polyps, neoplasms, adenoidal hypertrophy.
5. Foreign body.
6. Septal deviation, choanal atresia.

    G. Treatment.
1. Acute bacterial rhinosinusitis (ABRS) in children.
    a. Mild symptomatology and no antibiotics within past 4–6 weeks.
      • Amoxicillin (90 mg/kg/day) for 10 days.
      • High-dose amoxicillin-clavulanate ES: 90 mg/kg/day, (based on amoxicillin component) divided bid.
      • Cefpodoxime proxetil, cefuroxime axetil, cefdinir, cefprozil.
    b. Mild disease and *have* received antibiotics within previous 4–6 weeks or in moderate disease.
      • High-dose amoxicillin-clavulanate ES (same dose).

- Cefdinir if allergic.
- Azithromycin or clarithromycin if severely allergic.
  c. Consider switch in medications if no response in 72 hours.
2. Chronic sinusitis: may need to treat for 4 weeks.
3. Normal saline nasal sprays: assists drainage and ventilation.
4. Topical nasal steroids: may decrease swelling of turbinates and aid ostia to drain.
5. Mucolytics: may help mucous clearance.
6. Antihistamines: helpful if allergic component.
7. Decongestants: controversial benefit.
8. Humidified air.
9. Encourage fluids.
H. Follow up.
1. Patient to call if no response to medications in 72 hours.
2. Recheck in 2 weeks.
3. Referral to ENT or allergist if indicated or refractory.
I. Complications.

Brain abscess, 324	Orbital cellulitis, 376.01
Cavernous sinus thrombosis, 325	Osteomyelitis of maxilla or frontal bone, 730.28
Exacerbation of asthma, 493.92	Subdural empyema, 324.9
Optic neuritis, 377.3	

1. Orbital cellulitis.
2. Intracranial complications such as cavernous sinus thrombosis, subdural empyema, brain abscess.
3. Exacerbation of asthma.
4. Optic neuritis.
5. Osteomyelitis of maxilla or frontal bone.
J. Education.
1. Prevention: Avoid allergens and treat allergies when appropriate.
2. Encourage humidified air at home unless it exacerbates mildew, mold allergies.
3. Emphasize that most rhinitis and sinusitis are viral in etiology and antibiotics are not indicated.
4. Encourage compliance with prescribed antimicrobial agents.
5. Advise patient against diving (including scuba).

BIBLIOGRAPHY

American Academy of Pediatrics Subcommittee on Management of Sinusitis and Committee on Quality Improvement. Clinical practice guideline: management of sinusitis. *Pediatrics.* 2001;108(3):798-808.

American Academy of Pediatrics. *2009 red book: report of the Committee on Infectious Diseases.* 28th ed. Elk Grove Village, IL: American Academy of Pediatrics; 2009.

Choby B. Diagnosis and treatment of streptococcal pharyngitis. *Am Family Physician.* 2009;79(5):383-390.

Clark M, Krol D. *PACT module: protecting all children's teeth, oral health initiate.* Elk Grove Village, IL: American Academy of Pediatrics; 2009.

Dulin M. Management of cervical lymphadenopathy in children. *Am Family Physician.* 2008;78(9):1097-1098.

Ebell M. Epstein-Barr virus infectious mononucleosis. *Am Family Physician.* 2004;70(7):1279-1287.

Feder HM. Periodic fever, aphthous stomatitis, pharyngitis, adenitis: a clinical review of a new syndrome. *Clin Opin Pediatr.* 2000;12:233-236.

Florin T, Zaoutis T, Zaoutis L. Beyond cat scratch disease: widening spectrum of Bartonella henslae infection. *Pediatrics.* 2008;121:e1413-e1425.

Hayden G, Hendley J. An up-to-date approach to pharyngitis in children. *Resp Dis Pediatr J.* 2001;3:125-131.

Heims S. Foreign bodies in the ear, nose and throat. *Am Family Physician.* 2007;76(8):1185-1189.

Leung A, Robson L. Childhood cervical lymphadenopathy. *J Ped Health Care.* 2004;18:3-7.

Mahr T, Sheth K. Update on allergic rhinitis. *Pediatrics in Rev.* 2005;26:284-289.

Margileth M. Recent advances in the diagnosis and treatment of cat scratch disease. *Current Infectious Dis Rep.* 2000;2(2):141-146.

Ownby DR, et al. Exposure to dogs and cats in the first year of life and risk of allergic sensitization at 6 to 7 years of age. *JAMA.* 2002;288:963-972.

Platts-Mills TAE. Allergen avoidance in the treatment of asthma and rhinitis. *N Engl J Med.* 2003;349:207-208.

Sinus and Allergy Health Partnership. Antimicrobial treatment guidelines for acute bacterial rhinosinusitis. *Otolaryngol Head Neck Surgery J.* 2003;130(suppl):1-44.

Welch M. *Guide to your child's allergies and asthma.* Elk Grove Village, IL: American Academy of Pediatrics; 2010.

CHAPTER 24

Respiratory Disorders

Marti Michel

I. CROUP

Airway obstruction, severe, 519.8	Laryngotracheobronchitis, 490
Anxiety, 300	Laryngotracheobronchopneumonia, 485
Change in level of consciousness, 780.09	Mild erythema, 695.9
Croup, 464.4	Mild fever, 780.6
Croup, spasmodic, 478.78	Progressive restlessness, 799.2
Cyanosis, 782.5	Respiratory distress, 786.09
Edema of larynx, 478.6	Restlessness, 799.2
Edema of nasal mucosa, 478.25	Rhinorrhea, 478.1
Fatigue, 780.79	Sore throat, 462
Harsh, barking cough, 786.2	Suprasternal, 738.3
Hoarseness, 784.49	Tachycardia, 785
Hypoxemia, 799	Tachypnea, 786.06
Increased retractions, 786	Upper airway obstruction, acute, 519.8
Inspiratory stridor, 786.1	Wheezing, 786.07
Laryngotracheitis, 464.2	

A. Etiology.
  1. Acute upper airway obstruction in children, most often caused by viral infection.
     a. Most common form of viral croup is laryngotracheitis resulting from inflammation and edema of larynx, subglottic area.
        • Causative agents include parainfluenza 1, 2, 3 (parainfluenza 1 and 3 most common), influenza A and B, respiratory syncytial virus (RSV), adenovirus, measles.

    b. Spasmodic croup is similar to viral croup but is not associated with fever and symptoms, lasts only hours, not days.
- Onset typically occurs during night in a child who has been well.
- May represent allergic reaction to viral antigen.

    c. Laryngotracheobronchitis (LTB) and laryngotracheobronchopneumonia (LTBP) involve upper airway; also affect lower airway, specifically bronchi.
- Same viral agents are common to LTB and LTBP.
- Bacterial superinfection occurs more commonly in this croup variant; includes *Staphylococcus aureus, Streptococcus pyogenes, Streptococcus pneumoniae, Haemophilus influenzae, Corynebacterium diphtheria.*
  - i. Agents are infrequent causes but tend to cause more severe illness.

B. Occurrence.
1. Viral croup occurs at 6 months to 5 years of age, with peak in second year of life.
2. Affects boys more than girls.
3. Occurs in late fall, early winter; correlates with the activity of viral agents causing the syndrome.
4. Symptoms typically last 3–7 days.

C. Clinical manifestations.
1. Gradual onset with rhinorrhea, sore throat, mild fever.
2. Disease has wide spectrum from very mild illness to severe illness.
3. Harsh, "seal-like" barking cough.
4. Hoarseness.
5. Inspiratory stridor.
6. Increasing obstruction.
    a. Tachycardia, tachypnea—usually not > 50 breaths/min.
    b. Suprasternal, supraclavicular, substernal, and intercostal retractions.
    c. Paradoxical abdominal and chest wall movement.
    d. Progressive restlessness and anxiety correlates with hypoxemia.

D. Physical findings.
1. Normal or mildly elevated temperature.
2. Mild erythema and edema of nasal mucosa.
3. Inspiratory stridor.
4. Hoarseness.
5. Harsh, barky cough.
6. Nontoxic appearing.

      7. On auscultation, normal breath sounds except transmission of stridor.

      8. With increased obstruction: wheezing, prolonged expiration, decreased breath sounds.

E. Diagnostic tests.

      1. Diagnosis made on basis of history and clinical presentation.

      2. Imaging is not usually necessary in the ambulatory setting; posteroanterior neck X-ray.

          a. Classic "steeple sign": narrowed air column consistent with narrowing of subglottic space.

          b. Lateral view is useful in ruling out epiglottitis, retropharyngeal abscess, or radiopaque foreign body.

      3. If indicated, WBC normal or low with polymorphonucleotides (PMNs).

      4. Clinical croup score can classify severity of illness and aid in decision making regarding hospitalization.

F. Differential diagnosis.

Diphtheria, 032.9	Peritonsillar abscess, 475
Epiglottitis, 464.3	Retropharyngeal abscess, 478.24
Foreign obstruction, 933.1	

      1. Epiglottitis: toxic appearing, drooling, high fever, acute onset, age range typically 3–7 years.

      2. Laryngeal foreign body: history, age, abrupt onset, lack of preceding respiratory symptoms.

      3. Diphtheria: characteristic thin, gray membrane extends from tonsil to associated soft/hard palate.

      4. Retropharyngeal or peritonsillar abscess: severe throat pain, refusal to swallow or speak, fever to 105°F (40.6°C).

      5. Bacterial tracheitis: affects children of any age, acute onset with respiratory stridor, high fever, and copious and purulent secretions.

G. Treatment.

      1. Most children have mild airway obstruction that resolves without specific treatment.

      2. Supportive care at home includes making the child comfortable, avoiding fatigue and anxiety; encourage fluids and antipyretics for fever.

      3. Cool mist vaporizer may be used.

      4. Nebulized epinephrine has been beneficial for children with more severe croup in the emergency department or hospital setting.

5. Corticosteroids.
   a. Systemic or nebulized corticosteroids are mainstay of both outpatient and inpatient treatment.
   b. Decrease edema of laryngeal mucosa.
   c. Single dose 0.6 mg dexamethasone given orally or IM or 2 mg dose of nebulized budesonide.
   d. Clinical improvement in 6–12 hours.
   e. Efficacy did not vary according to route of administration
   f. Facilitates clinical improvement, decreases hospitalizations and fewer follow-up visits.
6. Criteria for hospitalization:
   a. Signs of moderate to severe airway obstruction.
   b. Increased work of breathing and respiratory distress.
   c. Hypoxemia.
   d. Restlessness, anxiety, or fatigue.
   e. Change in level of consciousness.
   f. Dehydration.
H. Follow up.
   1. Call healthcare provider immediately if signs of respiratory distress increase.
   2. Increased respiratory rate.
   3. Stridor at rest.
   4. Increased retractions.
   5. Change in level of consciousness, restlessness, or anxiety.
   6. Cyanosis.
I. Complications.
   1. Acute deterioration in respiratory status requires hospitalization/intubation.
J. Education.
   1. Croup usually lasts 3–7 days; typically worse at night.
   2. Give guidelines about oral intake (fluids) and urine output.
   3. Use of bathroom mist, cool night air, cool-mist vaporizer to relieve symptoms.
   4. Signs of increasing respiratory distress and hypoxemia.
   5. Good handwashing, containment of coughs/sneezes prevents spread of illness.
   6. Maintain calm, reassuring manner. Avoid situations that provoke stress or crying, which can worsen respiratory distress.
   7. Children may have repeated episodes of croup.

8. Antibiotics are not indicated for viral croup.
9. Avoid secondhand smoke exposure.

II. BRONCHIOLITIS

Apnea, 770.81	Poor appetite, 783
Atelectasis, 518	Poor feeding, 783.3
Bronchiolitis, 466.19	Respiratory syncytial virus, 079.6
Cough, 786.2	Rhinorrhea, 478.1
Dyspnea, 786.09	Sneezing, 784.9
Hypoxemia, 799	Subsegmental consolidation, 481
Irritability, 799.2	Tachypnea, 786.06
Lethargy, 780.79	Upper respiratory tract infection, 465.9
Low-grade fever, 780.6	Vomiting, 787.03
Nasal congestion, 478.1	Wheezing, 786.07

A. Etiology.
    1. Bronchiolitis is common viral illness.
        a. RSV, bronchiolitis is most common cause of acute lower respiratory infection (LRI) in first 2 years of life.
        b. Bronchiolitis is also caused by parainfluenza 1 and 3, adenovirus, rhinoviruses, influenza, and human metapneumovirus.
    2. Transmission.
        a. Highly contagious.
            • Virus shed 5–12 days and up to 30 days with underlying disease.
            • Virus spreads by large droplet aerosols generated by coughing, sneezing.
            • Transmitted by direct contact with nasopharyngeal secretions from infected person.
                i. Virus survives on skin approximately 20 minutes.
                ii. Virus survives on gowns/tissues approximately 30–60 minutes.
                iii. Virus survives on hard, nonporous surfaces approximately 6 hours.
            • High-risk factors for more severe disease: prematurity, chronic lung disease, congenital heart disease, immunosuppression.
        b. Reinfection occurs throughout life.

B. Occurrence.
1. Seasonal prevalence.
   a. Yearly epidemics in early winter/spring.
   b. In temperate climates, typically start in November and persist through April.
   c. Strains A and B circulated concurrently during outbreaks; strain A more dominant.
   d. By age 3, most children have been infected with RSV.
   e. Only 1–5% require hospitalization.
   f. Adolescents, adults with RSV have symptoms of upper respiratory tract infection.
C. Clinical manifestations.
1. Initial presentation.
   a. Mild upper respiratory infection (URI) with rhinorrhea and nasal congestion.
   b. Low-grade fever for 2–3 days.
   c. Poor appetite.
   d. Hoarse cough progresses to deep, wet cough.
      • Often paroxysmal.
      • Often associated with post-tussive vomiting.
      • Associated with wheezing.
2. Clinical progression.
   a. LRT involvement evident by:
      • Tachypnea: 60–80 breaths/minute.
      • Dyspnea.
      • Coughing, wheezing.
   b. Neonatal presentation.
      • Lethargy, irritability.
      • Poor feeding.
      • URI symptoms.
      • Apnea: occurrence is inversely proportional to age.
D. Physical findings.
1. Increased work of breathing.
   a. Nasal congestion with thick purulent secretions.
   b. Respirations rapid, shallow with accessory muscle use, retractions.
   c. Nasal flaring, grunting, head bobbing.
   d. Paroxysmal cough, wheezing, crackles.
   e. Prolonged expiratory phase, chest hyperexpansion and hyperresonance.
   f. Liver and spleen may be palpable secondary to chest hyperexpansion.

      g. Hypoxemia correlates with severity of tachypnea.
      h. Paradoxical abdominal and chest wall movement.
E. Diagnostic tests.
  1. Diagnosis often made on basis of clinical presentation, physical findings, epidemiology.
      a. Definitive diagnosis may not be necessary in infants with mild disease.
  2. Chest X-ray (CXR).
      a. Hyperinflation may be only abnormality: flattened diaphragms, increased lucency.
      b. Peribronchial thickening and increased interstitial markings.
      c. Subsegmental consolidation in upper and middle lobes: patchy atelectasis or consolidation due to atelectasis.
  3. Oximetry: to determine oxygenation status.
  4. Laboratory tests.
      a. Identification of virus or viral antigen in respiratory secretions.
        • Specimen obtained by nasal swab.
        • Rapid diagnostic tests detect antigen using immunofluorescence techniques or enzyme-linked immunoassays.
        • Viral culture.
F. Differential diagnosis.

Aspiration, 934.8	Hypoxemia, 799
Asthma, 493.9	Immunodeficiency, 279.3
Bacterial pneumonia, 482.9	*Mycoplasma pneumoniae,* 483
Cervical lymphadenopathy, 785.6	Nasal congestion, 478.1
Chlamydial infection, 079.98	Pneumonia, 486
Congenital heart disease, 746.9	Poor feeding, 783.3
Congestive heart failure, 428	Poor growth, 764.9
Cough, 786.2	Respiratory distress, 786.09
Cystic fibrosis, 277.02	Respiratory failure, 518.81
Fever, 780.6	Rhinitis, 477.9
Foreign body, 934.8	Tachypnea, 786.06
Heart murmur, 785.2	Upper respiratory infection, 465.9

  1. Cystic fibrosis: sweat test is gold standard for diagnosis.
  2. Pneumonia: viral URI symptoms and coryza with low-grade fever; bacterial pneumonia; abrupt onset with high fever; *Mycobacterium pneumoniae* (insidious onset and nontoxic appearance).

    3. Asthma: pattern of symptoms, absence of fever, inspiratory wheezing, prolonged expiratory phase.

    4. Foreign body aspiration: typically in toddler; may be detected on X-ray or by bronchoscopy.

    5. Aspiration: swallowing study to determine silent or free aspiration.

    6. Chlamydial infection: manifests from 3 to 19 weeks of age, afebrile, repetitive, staccato cough with tachypnea; wheezing is rare; cervical lymphadenopathy.

    7. Immunodeficiency: systemic illness following vaccination with live virus; severe, life-threatening illness with viral infection.

    8. Congenital heart disease: accompanied by heart murmur, signs of CHF, poor feeding, poor growth.

    9. Gastroesophageal reflux.

G. Treatment.

    1. Treatment is supportive, maintaining adequate hydration, oxygenation; monitor closely for increasing respiratory distress.

       a. Management of nasal congestion and rhinitis.

       b. Use of antipyretics.

       c. Guidelines for feeding and urine output.

       d. Recognition of signs of increasing respiratory distress.

       e. Patients have a worsening of clinical symptoms with peak at day 3–4 of illness.

       f. Bronchodilators are not routinely recommended.

       g. Consider a monitored trial of bronchodilator and continue only if a clinical response is documented.

    2. Criteria for hospitalization.

       a. Age (younger more likely).

       b. Tachypnea/hypoxemia.

       c. Hydration management.

H. Follow up.

    1. Most infants improve within 4–6 days.

       a. Guidelines for parents to call healthcare provider: increased respiratory distress, poor fluid intake, or low urine output.

       b. Close outpatient follow-up by telephone or visit may be indicated.

I. Complications.

Lung disease, chronic, 518.89	Respiratory syncytial virus, 079.6
Pneumothorax, spontaneous, 512.8	Wheezing, 786.07
Respiratory failure, 518.81	

1. Acute complications.
   a. Respiratory failure, apnea: rarely secondary bacterial infection.
   b. Spontaneous pneumothorax due to air trapping, airway narrowing.
   c. Worsening of chronic lung disease.
   d. Mortality 1–5% with higher rates in high-risk groups.
2. Long-term complications.
   a. Recurrent episodes of wheezing.
   b. Infants have airway hyperreactivity and impaired pulmonary function for up to 10 years after RSV infection.

J. Education.
  1. Avoid secondhand smoke exposure.
  2. Prevention.
     a. For high-risk populations passive immunity (monoclonal antibody technology) through monthly administration of palivizumab (Synagis) from October/November through April. Check current guidelines for recommended number of doses.
     b. Good handwashing, avoidance of ill contacts during bronchiolitis season.
  3. Post-illness.
     a. Reinfection common; having RSV offers no immunity to subsequent infections.
     b. May have period of prolonged wheezing after infection.
     c. Recurrent wheezing is common, especially with URIs.
     d. Cough and other signs resolve gradually over 1–2 weeks.

III. INFLUENZA

Abdominal pain, 789	Increased retractions, 786.9
Anxiety, 300	Influenza, 487.1
Atelectasis, 518	Irritability, 799.2
Change in level of consciousness, 780.09	Myalgia, 729.1
Change in mental status, 780.99	Nausea, 787.02
Chills, 780.99	Pharyngitis, 462
Conjunctivitis, 372.3	Pneumonia, 486
Cough, 786.2	Respiratory distress, 786.09
Croup, 464.4	Respiratory rate, increased, 786.01
Cyanosis, 782.5	Restlessness, 799.2

Diffuse myalgia, 729.1	Shortness of breath, 786.05
Dyspnea, 786.09	Tachycardia, 785
Extreme fatigue, 780.79	Tachypnea, 786.06
Fever, 780.6	Upper respiratory infection, 465.9
Generalized malaise, 780.79	Vomiting, 787.03
Headache, 784	Wheezing, 786.07

A. Etiology.
   1. Influenza is a highly contagious respiratory illness caused by influenza viruses.
      a. Influenza viruses are orthomyxoviruses.
      b. Type A and B are primary pathogens, responsible for community out-breaks.
      c. Influenza A viruses are subcategorized based on surface (H) and neur-aminidase (N).
         • Subtypes include H1N1, H1N2, and H3N2.
   2. Influenza is spread by large-particle respiratory droplet.
      a. Close contact with person with influenza.
      b Direct contact with articles contaminated with nasopharyngeal secre-tions.
      c. Virus is shed 1 day prior to developing symptoms.
         • Children may shed virus several days prior to developing symp-toms and can remain infectious more than 10 days.
         • Immunocompromised persons may shed virus for weeks to months.
      d. Incubation period is 1–4 days with average of 2 days after exposure.
B. Occurrence.
   1. Peak of flu season can occur from December through March.
   2. About 1% of children require hospitalization annually.
   3. Influenza can cause URI, croup, bronchiolitis, pneumonia.
C. Clinical manifestations.
   1. Abrupt onset of fever with rigors, chills.
   2. Pharyngitis.
   3. Cough.
   4. Diffuse myalgia.
   5. Extreme fatigue, headache, and generalized malaise.
   6. Gastrointestinal symptoms: abdominal pain, nausea, vomiting.
   7. Conjunctivitis.

8. With severe disease: irritability, change in mental status.
9. Symptoms progressively worsen over 12–24 hours.
10. May present with nonspecific signs of febrile illness, limited respiratory symptoms.
D. Physical findings.
  1. High fever.
  2. Tachycardia, tachypnea.
  3. Nonproductive cough.
  4. If lower respiratory tract infected, physical findings consistent with pneumonia or bronchiolitis.
E. Diagnostic tests.
  1. Identification of virus or viral antigen in nasopharyngeal secretions.
    a. Specimens should be obtained within 72 hours of illness, due to decrease in viral shedding after that time.
    b. Specimen obtained by swab, nasal aspirate, or wash.
    c. Viral culture.
    d. Rapid diagnostic tests via fluorescent antibody staining, enzyme-linked immunoassay, or optical immunoassay.
      • Rapid tests are more sensitive on pediatric specimens than adult specimens.
      • Some tests detect both influenza A and B; some detect only one strain.
    e. Reverse transcriptase-polymerase chain reaction (RT-PCR).
  2. Diagnosis of specific flu-related complications.
  3. Chest X-ray normal or areas of atelectasis.
F. Differential diagnosis.

Bronchiolitis, 466.19
Laryngotracheobronchitis, 490
Pneumonia, 486

  1. Other lower respiratory illness (e.g., bronchiolitis, laryngotracheobronchitis, pneumonia).
G. Treatment.
  1. Encourage fluids.
  2. Antipyretics for fever (never use salicylates in children or adolescents).
  3. Monitor for complications of influenza.
  4. Antiviral therapy.
    a. Recommendations for selection of antiviral drugs are made annually: www.cdc.gov.

    b. Must be administered within 48 hours of onset of illness.

    c. Relenza (Zanamivir): administered by inhalation for treatment of influenza A and B for children ≥ 7 years of age; side effects include dizziness, runny or stuffy nose, cough, diarrhea, or headache. Can cause bronchospasm; not recommended for use in persons with underlying lung disease such as asthma.

    d. Tamiflu (Oseltamivir): administered orally (liquid for children or capsule formulation) for treatment of influenza A and B for children and adults ≥ 1 year of age; adverse effects nausea, vomiting in first 2 days of treatment. Taking Tamiflu with food can reduce these side effects.

    e. Confusion and abnormal behavior have been reported with both antiviral drugs and may be more common in children.

H. Follow up.
1. Call healthcare provider immediately if signs of respiratory distress increase.
    a. Increased respiratory rate, shortness of breath.
    b. Increased retractions.
    c. Change in level of consciousness, restlessness, or anxiety.
    d. Cyanosis.
2. Close telephone follow up for those at high risk for flu-related complications.

I. Complications.

Asthma, 493.9	Dehydration, 276.5
Bacterial pneumonia, 482.9	Diabetes, 250
Chronic heart failure, 428	Viral pneumonia, 480.9

1. Viral and bacterial pneumonia.
2. Severe illness requiring hospitalization.
3. Dehydration.
4. Worsening of chronic illness, including CHF, asthma, or diabetes.
5. Death.

J. Education.
1. Prevention.
    a. Annual intranasal vaccine (LAIV—live attenuated intranasal vaccine) is an option for healthy children and adults 2–49 years of age.
    b. Yearly influenza vaccine in fall for all children 6 months to 18 years of age with special attention to those at high risk of complications and their close contacts.

- Trivalent inactivated vaccine is administered IM and is approved for children 6 months of age or older.
- Children younger than 9 years of age require 2 doses of vaccine in the first year they received the vaccine, administered 1 month apart to produce sufficient antibody response.

    c. Good handwashing, avoidance of ill contacts during influenza outbreaks.

2. Post-illness.

    a. Treat with antiviral agents within 48 hours after onset of symptoms to reduce duration of illness.

    b. Recognize signs of severe illness requiring medical intervention including shortness of breath, dyspnea, cyanosis, change in level of consciousness.

    c. Encourage fluids to maintain adequate hydration and urine output.

    d. Acetaminophen for treatment of myalgia, headache, fever.

    e. Recurrent wheezing is common, especially with URIs.

    f. Avoid secondhand smoke exposure.

IV. BRONCHITIS

Bacterial infection, 041.9	Mycoplasmal infection, 041.81
Bronchitis, 490	Pharyngitis, 462
Bronchitis, acute, 466	Pulmonary disease, chronic, 518.89
Bronchitis, chronic, 491.9	Respiratory syncytial virus, 079.6
Chest pain, 786.5	Rhinitis, 472
Cough, 786.2	Upper respiratory infection, 465.9
Fever, 780.6	Vomiting, 787.03
Fungal infection, 117.9	Wheezing, 786.07

A. Etiology.
1. Bronchitis is a common respiratory problem of childhood characterized by cough.
2. Most commonly occurs after viral infection.
    a. Rhinovirus, RSV, influenza, parainfluenza, adenovirus, coxsackievirus, paramyxoviruses can be etiologic agent.
3. May occur with bacterial, mycoplasmal, or fungal infection.

    4. May occur as result of inflammation caused by frequent viral infection, secondhand smoke exposure, and air pollution.

    5. Chronic bronchitis is poorly defined in children.

B. Occurrence.

    1. Peak months in young children are related to high RSV activity.

    2. Peak incidence is in winter months.

    3. Chronic/recurrent bronchitis: cough lasting > 1 month or 4 episodes within 1 year.

C. Clinical manifestations.

    1. Mild URI symptoms including rhinitis and pharyngitis.

    2. Dry hacking cough begins 3–4 days after onset of rhinitis.

    3. Cough often becomes productive after a few days.

    4. Older patients may complain of chest pain, worse with coughing.

    5. As cough progressively worsens, the child has more signs of generalized illness.

    6. Younger children may have post-tussive vomiting.

    7. Normal temperature or mild elevation.

D. Physical findings.

    1. Physical findings vary with phase of illness.

    2. Initially clear or mucopurulent nasal secretions.

    3. Auscultation initially may be normal.

    4. Cough is dry, hacking in nature.

    5. Normal or slightly elevated temperature.

    6. Over next week, cough becomes productive as condition progresses to include lower respiratory symptoms.

       a. Coarse crackles with variable wheezing may be present.

       b. Moderate to severe productive cough, chest pain.

       c. Post-tussive vomiting, thick yellow mucopurulent sputum.

    7. Elevated temperature is likely during this time.

E. Diagnostic tests.

    1. Diagnosis is often diagnosis of exclusion (see "Differential Diagnosis").

    2. Assessment of general health status including height, weight, signs of chronic pulmonary disease.

    3. Elevated neutrophil count or C-reactive protein is suggestive of bacterial etiology.

    4. CXR is usually normal, but may show peribronchial thickening.

    5. RSV wash for rapid testing.

F. Differential diagnosis.

Anorexia, 783	Headache, 784
Asthma, 493.9	Heart murmur, 785.2
Bronchiectasis, 494	Immunodeficiency, 279.3
Bronchopulmonary dysplasia, 770.7	Irritability, 799.2
Chronic pulmonary disorders, other, 518.89	Poor feeding, 783
Congenital heart disease, 746.9	Poor growth, 764.9
Congestive heart failure, 428	Purulent rhinitis, 472
Digital clubbing, 781.5	Sinusitis, 473.9
Foreign body aspiration, 934.8	Wheezing, 786.07
Gastroesophageal reflux, 530.81	

1. Asthma: pattern of symptoms, absence of fever, expiratory wheezing, prolonged expiratory phase.
2. Bronchiectasis: recurrent pulmonary infections, anorexia, irritability, poor growth, digital clubbing, rule out other chronic pulmonary disorders.
3. Bronchopulmonary dysplasia: history of prematurity, treatment with oxygen therapy, and/or mechanical ventilation during neonatal period.
4. Immunodeficiency: systemic illness following vaccination with live virus; severe life-threatening illness with viral infection.
5. Gastroesophageal reflux: barium swallow demonstrates reflux of barium into esophagus; esophageal pH monitoring.
6. Congenital heart disease: accompanied by heart murmur, signs of CHF, poor feeding, poor growth.
7. Sinusitis: purulent rhinitis lasting 2 weeks, facial/dental pain, headache, pressure over affected area.
8. Foreign body aspiration: typically in toddler, unilateral physical findings, X-ray or by bronchoscopy.

G. Treatment.
1. Treatment is supportive.
2. Cough suppressants should be avoided in children with productive cough.
3. Rest as needed.
4. Avoidance of environmental irritants.

5. Empiric trial of bronchodilator therapy.
6. Acetaminophen for chest pain, fever.
7. Antibiotic therapy may be considered if bacterial infection is strongly suspected (prolonged symptoms, patient's age, high fever).
8. Humidification of air promotes comfort.
9. Chest physiotherapy may be indicated if productive cough, coarse crackles on exam.

H. Follow up.
1. If cough for 2 weeks or worsens, fever, or signs of respiratory distress: contact healthcare provider.

I. Complications.

Otitis media, chronic, 382.9

Pneumonia, 486

Sinusitis, 473.9

1. In healthy children, bronchitis is not a serious illness.
2. In chronically ill children, may develop concurrent otitis, sinusitis, pneumonia.

J. Education.
1. Avoid large daycare settings for young children to minimize frequency of viral infection.
2. Avoid secondhand smoke exposure.
3. Bronchitis is usually caused by viral infection; antibiotics are not effective.
4. Acute bronchitis is a benign, self-limited illness usually lasting 2 weeks.
5. Should consult with healthcare providers before administering cough suppressants.
6. If child has signs of respiratory distress, contact healthcare provider.
7. If cough does not resolve within 2 weeks or worsens or fever recurs, contact healthcare provider.

V. PERTUSSIS

Apnea, 770.81	Lymphocytosis, 288.8
Atelectasis, 518	Pertussis, 033.9
Choking, 784.9	Petechiae, 782.7
Cough, 786.2	Pneumonia, 486
Cough, paroxysmal, 780.2	Rhinorrhea, 478.1

Cyanosis, 782.5	Sneezing, 784.9
Exhaustion, 780.79	Subconjunctival hemorrhages, 372.72
Fever, 780.6	Upper respiratory infection, 065.9
Lacrimation, 375.2	Vomiting, 787.03
Leukocytosis, 288.8	Whooping cough, 033.9

A. Etiology.
   1. Pertussis: highly contagious, vaccine-preventable bacterial infection caused by *Bordetella pertussis,* less commonly by *B. parapertussis* (Gram-negative coccobacillus).
   2. Transmission: airborne, occurs by contact with respiratory droplets of infected person or by indirect contact with contaminated surfaces.
   3. Disease is endemic in United States, with all 50 states reporting cases annually.
   4. Most cases in United States occur between June and October.
B. Occurrence.
   1. Pertussis causes disease in every age group.
      a. Significantly impacts nonimmunized or partially immunized young children; can cause severe disease. Highest mortality in infants younger than 6 months of age.
   2. Incubation period is 7–10 days with a range of 5–21 days.
   3. Persons with pertussis are considered infectious from 7 days after exposure to 3 weeks after person enters paroxysmal stage.
      a. Pertussis is most contagious from catarrhal stage until 2 weeks after onset of cough without appropriate therapy.
C. Clinical manifestations.
   1. Pertussis is lengthy disease lasting 6–10 weeks, divided into 3 stages.
      a. Catarrhal stage lasts 1–2 weeks, may not be recognized in infants younger than 3 months.
         • Characterized by URI symptoms such as rhinorrhea, sneezing, mild cough, low-grade fever.
      b. The paroxysmal stage lasts 2–4 weeks or longer.
         • Characterized by paroxysmal cough/bouts of rapid cough, sudden coughing.
         • Have color change, bulging eyes, tearing, tongue protrusion.
         • May be triggered by feeding, crying, excitement, activity.
         • May have multiple episodes each hour during peak but appear well between episodes.
         • May have characteristic whoop during forceful inspiration.

- Post-tussive vomiting, exhaustion are common following episode.
- Infants younger than 3 months of age have apnea, choking, gasping.
    c. Convalescent stage lasts 1–2 weeks, but cough can persist for several months. During this stage, cough and post-tussive vomiting decrease.
D. Physical findings.
    1. Cough.
        a. Catarrhal stage: mild.
        b. Paroxysmal cough: associated with cyanosis, lacrimation, exhaustion, post-tussive vomiting.
        c. Subconjunctival hemorrhages and petechiae on head and neck.
    2. Breath sounds are normal, unless significant atelectasis or pneumonia.
E. Diagnostic tests.
    1. Consider in cases of prolonged cough with history of post-tussive vomiting, whoop, paroxysmal cough.
    2. Culture is "gold standard" for laboratory diagnosis.
        a. Most likely to be positive during catarrhal stage to peak of paroxysmal stage.
        b. Use calcium alginate or Dacron swab of posterior nasopharynx for 15–30 seconds or by nasal wash and plate on specialized media, incubate for 7 days.
    3. Rapid testing by nasal wash for direct fluorescent antibody (DFA) or polymerase chain reaction (PCR).
        a. Do not use calcium alginate swabs for PCR as it is inhibitory to PCR.
    4. Serology.
        a. Enzyme immunoassay detects antibody to B pertussis in acute and convalescent samples: not helpful during acute illness and difficult to interpret in immunized persons.
    5. CBC: leukocytosis with lymphocytosis in catarrhal and early paroxysmal stages.
        a. Present in infants and young children but not in adolescents.
F. Differential diagnosis.

Adenoviral infection, 079	Chlamydial infection, unspecified, 079.98
Bordetella parapertussis infection, 033.1	Cytomegalovirus, 078.5

1. Adenoviral infection: presence of fever distinguishes from pertussis.
2. *Mycoplasma* infection: causes prolonged cough but fever, systemic symptoms, crackles on auscultation help differentiate from pertussis.
3. *B. parapertussis* infection: less severe illness.
4. In infancy, consider chlamydia, cytomegalovirus (CMV).

G. Treatment.
1. Most children beyond infancy can be managed at home.
2. Macrolides are treatment of choice for infected persons and close contacts.
3. Azithromycin, erythromycin, or clarithromycin are first-line agents for treatment and prophylaxis.
   a. Do not use in young infants because of association with infantile hypertrophic pyloric stenosis (IFPS).
4. Dosing.
   a. Less than 30 days of age:
      - Azithromycin 10 mg/kg/day as single daily dose for 5 days.
      - All infants younger than 30 days of age who receive macrolides should be monitored for IFPH during and for 1 month following completion of course.
   b. 1–5 months of age.
      - Azithromycin 10 mg/kg/day as single daily dose for 5 days OR
      - Erythromycin 40–50 mg/kg/day in 4 divided doses for 14 days OR
      - Clarithromycin 15 mg/kg/day in 2 divided doses for 7 days.
   c. Infants 6 months of age or older and children.
      - Azithromycin 10 mg/kg/day as single daily dose on day 1 (maximum dose 500 mg), then 5 mg/kg/day (maximum dose 250 mg) on days 2–5 OR
      - Erythromycin 40–50 mg/kg/day in 4 divided doses for 14 days OR
      - Clarithromycin 15 mg/kg/day in 2 divided doses for 7 days.
   d. Adults.
      - Azithromycin 500 mg as single daily dose on day 1, then 250 mg on days 2–5 OR
      - Erythromycin 2 g/day in 4 divided doses for 14 days OR
      - Clarithromycin 1 g/day in 2 divided doses for 7 days.
5. Alternatively use trimethoprim-sulfamethoxazole (TMP-SMX), 8–12 mg/kg/day divided every 12 hours for 14 days, if unable to take macrolides or culture resistant to macrolides.
6. Those with pertussis should be considered contagious until treatment with appropriate therapy for 5 days.

7. Treat all household and close contacts including daycare and school regardless of age, immunization status, symptoms.
8. In addition to chemoprophylaxis, for children younger than 7 years of age who are not immunized or partially immunized, follow schedule for accelerated vaccination.
9. Reportable disease to local and state health departments.

H. Follow up.

1. Guidelines for parents to call healthcare provider for poor fluid intake, low urine output, change in level of consciousness, cyanosis, or respiratory distress.
2. Close outpatient follow up by telephone to monitor and reassure family.

I. Complications.

Apnea, 770.81	Fluid and electrolyte imbalances, 276.9
Bacterial pneumonia, 482.9	Otitis media, 382.9
Conjunctival hemorrhage, 372.72	Petechiae, 782.7
Encephalopathy, 348.3	Seizures, 780.39
Epistaxis, 784.7	Viral pneumonia, 480.9

1. Infants younger than 6 months of age have highest rate of hospitalization, secondary pneumonia, and seizures.
2. Children with history of prematurity or underlying chronic heart, pulmonary, or neurologic disease are at high risk for severe disease.
3. Apnea.
4. Secondary infection causing viral or bacterial pneumonia or otitis media.
   a. Secondary bacterial pneumonia causes most pertussis-related deaths.
5. Neurologic complications include encephalopathy and seizures.
6. Sequelae of violent coughing including conjunctival hemorrhage, CNS hemorrhage, pneumothorax, epistaxis, petechiae.
7. Fluid and electrolyte imbalances.
8. Death: Infants younger than 1 year of age are at highest risk.

J. Education.

1. Very contagious and spread by direct or indirect contact with respiratory droplets.
2. Good handwashing, containment of coughs/sneezes prevents spread of illness.
3. Guidelines about adequate hydration and nutrition.
4. Children may continue to have cough for several months.
5. Provide adequate rest and avoid activity that triggers cough.

6. Need for antibiotic treatment of all household and close contacts.
7. Household and close contacts are considered contagious until completed 5 days of erythromycin therapy.
8. Need for accelerated immunization for contacts younger than 7 years of age partially immunized/not immunized.
9. Avoid secondhand smoke exposure.

VI. ASTHMA

Airflow obstruction, episodic, 519.8	Family history of eczema, dermatitis, V19.4
Allergens, inhalant, 477.9	Fatigue, 780.79
Allergens, outdoor, 477.9	Itching, 698.9
Animal allergens, house-dust mites, cockroach allergens, molds, 477.8	Mucosal swelling, 784.2
	Nasal polyps, 471.9
Asthma, 493.9	Otitis, 382.9
Bronchiolitis, recurrent, 466.19	Pneumonia, 486
Bronchitis, allergic, 493.9	Rhinitis, 472
Chest pain, 786.5	Rhinorrhea, clear, 478.1
Chest tightness, 786.59	Shortness of breath, 786.05
Conjunctivitis, 372.3	Sinusitis, 473.9
Cough, 786.2	Sleep disturbances, 780.5
Eczema, 691.8	Sneezing, 784.9
Family history of allergy, V19.6	Upper respiratory infection, 465.9
Family history of asthma, V17.5	Wheezing, 786.07

A. Etiology.
  1. Asthma is chronic inflammatory disorder of airways in which many cells and cellular elements play a role.
     a. Mast cells, eosinophils, T-lymphocytes, neutrophils.
  2. May have genetic predisposition (with critical interaction with environment).
  3. The characteristics of asthma are:
     a. Symptoms of episodic airflow obstruction that is reversible.
     b. Airway inflammation.
     c. Increased airway responsiveness to variety of stimuli.

    4. Hyperresponsiveness.
      a. Chronically inflamed airways are hyperresponsive.
      b. When exposed to "triggers," there is bronchoconstriction and airflow limitation.
      c. Inflammation contributes to airway edema and increased mucous production.
      d. Cough and wheeze are characteristic of asthma but are also common nonspecific symptoms associated with many other clinical entities.
    5. Common triggers.
      a. Inhalant allergens: animal allergens, house dust mites, cockroach allergens, molds, outdoor allergens.
      b. Irritants: active/passive tobacco smoke exposure, indoor and outdoor air pollution, strong odors, chemical cleaning products.
      c. Viral illness.
        • URI, sinusitis, rhinitis, otitis, lower respiratory infection.
        • Viral illness is primary trigger for asthma in young children.
      d. Weather: rapid change in weather; hot, humid weather; or cold air.
      e. Exercise.
      f. Emotions or stress.
      g. Occupational exposures: farm and barn exposures, formaldehydes, paint fumes, smoke, strong odors.
      h. Aspirin sensitivity (more common in adults): includes other NSAIDs.
      i. Sulfite sensitivity: in many processed foods, dried fruit, salad bars, beer, wine.
      j. Risk factors.
        • Atopy: family history or eczema.
        • Gender: preadolescent boys are at higher risk.
        • Smoking: history of mother smoking perinatally.
        • Respiratory viral disease.
      k. Aggravating factors: smoking, gastroesophageal reflux, sinusitis.
  B. Occurrence.
    1. Most common serious chronic illness among children.
    2. Onset at any age from infancy to old age; 50–80% of children with asthma develop symptoms before 5 years of age.
  C. Clinical manifestations.
    1. Recurrent wheezing.
    2. Dry, persistent cough, nocturnal cough.
    3. Recurrent chest tightness or shortness of breath, chest pain.
    4. Sputum production.
    5. Exercise-induced cough, wheezing, shortness of breath, or chest tightness.

6. In younger children, difficulty keeping up with peers.
7. Atopic profile.
   a. Eczema.
   b. Seasonal or perennial allergy symptoms.
   c. Rhinitis, sneezing, itching and rubbing of nose, throat clearing.
   d. Conjunctivitis.
8. Fatigue secondary to sleep disturbance.
9. Poor school performance secondary to sleep disturbance.

D. Physical findings.
   1. Upper respiratory tract.
      a. Allergic shiners, "allergic salute" (characteristic crease at bridge of nose due to chronic rhinitis).
      b. Conjunctivitis.
      c. Boggy, pale nasal mucosa, mucosal swelling, clear rhinorrhea, nasal polyps, nasal flaring.
      d. Grunting.
   2. Chest exam.
      a. Normal chest examination does not rule out asthma.
      b. Bilateral wheezing, end-expiratory wheezing on forced expiration.
      c. Prolonged expiratory phase; rapid, shallow respirations.
      d. Hyperresonance to percussion.
      e. Hyperexpansion of chest, increased anterior–posterior diameter.
      f. Intercostal, suprasternal, and/or subcostal retractions.
      g. In infants, paradoxical breathing.
      h. In young children, pushing with abdominal musculature on expiration.
      i. Dry, tight-sounding cough.

E. Diagnostic tests.
   1. Detailed medical history.
      a. Family history of allergy, asthma, eczema, dermatitis.
      b. Identify symptoms consistent with asthma.
      c. Identify pattern of symptoms that occur or worsen in presence of specific triggers.
         • Consider diagnosis after 3 episodes of cough and/or wheezing, once alternative diagnoses are excluded.
   2. Focused physical examination with special attention on the upper respiratory tract, chest, and skin.
   3. Laboratory procedures.
      a. Spirometry.
         • Age limited; difficult to accurately test children younger than 5–7 years of age in most settings.

- Pre- and postbronchodilator to validate reversibility.
  i. May be normal.
  ii. Essential for diagnosis.
  iii. Test annually to establish baseline pulmonary function.
  b. Peak flow is monitoring tool, not diagnostic tool.
4. Chest X-ray: important in newly diagnosed asthmatic, rules out alternative diagnoses.
5. Special studies.
  a. Sinus X-rays or CT to evaluate sinusitis.
  b. pH probe or barium swallow to evaluate gastroesophageal reflux (GER).
  c. Allergy testing.
    - Referral to board-certified allergist to administer skin tests and interpret.
    - RAST testing: not as sensitive as skin testing, results not immediate.
    - Allergic bronchitis, wheezy bronchitis.
    - Recurrent bronchiolitis or pneumonia.
      i. Even children with mild persistent asthma have significant airway inflammation.
      ii. Without adequate anti-inflammatory therapy, there may be airway remodeling or irreversible changes in asthma airway.
6. Asthma classification.
  a. Severity: intrinsic to the disease process.
    - First step in initiating therapy for patient who has not been taking long-term controller medication.
  b. Control: fluctuates over time.
  c. Impairment: assessment component for severity and control; effect of asthma on quality of life and functional capacity.
  d. Risk: assessment component for severity and control; refers to future impact on quality of life and functional capacity.
  e. Four categories: intermittent, mild persistent, moderate persistent, and severe persistent.
    - Symptoms > 2 times per week, nighttime symptoms > 2 times a month.
    - Asymptomatic and normal peak flow between exacerbations.
    - Exacerbations brief; intensity may vary.
    - May have severe or lethal episodes.
  f. Mild persistent asthma.
    - Symptoms 2 times per week but less than daily. Nighttime symptoms 2 times a month.

- Exacerbations may affect activity.
- Nighttime symptoms 2 times per month.
- g. Moderate persistent asthma.
  - Daily symptoms, daily use of inhaled quick-relief bronchodilators.
  - Nighttime symptoms 1 time a week.
  - Exacerbations affect activity, occur 2 times per week; may last days.
- h. Severe persistent.
  - Continual symptoms; frequent exacerbations, nighttime symptoms.
  - Limited physical activity.
F. Differential diagnosis.

Bronchiolitis, viral, 466.19	Malabsorption, 579.9
Bronchopulmonary dysplasia, 770.7	Poor growth, 764.9
Cystic fibrosis, 277	Pulmonary infection, chronic, 518.89
Foreign body aspiration, 934.8	Tracheoesophageal fistula, 530.84
Gastroesophageal reflux, 530.81	

1. Vocal cord dysfunction: paradoxical adduction of vocal cords during inspiration (often in adolescent girls). Symptoms of distress including inspiratory wheezing and are out of proportion to clinical exam, including normal oxygen saturations. Diagnosis established by direct visualization of vocal cords using flexible rhinolaryngoscopy or flexible laryngoscopy.
2. Congenital pulmonary malformations: radiologic testing, bronchoscopy to rule out abnormality.
   a. Tracheoesophageal fistula.
   b. Vascular ring, sling, or extrinsic mass.
3. Foreign body aspiration: focal findings on auscultation; medical history key.
4. Bronchopulmonary dysplasia: history of prematurity, treatment with oxygen therapy, mechanical ventilation during neonatal period.
5. Viral bronchiolitis: virus may be identified by antigen testing or culture; may be trigger for asthma. Asthma differentiated by pattern of symptoms over time.
6. Gastroesophageal reflux: reflux of barium into esophagus by barium swallow or esophageal pH monitoring. Can be aggravating factor in asthma control.
7. Cystic fibrosis: genetic disease characterized by excessive production of thick, tenacious respiratory secretions, chronic pulmonary infection, malabsorption, subsequent poor growth.

G. Treatment.
   1. Goals of treatment.
      a. No coughing, shortness of breath/rapid breathing, wheezing, chest tightness.
      b. No waking up at night because of asthma symptoms.
      c. Normal activities including play, sports, exercise.
      d. No absences from school or activities or work (for parent or caregiver).
      e. Normal lung function.
   2. Key principles.
      a. Prevent airway inflammation by eliminating or avoiding triggers.
      b. Asthma can be controlled, not cured.
      c. Reverse and suppress inflammation.
   3. Nonpharmacologic therapy.
      a. Patient education.
      b. Objective measures of lung function using peak flow monitoring and follow-up spirometry.
      c. Control or avoid aggravating factors.
   4. Pharmacologic therapy.
      a. Simplify treatment plan whenever possible.
      b. Classification of severity guides choice and frequency of therapy.
      c. Persistent asthma is most effectively controlled with daily anti-inflammatory medications.
      d. National Asthma Education and Prevention guidelines support aggressive therapy to achieve rapid control of symptoms and then step down to lowest level of therapy to maintain control.
      e. Goals in treatment of acute episode are:
         • Rapid reversal of acute airway obstruction.
         • Identify causes of asthma episode.
         • Adjust chronic maintenance to prevent recurrence of asthma flare.
         • Inhaled beta2-agonist is quick-relief medication for all levels of severity and treatment of choice for prevention of exercise-induced asthma.
         • Short "burst" of oral glucocorticoids is used to reduce inflammation during acute episode.
   5. Build child/family and healthcare provider partnership.
      a. Understand and address reasons for adherence problems in asthma.
      b. Explore patient/family misconceptions about asthma.
      c. Agree on goals and expectations of treatment.
      d. Jointly develop treatment plan.

H. Follow up.
   1. Before increasing medications, investigate reasons for poor asthma control.
      a. Improper inhaler technique.
      b. Adherence issues, knowledge deficit.
      c. Environmental exposures.
      d. Exacerbation of aggravating conditions (e.g., GER, sinusitis).
   2. Many children have multiple caretakers.
      a. Each caretaker must have access to medications, appropriate devices, asthma action plan.
      b. Provide information to all caregivers including daycare providers, teachers, coaches, school nurses.
      c. Ensure reliable, immediate access to medications in all settings including school.
   3. Regular use of quick-relief medicine indicates deterioration in control of asthma and need to assess maintenance therapy.
   4. Regular follow-up visits are encouraged to achieve and maintain control with appropriate intensity of therapy.
   5. Monitor child for side effects of medications.
   6. Refer to asthma specialist for difficult-to-control asthma in children older than 5 years of age: consider at step 3; refer at step 4. (See **Figures 24-5 through 24-8**).
   7. For children younger than 5 years of age: consider referral at step 2; refer at steps 3 and 4. (See **Figures 24-5 through 24-8**).
   8. Peak flow monitoring to establish personal best: more specific than predicted value.
   9. At each encounter, reassess concerns and correct misconceptions.
   10. Monitor quality of life on regular basis.
   11. Recognize and address barriers to asthma self-management.
   12. Assess source of social support for child and family.
   13. Assess child and family satisfaction with asthma care.
   14. Yearly influenza vaccine for child and household contacts.
I. Complications.

Pneumonia, 486

Pneumothorax, 512.8

---

   1. Pneumothorax, pneumonia.
   2. Acute exacerbation requiring hospitalization, intubation, mechanical ventilation.
   3. Death.

J. Education.
1. Asthma education should begin at diagnosis and continue at every encounter: include child as developmentally appropriate and all caregivers.
2. Key components.
   a. Basic asthma facts to enable child and family to understand rationale for treatment decisions and asthma self-management.
   b. Roles of medications in treating acute symptoms and achieving/maintaining asthma control.
   c. Environmental avoidance and control measures.
   d. Teach relevant skills: how to use devices such as spacers, other medication-delivery devices, peak-flow meter; have child demonstrate relevant skills at each encounter.
   e. Provide asthma action plan: daily maintenance therapy including avoidance of triggers, plan for recognizing and treating worsening asthma, and when to seek medical attention.
3. Establish goals of therapy jointly and monitor child and family's perception of progress toward reaching goals.

VII. PNEUMONIA

Abdominal distention, 787.3	Pleural effusion, 511.9
Anorexia, 783	Pleuritic pain, 786.52
Arthritic symptoms, transient, 716.4	Pneumonia, 486
Arthropathy, 716.9	Pneumonia, bacterial, 482.9
Cervical lymphadenopathy, 785.6	Pneumonia, bronchopneumonia, 485
Conjunctivitis, unilateral, 372.3	Pneumonia, interstitial, 516.8
Coryza, 460	Pneumonia, lobar, 481
Cough, 786.2	Pneumonia, mycoplasma, 483
Cyanosis, 782.5	Pneumonia, *Staphylococcus aureus*, 482.41
Dehydration, 276.5	Pneumonia, viral, 480.9
Diarrhea, 787.9	Respiratory distress, 786.09
Drowsiness, 780.09	Respiratory syncytial virus, 079.6
Dyspnea, 786.09	Restlessness, 799.2
Ear pain, 388.7	Retractions, substernal, 738.3

Empyema, 510.9

Fever, 780.6

Headache, 784

Hoarseness, 784.49

Hypoxemia, 799

Lethargy, 780.79

Leukocytosis, 288.8

Malaise, 780.79

Meningismus, 781.6

Mycoplasma pneumoniae, 483

Nasal congestion, 478.1

Nausea, 787.02

Nuchal rigidity, 781.6

Otitis media, 382.9

Parainfluenza infection, 480.2

Retractions, suprasternal, 738.8

Rhinitis, 472

Rigors, 780.99

Seizure, 780.39

Sneezes, 7884.9

Sore throat, 462

Staphylococcus pneumoniae, 482.3

Tachycardia, 785

Tachypnea, 786.06

Tactile fremitus, 785.3

Upper respiratory infection, 465.9

Urticaria, 708.9

Vomiting, 787.03

Wheezing, 786.07

A. Etiology.
1. Pneumonia is inflammation and infection of lung parenchyma due to infectious pathogens.
2. It represents wide spectrum of signs/symptoms and disease severity.
3. Pathogens vary depending on age of patient.
4. Classification.
   a. By pathogen (bacterial, including mycoplasma or viral).
   b. By anatomic location: lobar, interstitial, bronchopneumonia.
5. Common viral pathogens.
   a. RSV; adenovirus; parainfluenza 1, 2, 3; influenza A and B; rhinovirus.
   b. Transmission: highly contagious.
      • Transmitted by direct contact with nasopharyngeal secretions from infected person.
      • Pneumonia results from spread of infection along airways.
         i. Causes direct injury to respiratory epithelium, resulting in airway obstruction, abnormal secretion and necrotic debris in airway lumen and lymphocytic infiltrations of interstitium and lung parenchyma.
         ii. Small airways are obstructed, resulting in poor oxygenation and air trapping, which leads to ventilation and perfusion mismatch.

6. Common bacterial pathogens.
   a. *Streptococcus pneumoniae, Mycoplasma pneumoniae, Streptococcus* (group A) *pyogenes, Staphylococcus aureus.*
   b. Transmission: contagious.
      • Bacterial pathogens may be aspirated or inhaled, rarely by hematogenous spread.
      • Transmitted via person-to-person contact by large droplet aerosolization during coughing/sneezing.
      • Viral infection damages host's normal airway defense mechanisms, facilitating secondary bacterial infection.
   c. *S. pneumoniae.*
      • Many have *S. pneumoniae* colonization in upper respiratory tract.
      • Gram-positive encapsulated diplococci produce local edema.
         i. Organism is distributed into adjacent areas of lung, resulting in typical focal lobar consolidation.
         ii. More than 90 serotypes exist.
   d. *S. aureus.*
      • Gram-positive organism; beta-lactamase producer.
      • Produces exoproducts, enzymes, toxins, which contribute to virulence of this organism.
      • Causes confluent bronchopneumonia; often unilateral with areas of hemorrhagic necrosis, cavitation of lung parenchyma, resulting in formation of pneumatocele, empyema, or bronchopulmonary fistula.
   e. *M. pneumoniae.*
      • Smallest self-replicating bacterium; lacks cell wall, dependent on host.
      • Binds to ciliated respiratory epithelium and inhibits ciliary action.
      • Airways and areas surrounding are filled with infiltrates.
      • Causes cellular destruction and inflammatory response.
B. Occurrence.
   1. Acute childhood respiratory infections result in 4.5 million deaths/year.
      a. 70% are pneumonia-related deaths.
      b. Bacterial pneumonia less common than viral pneumonia, but has highest mortality.
   2. Viral pneumonia.
      a. Peak attack rate between 2–3 years of life.
      b. More common in fall and winter.
         • Fall: parainfluenza infection causing croup.
         • Winter: RSV and influenza.

- Viral pneumonia can be complicated by secondary bacterial infection.

3. Bacterial pneumonia.
   a. More common in children older than 5 years of age.
   b. Occurs in winter to early spring.
   c. Organisms vary according to age of child.
      - *S. pneumoniae.*
        i. Children younger than 4 years of age at highest risk.
        ii. Risks factors: male > female, daycare attendance, frequent otitis media (3 times in 6 months), frequent URIs (3 infections in 6 months), prematurity, and previous hospitalization for respiratory disease.
        iii. Incubation period varies by serotype but generally short: 1–3 days.
      - *M. pneumoniae.*
        i. Leading cause of pneumonia in school-age children, adolescents.
        ii. Occurs year round. Incubation period: 2–3 weeks (range: 1–4 weeks).
        iii. Rarely severe enough to warrant hospitalization.
      - *S. aureus:* children younger than 2 years of age at highest risk.

C. Clinical manifestations.
   1. Viral pneumonia: symptoms variable depending on age.
      a. Onset may be acute or gradual but typically progresses more slowly than bacterial infection.
      b. Nasal congestion and coryza.
      c. Lower respiratory symptoms develop insidiously.
      d. Temperature variable depending on causative agent.
      e. Nontoxic appearing.
      f. History of URI symptoms, rhinitis, cough.
      g. Hoarseness, wheezing, rapid/shallow respirations.
   2. Bacterial pneumonia.
      a. *S. pneumoniae.*
         - Infants initially.
           i. Mild URI symptoms, unilateral conjunctivitis or OM.
           ii. Abrupt onset of fever to 104ºF. May have seizure due to abrupt spike in temperature.
           iii. Mild cough; may have diarrhea, vomiting.
         - Infant progress.
           i. Restlessness, apprehension.

          ii. Nasal flaring; rapid, shallow respiration; grunting.

          iii. Abdominal distention.

          iv. Cough may be absent.

          v. Circumoral cyanosis.

        • Older children and adolescents.

          i. Onset abrupt with rigors followed by temperature 102–104°F.

          ii. Appears ill.

          iii. Headache.

          iv. Anorexia, nausea, vomiting, diarrhea, abdominal pain.

          v. Dyspnea, pleuritic pain, and cough; cough may be productive.

          vi. Alternating restlessness and drowsiness.

   3. *M. pneumoniae.*

     a. Slow onset.

     b. Malaise, transient arthritic symptoms.

     c. Persistent dry, hacking cough; sore throat often followed by hoarseness.

     d. Low-grade temperature and chills.

     e. May have ear pain.

D. Physical findings.

   1. Viral pneumonia: symptoms dependent on causative agent and age of child.

     a. Nontoxic appearing.

     b. Tachypnea, cough, diffuse bilateral wheezing, decreased breath sounds throughout lung fields.

     c. Suprasternal, intercostal, substernal retractions.

     d. Cyanosis.

   2. Bacterial pneumonia.

     a. *S. pneumoniae.*

       • Infants.

         i. Tachypnea; nasal flaring, grunting, retractions; diminished breath sounds; crackles, wheezing.

         ii. Fever.

         iii. Tachycardia.

         iv. Palpable liver or spleen secondary to abdominal distention.

         v. Air hunger and cyanosis.

       • Older children and adolescents.

         i. Diminished breath sounds over affected area of lung.

         ii. Dullness to percussion over area of consolidation.

         iii. Increased tactile fremitus over area of consolidation.

      iv. Cough productive of bloody or rust-tinged sputum.

      v. Crackles, wheezing, splinting of respirations on affected side.

      vi. Fever.

      vii. Nuchal rigidity and other signs of meningeus may be present if upper lobes are involved.

      viii. Drowsiness, restlessness.

      ix. Respiratory distress and hypoxemia are variable or mild without widespread disease or pleural effusion.

   3. *M. pneumoniae.*

      a. Fever.

      b. Diminished breath sounds; coarse, harsh breath sounds.

      c. May have macular rash, erythematous macular rash, urticaria.

      d. Cervical lymphadenopathy.

      e. Conjunctivitis, otitis media.

      f. Arthropathy.

E. Diagnostic tests.

   1. Viral pneumonia.

      a. Definitive diagnosis: viral isolation/viral antigens in respiratory tract infection.

      b. CXR: typically shows bilateral, diffuse infiltrates.

      c. WBC: normal or leukocytosis (not usually 20,000) with lymphocytosis.

   2. Bacterial pneumonia.

      a. No "gold standard" definitive test.

      b. Blood cultures are positive for the causative agent only about 10% of the time.

      c. WBC: leukocytosis (15,000–40,000) with granulocytosis.

      d. CXR.

- *S. pneumoniae:* lobar consolidation; typically single focus but may be multiple foci; "spherical" infiltrate or round pneumonia; right lobes are preferentially affected.
- *S. aureus:* bronchopneumonia (multiple, central segmental infiltrates become confluent and diffuse); these infiltrates lead to necrosis, cavitation, pneumatoceles, and abscess formation.

   3. *M. pneumoniae.*

      a. Clinical manifestation and physical exam are essential to diagnosis.

- Insidious onset, nontoxic.
- Child older than 5 years of age.
- Low-grade fever.

b. *M. pneumoniae* detected by polymerase chain reaction (PCR) technology.

c. Cold agglutinins (during acute phase) with titer 1:64 or greater are predictive of *M. pneumoniae.*

d. WBC: normal.

F. Differential diagnosis.

Aspirations, 934.8	Foreign body aspiration, 934.8
Asthma, 493.9	*Mycoplasma pneumoniae,* 483
Bronchiolitis, 466.49	Pneumonia, viral, 480.9
Coryza, 460	Tracheoesophageal fistula, 530.84
Cystic fibrosis, 277	Upper respiratory infection, 465.9
Fever, 780.6	

1. Viral pneumonia: URI symptoms and coryza with low-grade fever; bacterial pneumonia: abrupt onset with high fever; *M. pneumoniae:* insidious onset and nontoxic appearance.
2. Foreign body aspiration: may be detected on X-ray or by bronchoscopy.
3. Cystic fibrosis: sweat test is definitive diagnostic test.
4. Asthma: pattern of symptoms, absence of fever; inspiratory wheezing; prolonged expiratory phase.
5. Aspiration: swallowing study to determine silent or free aspiration.
6. Tracheoesophageal fistula: gas-filled bowel on X-ray in an infant with respiratory problems and drooling at birth.
7. Bronchiolitis: rapid testing for viral antigen.
8. Right lower lobe pneumonia can present as GI process; X-ray can differentiate.
9. Right upper lobe pneumonia can present as meningitis, severity of illness, lumbar puncture.

G. Treatment.
   1. Viral pneumonia.
      a. Supportive care; typically mild illness and can be managed at home; young infant at risk for respiratory fatigue and more severe symptoms.
   2. Bacterial pneumonia.
      a. Dependent on bacteria; dependent on condition of child (oxygenation, hydration status, age: infants younger than 4–6 months are usually hospitalized).
      b. Acetaminophen for fever and chest pain.
      c. Antibiotic treatment is generally 7–10 days.

      d. Amoxicillin is outpatient drug of choice; alternative choices are clarithromycin for children 6 weeks to 4 years of age; erythromycin for children older than 4 years of age.

      e. With high level of penicillin-resistant pneumococci present in community, consider cefuroxime, amoxicillin-clavulanate (Augmentin), or azithromycin.

  3. *M. pneumoniae.*

      a. Usually mild disease that can be managed at home.

      b. Erythromycin is drug of choice.

      c. Antibiotic treatment is generally 7–10 days.

      d. Acetaminophen for fever.

H. Follow up.

  1. Follow-up X-ray not needed in most cases of community-acquired pneumonia.

      a. Exceptions include severe illness requiring hospitalization, complications such as abscess, empyema, pleural effusion.

      b. May take up to 6 weeks for significant improvement.

  2. Daily contact with healthcare provider may be indicated with more serious illness, in children with underlying conditions, and in very young children.

  3. Recheck child if no improvement after 48 hours of treatment or if worsening occurs.

  4. Follow-up visit at 10–14 days; occasional relapse may occur.

I. Complications.

Empyema, 510.9	Pleural effusion, 511.9
Encephalopathy, 248.3	Pulmonary abscess, 513
Guillain-Barré syndrome, 357	*Staphylococcus aureus,* 041.11
Meningoencephalitis, 323.9	Stevens-Johnson syndrome, 695.1
Mycoplasma pneumoniae, 483	Toxic shock syndrome, 040.82
Pericarditis, 423.9	Transverse myelitis, 323.9

  1. Severe disease requiring hospitalization and ventilatory support.

  2. Empyema, pulmonary abscess, pleural effusion, pericarditis.

  3. *S. aureus:* toxic shock syndrome.

  4. *M. pneumoniae:* Stevens-Johnson syndrome, transverse myelitis, meningoencephalitis, encephalopathy, Guillain-Barré syndrome.

J. Education.

  1. Immunizations are essential to decrease individual morbidity and mortality associated with pneumonia but also to reduce incidence in community.

2. Understand symptoms that warrant immediate attention (lethargy, seizure, severe respiratory distress) and symptoms that require follow up (no improvement 48 hours after starting antibiotics, worsening of respiratory symptoms, signs of dehydration).

Figure 24-1 Assessing asthma control and adjusting therapy in children 0–4 years of age.

Components of Control		Classification of Asthma Control (0–4 years of age)		
		Well Controlled	**Not Well Controlled**	**Very poorly Controlled**
Impairment	Symptoms	≤ 2 days/week	> 2 days/week	Throughout the day
	Nighttime awakenings	≤ 1x/month	> 1x/month	> 1x/week
	Interference with normal activity	None	Some limitation	Extremely limited
	Short-acting beta₂-agonist use for symptom control (not prevention ot EIB)	≤ 2 days/week	> 2 days/week	Several times per day
Risk	Exacerbations requiring oral systemic corticosteroids	0–1/year	2–3/year	> 3/year
	Treatment-related adverse effects	Medication side effects can vary in intensity from none to very troublesome and worrisome. The level of intensity does not correlate to specific of control but should be considered in the overall assessment of risk.		
Recommended Action for Treatment		• Maintain current treatment. • Regular follow up every 1–6 months. • Consider step down if well controlled for at least 3 months.	• Step up (1 step) and • Reevaluate in 2–6 weeks. • If no clear benefit in 4–6 weeks, consider alternative diagnosis or adjusting therapy. • For side effects, consider alternative treatment options.	• Consider short course of oral systemic corticosteroids, • Step up (1–2 steps), and • Reevaluate in 2 weeks. • If no clear benefit in 4–6 weeks, consider alernative diagnosis or adjusting therapy. • For side effects, consider alternative treatment options.

Key: EIB, exercise-induced bronchospasm.

Notes :

■ The stepwise approach is meant to assist, not replace, the clinical decision making required to meet individual patient needs.

■ The level of control is based on the most severe impairment or risk category. Assess impairment domain by caregiver's recall of previous 2–4 weeks. Symptom assessment for longer periods should reflect a global assessment such as inquiring whether the patient's asthma is better or worse since the last visit.

■ At present, there are inadequate data to correspond frequencies of exacerbations with different levels of asthma control. In general, more frequent and intense exacerbations (i.e., requiring urgent, unscheduled care, hospitalization, or ICU admission) indicate poorer disease control. For treatment purposes, patients who had ≥ 2 exacerbations requiring oral systemic corticosteroids in the past year may be considered the same as patients who have not-well-controlled asthma, even in the absence of impairment levels consistent with not-well-contolled asthma.

■ Before step up in therepy:

— Review adherence to medications, inhaler technique, and environmental control.

— If alternative treatment option was used in a step, discontinue it and use preferred treatment for that step.

3. Need to give antibiotic as prescribed for full course.
4. Careful handwashing, containment of coughs/sneezes reduces spread of disease.
5. *M. pneumoniae:* common for close household contacts to develop illness.

Figure 24-2 Assessing asthma control and adjusting therapy in children 5–11 years of age.

Components of Control		Classification of Asthma Control (5–11 years of age)		
		Well Controlled	Not Well Controlled	Very Poorly Controlled
Impairment	Symptoms	≤ 2 days/week but not more than once on each day	> 2 days/week or multiple times on ≤ 2 days/week	Throughout the day
	Nighttime awakenings	≤ 1x/month	≥ 2x/month	≥ 2x/week
	Interference with normal activity	None	Some limitation	Extremely limited
	Short-acting beta$_2$-agonist use for symptom control (not prevention of EIB)	≤ 2 days/week	> 2 days/week	Several times per day
	Lung function • FEV$_1$ or peak flow • FEV$_1$/FVC	> 80% predicted/personal best > 80%	60–80% predicted/personal best 75–80%	< 60% predicted/personal best < 75%
Risk	Exacerbations requiring oral systemic corticosteroids	0–1/year	≥ 2/year (see note)	
		Consider severity and interval since last exacerbation		
	Reduction in lung growth	Evaluation requires long–term follow up.		
	Treatment-related adverse effects	Medication side effects can vary in intensity from none to very troublesome and worrisome. The level of intensity does not correlate to specific levels of control but should be considered in the overall assessment of risk.		
Recommended Action for Treatment		• Maintain current step. • Regular follow up every 1–6 months. • Consider step down if well controlled for at least 3 months.	• Step up at least 1 step and • Reevaluate in 2–6 weeks. • For side effects consider alternative treatment options.	• Consider short course of oral systemic corticosteroids, • Step up (1–2 steps), and • Reevaluate in 2 weeks. • For side effects, consider alternative treatment options.

Key: EIB, exercise-induced bronchospasm; FEV$_1$, forced expiratory volume in 1 second; FVC, forced vital capacity.

Notes :

■ The stepwise approach is meant to assist, not replace, the clinical decision making required to meet individual patient needs.

■ The level of control is based on the most severe impairment or risk category. Assess impairment domain by patient's/caregiver's recall of previous 2–4 weeks and spirometry/or peak flow measures. Symptom assessment for longer periods should reflect a global assessment such as inquiring whether the patient's asthma is better or worse since the last visit.

■ At present, there are inadequate data to correspond frequencies of exacerbations with different levels of asthma control. In general, more frequent and intense exacerbations (i.e., requiring urgent, unscheduled care, hospitalization, or ICU admission) indicate poorer disease control. For treatment purposes, patients who had ≥ 2 exacerbations requiring oral systemic corticosteroids in the past year may be considered the same as patients who have persistent asthma, even in the absence of impairment levels consistent with persistent asthma.

■ Before step up in therepy:

— Review adherence to medications, inhaler technique, and environmental control, and comorbid conditions.

— If alternative treatment option was used in a step, discontinue it and use prefferred treatment for that step.

Figure 24-3 Assessing asthma control and adjusting therapy in youths ≥ 12 years of age and adults.

Components of Control		Classification of Asthma Control (≥ 12 years of age)		
		Well Controlled	**Not Well Controlled**	**Very Poorly Controlled**
Impairment	Symptoms	≤ 2 days/week	> 2 days/week	Throughout the day
	Nighttime awakenings	≤ 2x/month	1–3x/week	≥ 4x/week
	Interference with normal activity	None	Some limitation	Extremely limited
	Short-acting beta$_2$-agonist use for symptom control (not prevention of EIB)	≤ 2 days/week	> 2 days/week	Several times per day
	FEV$_1$ or peak flow	> 80% predicted/ personal best	60–80% predicted/ personal best	< 60% predicted/ personal best

	Validated questionnaires
	  ATAQ
	  ACQ
	  ACT
		0
		≤ 0.75*
		≥ 20
			1–2
			≥ 1.5
			16–19
				3–4
				N/A
				≤ 15

Risk	Exacerbations requiring oral systemic corticosteroids	0–1/year	≥ 2/year (see note)	
		Consider severity and interval since last exacerbation		
	Progressive loss of lung function	Evaluation requires long-term follow up care		
	Treatment-related adverse effects	Medication side effects can vary in intensity from none to very troublesome and worrisome. The level of intensity does not correlate to specific levels of control but should be considered in the overall assessment of risk.		
Recommended Action for Treatment		• Maintain current step. • Regular followups every 1–6 months to maintain control. • Consider step down if well controlled for at least 3 months.	• Step up 1 step and • Reevaluate in 2–6 weeks. • For side effects consider alternative treatment options.	• Consider short course of oral systemic corticosteroids. • Step up 1-2 steps, and • Reevaluate in 2 weeks. • For side effects, consider alternative treatment options.

*ACQ values of 0.76–1.4 are inderminate regarding well-controlled asthma.
Key: EIB, exercise-induced bronchospasm; ICU, intensive care unit

Notes :

■ The stepwise approach is meant to assist, not replace, the clinical decision making required to meet individual patient needs.

■ The level of control is based on the most severe impairment or risk category. Assess impairment domain by patient's recall of previous 2–4 weeks and by spirometry/or peak flow measures. Symptom assessment for longer periods should reflect a global assessment, such as inquiring whether the patient's asthma is better or worse since the last visit.

■ At present, there are inadequate data to correspond frequencies of exacerbations with different levels of asthma control. In general, more frequent and intense exacerbations (i.e., requiring urgent, unscheduled care, hospitalization, or ICU admission) indicate poorer disease control. For treatment purposes, patients who had ≥ 2 exacerbations requiring oral systemic corticosteroids in the past year may be considered the same as patients who have not-well-controlled asthma, even in the absence of impairment levels consistent with not-well-controlled asthma.

■ Validated questionnaires for the impairment domain (the questionnaires do not asses lung function or the risk domain):
　ATAQ = Asthma Therapy Assessment Questionnaire© (See sample in "Component 1: Measures of Asthma Assessment and Monitoring.")
　ACQ = Asthma Control Questionnaire© (user package may be obtained at www.qoltech.co.uk or juniper@qoltech.co.uk)
　ACT = Asthma Control Test™ (See sample in "Component 1: Measures of Asthma Assessment and Monitoring.") Minimal Important Difference: 1.0 for the ATAQ; 0.5 for the ACQ; not determined for the ACT.

■ Before step up in therapy:
— Review adherence to medications, inhaler technique, and environmental control, and comorbid conditions.
— If an alternative treatment option was used in a step, discontinue and use the preferred treatment for that step.

Figure 24-4a Classifying asthma severity and initiating treatment in children 0–4 years of age.

Assessing severity and initiating therapy in children who are not currently taking long-term control medication

Components of Severity		Classification of Asthma Severity (0–4 years of age)			
			Persistent		
		Intermittent	Mild	Moderate	Severe
Impairment	Symptoms	≤ 2 days/week	> 2 days/week but not daily	Daily	Throughout the day
	Nighttime awakenings	0	1–2x/month	3–4x/month	> 1x/week
	Short-acting beta$_2$-agonist use for symptom control (not prevention ot EIB)	≤ 2 days/week	> 2 days/week but not daily	Daily	Several times per day
	Interference with normal activity	None	Minor limitation	Some limitation	Extremely limited
Risk	Exacerbations requiring oral systemic corticosteroids	0–1/year	≥ 2 exacerbations in 6 months requiring oral systemic corticosteroids, or ≥ 4 wheezing episodes/1 year lasting > 1 day AND risk factors for persistent asthma		
		Consider severity and interval since last exacerbation. ◄─── Frequency and severity may fluctuate over time. ───► Exacerbations of any severity may occur in patients in any severity category.			
Recommended Step for Initiating Therapy		Step 1	Step 2	Step 3 and consider short course of oral systemic corticosteriods	
		In 2–6 weeks, depending on severity, evaluate level of asthma control that is achieved. If no clear benefit is observed in 4–6 weeks, consider adjusting therapy or alternative diagnosis.			

Key: EIB, exercise-included bronchospasm

Notes:

- The stepwise approach is meant to assist, not replace, the clinical decision making required to meet individual patient needs.

- Level of severity is determined by both impairment and risk. Assess impairment domain by patient's/caregiver's recall of previous 2–4 weeks. Symptom assessment for longer periods should reflect a global assessment such as inquiring whether the patient's asthma is better or worse since the visit. Assign severity to most severe category in which any feature occurs.

- At present, there are inadequate data to correspond frequencies of exacerbations with different levels of asthma severity. For treatment purposes, patients who had ≥ 2 exacerbations requiring oral systemic corticosteroids in the past 6 months, or ≥ 4 wheezing episodes in the past year, and who have risk factors for persistent asthma may be considered the same as patients who have persistent asthma, even in the absence of impairment levels consistent with persistent asthma.

Figure 24-4b Classifying asthma severity and initiating treatment in children 5–11 years of age.

Assessing severity and initiating therapy in children who are not currently taking long-term control medication

Components of Severity		Classification of Asthma Severity (5–11 years of age)			
		Intermittent	Persistent		
			Mild	Moderate	Severe
Impairment	Symptoms	≤ 2 days/week	> 2 days/week but not daily	Daily	Throughout the day
	Nighttime awakenings	≤ 2x/month	3–4x/month	> 1x/week but not nightly	often 7x/week
	Short-acting beta₂-agonist use for symptom control (not prevention ot EIB)	≤ 2 days/week	> 2 days/week but not daily	Daily	Several times per day
	Lung function	• Normal FEV₁ between exacerbations • FEV₁ > 80% predicted • FEV₁/FVC > 85%	• FEV₁ = > 80% predicted • FEV₁/FVC > 80%	• FEV₁ = 60–80% predicted • FEV₁/FVC = 75–80%	• FEV₁ < 60% predicted • FEV₁/FVC < 75%
Risk	Exacerbations requiring oral systemic corticosteroids	0–1/year (see note)	≥ 2/year (see note) ⟶		
		⟵ Consider severity and interval since last exacerbation. ⟶ Frequency and severity may fluctuate over time for patients in any category.			
		Relative annual risk of exacerbations may be FEV₁.			
Recommended Step for Initiating Therapy		Step 1	Step 2	Step 3, medium dose ICS option	Step 3, medium dose ICS option, or step 4
				and consider short course of oral systemic corticosteroids	
		In 2–6 weeks, evaluate level of asthma control that is achieved, and adjust therapy accordingly.			

Key: EIB, exercise-included bronchospasm; FEV₁, forced expiratory volume in 1 second; FVC, forced vital capacity; ICS, inhaled corticosteroids

Notes:

■ The stepwise approach is meant to assist, not replace, the clinical decision making required to meet individual patient needs.

■ Level of severity is determined by both impairment and risk. Assess impairment domain by patient's/caregiver's recall of previous 2–4 weeks and spirometry. Assign severity to the most severe category in which any feature occurs.

■ At present, there are inadequate data to correspond frequencies of exacerbations with different levels of asthma severity. In general, more frequent and intense exacerbations (i.e., requiring urgent, unscheduled care, hospitalization, or ICU admission) indicate greater underlying disease severity. For treatment purposes, patients who had ≥ 2 exacerbations requiring oral systemic corticosteroids in the past year may be considered the same as patients who have persistent asthma, even in the absence of impairment levels consistent with persistent asthma.

Figure 24-5 Classifying asthma severity and initiating treatment in youths ≥ 12 years of age adults.

Assessing severity and initiating treatment for patients who are not currently taking long-term control medications

Components of Severity		Classification of Asthma Severity ≥ 12 years of age			
		Intermittent	Persistent		
			Mild	Moderate	Severe
Impairment Normal FEV₁/FVC: 8–19 yr 85% 20–39yr 80% 40–59yr 75% 60–80yr 70%	Symptoms	≤ 2 days/week	> 2 days/week but not daily	Daily	Throughout the day
	Nighttime awakenings	≤ 2x/month	3–4x/month	> 1x/week but not nightly	often 7x/week
	Short-acting beta₂-agonist use for symptom control (not prevention ot EIB)	≤ 2 days/week	> 2 days/week but not daily, and not more than 1x on any day	Daily	Several times per day
	Interference with normal activity	None	Minor limitation	Some limitation	Extremely limited
	Lung function	• Normal FEV₁ between exacerbations • FEV₁ > 80% predicted` • FEV₁/FVC normal	• FEV₁ = > 80% predicted • FEV₁/FVC > 80%	• FEV₁ > 60% but <80% predicted • FEV₁/FVC reduced 5%	• FEV₁ < 60% predicted • FEV₁/FVC reduced > 5%
Risk	Exacerbations requiring oral systemic corticosteroids	0–1/year (see note)	≥ 2/year (see note) ⟶		
		⟵ Consider severity and interval since last exacerbation. ⟶ Frequency and severity may fluctuate over time for patients in any severity category.			
		Relative annual risk of exacerbations may be related to FEV₁.			
Recommended Step for Initiating Treatment		Step 1	Step 2	Step 3 and consider short course of oral systemic corticosteroids	Step 4 or 5
		In 2–6 weeks, evaluate level of asthma control that is achieved, and adjust therapy accordingly.			

Key: FEV₁, forced expiratory volume in 1 second; FVC, forced vital capacity; ICU, intensive care unit

Notes:

- The stepwise approach is meant to assist, not replace, the clinical decision making required to meet individual patient needs.

- Level of severity is determined by assessment of both impairment and risk. Assess impairment domain by patient's/caregiver's recall of previous 2–4weeks and spirometry. Assign severity to the most severe category in which any feature occurs.

- At present, there are inadequate data to correspond frequencies of exacerbations with different levels of asthma severity. In general, more frequent and intense exacerbations (i.e., requiring urgent, unscheduled care, hospitalization, or ICU admission) indicate greater underlying disease severity. For treatment purposes, patients who had ≥ 2 exacerbations requiring oral systemic corticosteroids in the past year may be considered the same as patients who have persistent asthma, even in the absence of impairment levels consistent with persistent asthma.

Figure 24-6 Estimated comparative daily dosages for inhaled corticosteroids in children.

Drug	Low Daily Dose Child 0–4	Low Daily Dose Child 5–11	Median Daily Dose Child 0–4	Median Daily Dose Child 5–11	High Daily Dose Child 0–4	High Daily Dose Child 5–11
Beclomethasone HFA						
40 or 80 mcg/puff	NA	80–160 mcg	NA	> 160–320 mcg	NA	> 320 mcg
Budesonide DPI						
90, 180, or 200 mcg/inhalation	NA	180–400 mcg	NA	> 400–800 mcg	NA	> 800 mcg
Budesonide inhaled						
inhalation suspension for nebulization (child dose)	0.25–0.5 mg	0.5 mg	> 0.5–1.0 mg	1.0 mg	> 1.0 mg	2.0 mg
Flunisolide						
250 mcg/puff	NA	500–750 mcg	NA	1,000–1,250 mcg	NA	> 1,250 mcg
Flunisolide HFA						
80 mcg/puff	NA	160 mcg	NA	320 mcg	NA	≥ 640 mcg
Fluticasone						
HFA/MDI: 44, 110, or 220 mcg/puff	176 mcg	88–176 mcg	> 176–352 mcg	> 176–352 mcg	> 352 mcg	> 352 mcg
DPI: 50,100, or 250 mcg/inhalation	NA	100–200 mcg	NA	> 200–400 mcg	NA	> 400 mcg
Mometasone DPI						
200 mcg/inhalation	NA	NA	NA	NA	NA	NA
Triamcinolone acetonide						
75 mcg/puff	NA	300–600 mcg	NA	> 600–900 mcg	NA	> 900 mcg

Key: HFA, hydrofluoroalkane; NA, not approved and no data available for this age group

Notes:

- The most important determinant of appropriate dosing is the clinician's judgment of the patient's response to therapy. The clinician must monitor the patient's response on several clinical parameters and adjust the dose accordingly. The stepwise approach to therapy emphasizes that once control of asthma is achieved, the dose of medication should be carefully titrated to the minimum dose required to maintain control, thus reducing the potential for adverse effect.

- Some doses may be outside package labeling, especially in the high-dose range. Budesonide nebulizer suspension is the only ICS with FDA approved labeling for children < 4 years of age.

- Metered-dose inhaler (MDI) dosages are expressed as the actuator dose (the amount of the drug leaving the actuator and delivered to the patient), which is the labeling required in the United States. This is different from the dosage expressed as the valve dose (the amount of the leaving the valve, not all of which is available to the patient), which is used in many European countries and in some scientific literature. Dry powder inhaler (DPI) doses are expressed as the amount of drug in the inhaler following activation.

- For children < 4 years of age: The safety and efficacy of ICS in children < 1 year has not been established. Children < 4 years of age generally require delivery of ICS (budesonode and fluticssone HFA) through a face mask that should fit snugly over nose and avoid nebulizing in the eyes. Wash face after each treatment to prevent local corticosteroid side effects. For budesonide, the dose may be administered 1–3 times daily. Budesonide suspension is compatible with albuterol, ipratropium, and levalbuterol nebulizer solutions in the same nebulizer. Use only jet nebulizers, as ultrasonic nebulizers are ineffective for suspensions.

- For fluticasone HFA, the dose should be divided 2 times daily: the low dose for children < 4 years is higher than for children 5–11 years of age due to lower dose delivered with face mask and data on efficacy in young children.

Figure 24-7a Stepwise approach for managing asthma in children 0–4 years of age.

Intermittent Asthma	**Persistent Asthma : Daily Medication** Consul with asthma specialist if step 3 care or higher is required. Consider consultation at step 2.

Step 1
Preferred:
SABA PRN

Step 2
Preferred:
Low-dose ICS
Alternative:
Cromolyn or montelukast

Step 3
Preferred:
Medium-dose ICS

Step 4
Preferred:
Medium-dose ICS + either LABA or montelukast

Step 5
Preferred:
High-dose ICS + either LABA or montelukast

Step 6
Preferred:
High-dose ICS + either LABA or montelukast
Oral systemic corticosteroids

Step up if needed
(first, check adherence, inhaler technique, and environmental control)

Assess control

Step down if possible
(and asthma is well controlled at least 3 months)

Patient Education and Environmental Control at Each Step

Quick-Relief Medication for All Patients

- SABA as needed for symptoms. Intensity of treatment depends on severity of syptoms.
- With viral respiratory infection: SABA q 4–6 hours up to 24 hours (longer with physician consult). Consider short course of oral systemic corticosteroids if exacerbation is severe or patient has history of previous severe exacerbations.
- Caution: Frequent use of SABA may indicate the need to step up treatment. See text for recommendations on initiating daily long-term control therapy.

Key: Alphabetical order is used when more than one treatment option is listed within either preferred or alternative therapy. ICS, inhaled corticosteroid; LABA, inhaled long-acting beta$_2$-agonist; SABA, inhaled short-acting beta$_2$-agonist

Notes:

- The stepwise approach is meant to assist, not replace, the clinical decision making required to meet individual patient needs.

- If alternative treatment is used and response inadequate, discontinue it and use the preferred treatment before stepping up.

- If clear benefit is not observed within 4–6 weeks and patient/family medication technique and adherence are satisfactory, consider adjusting therapy or alternative diagnosis.

- Studies on children 0–4 years of age are limited. Step 2 preferred therapy is based on Evidence A. All other recommendations are based on expert opinion and extrapolation from studies in older children.

Figure 24-7b Stepwise approach for managing asthma in children 5–11 years of age.

Intermittent Asthma	Persistent Asthma : Daily Medication
	Consul with asthma specialist if step 4 care or higher is required. Consider consultation at step 3.

Step 1
Preferred:
SABA PRN

Step 2
Preferred:
Low-dose ICS
Alternative:
Cromolyn, LTRA, Nedocromil, or theophylline

Step 3
Preferred:
EITHER:
Low-dose ICS + either LABA, LTRA or theophylline
OR
Medium-dose ICS

Step 4
Preferred:
Medium-dose ICS + LABA
Alternative:
Medium-dose ICS + either LTRA or theophylline

Step 5
Preferred:
High-dose ICS + LABA
Alternative:
High-dose ICS + either LTRA or theophylline

Step 6
Preferred:
High-dose ICS + LABA + oral systemic corticosteroid
Alternative:
High-dose ICS + either LTRA or theophylline + oral systemic corticosteroid

Step up if needed
(first, check adherence, inhaler technique, environmental control, and comordid conditions)
Assess control
Step down if possible
(and asthma is well controlled at least 3 months)

Each step: Patient education, environmental control, and management of comorbidities.

Steps 2–4: Consider subcutaneous allergen immunotherapy for patients who have allergic asthma (see notes).

Quick-Relief Medication for All Patients

- SABA as needed for symptoms. Intensity of treatment depends on severity of symptom: up to 3 treatments at 20-minute intervals as needed. Short course of oral systemic corticosteroids may be needed.
- Caution: Increasing use of SABA or use > 2 days a week for symptom relief (not prevention of EIB) generallly indicates inadequate control and the need to step up treatment.

Key: Alphabetical order is used when more than one treatment option is listed within either preferred or alternative therapy. ICS, inhaled corticosteroid; LABA, inhaled long-acting beta$_2$-agonist; LTRA, leukotriene receptor antagonist; SABA, inhaled short-acting beta$_2$-agonist

Notes:

- The stepwise approach is meant to assist, not replace, the clinical decision making required to meet individual patient needs.

- If alternative treatment is used and response inadequate, discontinue it and use the preferred treatment before stepping up.

- Step 1 and step 2 medications are based on Evidence A. Step 3 ICS + adjunctive therapy and ICS are based on Evidence B for efficacy of each treatment and extrapolation from comparator trials in older children and adults—comparator trials are not available for this age group; steps 4–6 are based on expert and extrapolation from studies in older children and adults.

- Immunotherapy for steps 2–4 is based on Evidence B for house-dust mites, animal danders, and pollens; evidence is weak or lacking for molds and cockroaches. Evidence is strongest for immunotherapy with single allergens. The role of allergy in asthma is greater in children than in adults. Clinicians who administer immunotherapy should be prepared and equipped to identify and treat anaphylaxis that may occur.

Figure 24-8 Stepwise approach for managing asthma in youths ≥ 12 years of age and adults.

Intermittent Asthma	Persistent Asthma : Daily Medication
	Consul with asthma specialist if step 4 care or higher is required. Consider consultation at step 3.

Step 1
Preferred:
SABA PRN

Step 2
Preferred:
Low-dose ICS
Alternative:
Cromolyn, LTRA, nedocromil,or theophylline

Step 3
Preferred:
Low-dose ICS + LABA
OR
Medium-dose ICS
Alternative:
Low-dose ICS + either LTRA or theophylline, or zileuton

Step 4
Preferred:
Medium-dose ICS + LABA
Alternative:
Medium-dose ICS + either LTRA or theophylline, or zileuton

Step 5
Preferred:
High-dose ICS + LABA
AND
Consider omalizumab for patients who have allergies

Step 6
Preferred:
High-dose ICS + LABA + oral corticosteroid
AND
Consider omalizumab for patients who have allergies

Step up if needed
(first, check adherence, environmental control, and comordid conditions)

Assess control

Step down if possible
(and asthma is well controlled at least 3 months)

Each step: Patient education, environmental control, and management of comorbidities.

Steps 2–4: Consider subcutaneous allergen immunotherapy for patients who have allergic asthma (see notes).

Quick-Relief Medication for All Patients
- SABA as needed for symptoms. Intensity of treatment depends on severity of symptoms: up to 3 treatments at 20-minute Intervals as needed. Short course of oral systemic corticosteroids may be needed.
- Use of SABA > 2 days a week for symptom relief (not prevention of EIB) generallly indicates inadequate control and the need to step up treatment.

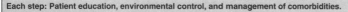

Key: Alphabetical order is used when more than one treatment option is listed within either preferred or alternative therapy. EIB, excercise-induced bronchospasm; ICS, inhaled corticosteroid; LABA, long-acting inhaled beta$_2$-agonist; LTRA, leukotriene receptor antagonist; SABA, inhaled short-acting beta$_2$-agonist

Notes:

- The stepwise approach is meant to assist, not replace, the clinical decision making required to meet individual patient needs.

- If alternative treatment is used and response inadequate, discontinue it and use the preferred treatment before stepping up.

- Zileuton is a less desirable alternative due to limited studies as adjunctive therapy and the perferred treatment before function. Theophylline requires monitoring of serum concentration levels.

- In step 6, before oral systemic corticosteroids are introduced, a trail of high-dose ICS + LABA + either LTRA, theophylline, or zileuton may be considered, although this approach has not been studied in clinical trials.

- Step 1, 2, and 3 perferred therapies are based on Evidence A; step 3 alternative therapy is based on Evidence A for LTRA, Evidence B for theophylline, and Evidence D for zileuton. Step 4 preferred therapy is based on Evidence B, and alternative therapy is based on Evidence B for LTRA and theophylline and Evidence D for zileuton. Step 5 perferred therapy is based on Evidence B. Step 6 perferred therapy is based on (EPR—2 1997) and Evidence B for omalizumab.

- Immunotherapy for steps 2–4 is based on Evidence B for house-dust mites, animal danders, and pollens; evidence is weak or lacking for molds and cockroaches. Evidence is strongest for immunotherapy with single allergens. The role of allergy in asthma is greater in children than in adults.

- Clinicians who administer immunotherapy or omalizumab should be prepared and equipped to identify and treat anaphylaxis that may occur.

BIBLIOGRAPHY

Behrman R, Kliegman R, Jenson H. *Nelson textbook of pediatrics.* 17th ed. Philadelphia, PA: W.B. Saunders; 2004.

CDC fact sheet: influenza technical information. Atlanta, GA: Centers for Disease Control and Prevention; 2003.

CDC fact sheet: pertussis technical information. Atlanta, GA: Centers for Disease Control and Prevention; 2003.

Klassen T, et al. Nebulized budesonide and oral dexamethasone for treatment of croup: a randomized controlled trial. *J Am Med Assoc.* 1998;279(20):1635.

Long S, Pickering L, Prober C. *Principles and practice of pediatric infectious diseases.* 2nd ed. Philadelphia, PA: Churchill Livingstone; 2003.

Michael M. Scope and impact of pediatric asthma. *Nurse Pract.* 2002;27(S):7.

National Heart, Lung, and Blood Institute, Global Initiative for Asthma. *Global burden of asthma* (NIH Publication No 02-3659:3) Bethesda, MD: National Institutes of Health; 2003.

National Heart, Lung, and Blood Institute, National Asthma Education and Prevention Program. *NAEPP expert panel report guidelines for the diagnosis and management of asthma, update on selected topics 2002* (NIH Publication No 02-5075). Bethesda, MD: National Institutes of Health; 2002.

National Heart, Lung, and Blood Institute, National Asthma Education and Prevention Program. *Practical guide for the diagnosis and management of asthma* (NIH Publication No 97-4053). Bethesda, MD: National Institutes of Health; 1997.

Pickering L. Influenza diagnosis and treatment in children: a review of studies on clinically useful test and antiviral treatment for influenza. *Pediatr Infect Dis J.* 2003;22(2):170.

Pickering L. *Red book.* 26th ed. Elk Grove Village, IL: American Academy of Pediatrics; 2003; p. 383.

Storch G. Rapid diagnostic tests for influenza. *Curr Opin Pediatr.* 2003;15:79.

Taussig M, Landau L. *Pediatric respiratory medicine.* St. Louis: Mosby; 1999; p. 565.

CHAPTER 25

Cardiovascular Disorders

Karen M. Corlett

I. CHEST PAIN

Asthma, 493.81	Musculoskeletal, 786.59
Asthma, exercise-induced, 493.9	Myocarditis, 429
Cardiac murmur, 782.2	Obesity, 278
Cardiomegaly, 429.3	Palpitations, 785.1
Cardiomyopathy, 425.4	Pericarditis, 423.9
Chest pain, 786.5	Pneumonia, 486
Chest pain, noncardiac, 786.59	Pneumothorax, 512.8
Congenital heart disease, 746.9	Presyncope, 780.2
Congestive heart failure, 428	Pulmonary, 786.52
Coronary artery anomalies, 746.9	Pulmonary embolus, 415.19
Coronary artery disease, 414.9	Rheumatic fever, 391.9
Dizziness, 780.4	Supraventricular tachycardia, 427.89
Dysrhythmias, 427.9	Syncope, 780.2
Enlarged liver, 789.1	Tachycardia, 785
Gastroesophageal reflux, 530.81	Tachypnea, 786.06
Heart disease, acquired, 429.9	Turner syndrome, 758.6
Heart murmur, 785.2	Valvular defects, 424
Kawasaki disease, 446.1	Ventricular tachycardias, 427.1
Marfan syndrome, 759.82	Weak peripheral pulses, 785.9

A. Etiology.
  1. Classes of chest pain.
     a. Severe, acute, unremitting chest pain: Refer immediately to pediatrician or urgent/emergent care facility. Rare and most often due to cardiac, pulmonary, or gastrointestinal causes.

        b. Chronic or recurrent chest pain: more likely.
- Typically patient has had several episodes of chest pain before medical attention is sought.
- Many times, physical exam may be normal.
- Patient history is crucial in elucidating etiology of chest pain although large percentage of chest pain in children will never have etiology determined.
- Chest pain is distressing to patients, families: chest pain in adult friends, relatives typically signifies cardiac event, most chest pain in childhood is noncardiac in origin.
- Thorough history and physical can rule out serious causes for chest pain.

   2. Chest pain, cardiac in origin.
     a. Coronary artery disease.
     b. Congenital heart disease.
     c. Typically have murmur.
     d. Acquired heart disease.
     e. Infectious etiologies.
     f. Cardiomyopathy, pericarditis, Kawasaki disease, rheumatic fever.
     g. Myocardial issues, myocarditis.
     h. Cardiomyopathies.
     i. Dysrhythmias.
     j. Supraventricular or ventricular tachycardias.

   3. Chest pain, noncardiac in origin: most common.
     a. Musculoskeletal.
     b. Pulmonary.
     c. Gastrointestinal.
     d. Psychogenic.

B. Occurrence.
   1. Few studies of overall incidence of chest pain in pediatric population due to wide range of specialists to whom these patients are referred.
   2. Incidence, particularly in adolescents, is significant.

C. Clinical manifestations.
   1. Chronic or recurrent intermittent chest pain.
     a. Most often occurs in adolescent population.
     b. May or may not limit activities.
     c. Usually chest pain has been long standing before treatment is sought.

   d. Important to elucidate inciting factors and relieving factors.
    • Relationship of pain to activity varies.
   e. Associated symptoms.
    • Syncope, presyncope, dizziness, palpitations.
   f. Congenital heart disease or previous cardiac surgery is important factor in determining cardiac origin of chest pain; also increases likelihood of dysrhythmia as origin for chest pain.

D. Physical findings.
  1. Most commonly patients will have no significant physical exam findings. Physical exam findings may be clues to origin of chest pain.
  2. Stigmata of certain syndromes: Marfan, Turner.
  3. Cardiac murmur.
  4. Evidence of congestive heart failure.
   a. Tachypnea, increased work of breathing, retractions, flaring, tachycardia, weak peripheral pulses, cool extremities, delayed capillary refill, rales, enlarged liver, easily fatigued, edema.
  5. Obesity: increased incidence of gastroesophageal reflux (GER).
  6. Reproducible pain with palpation.
  7. Signs of trauma to chest wall.
  8. Decreased breath sounds.

E. Diagnostic tests.
  1. Refer to pediatrician/specialist if chest pain of cardiac origin is suspected; may conduct the following tests as part of evaluation.
  2. Chest X-ray (CXR).
   a. Evaluate for cardiomegaly. May also reveal rib fractures or pneumonia.
  3. Electrocardiogram.
   a. Clue to cardiac origins: hypertrophied atria or ventricles, long QT syndrome, congenital heart disease, infarcts, dysrhythmias.
  4. Echocardiography.
   a. Structural abnormalities.
   b. Coronary artery anatomy.
   c. Cardiac function.
  5. Exercise testing.
   a. ST segment response to exercise.
   b. May provoke dysrhythmias.
   c. May provoke exercise-induced asthma.
  6. May reassure patient and parents if normal.

F. Differential diagnosis.

Acute pancreatitis, 577	Peptic ulcer disease, 533.9
Asthma, 493.9	Pleural pain, 786.52
Asthma, exercise-induced, 493.81	Pleuritis, 511
Biliary colic, 574.2	Pneumonia, 486
Costochondritis, 733.6	Pneumothorax, 512.8
Esophagitis, 530.1	Precordial catch, 786.51
Gastroesophageal reflux, 530.81	Pulmonary embolus, 415.19
Muscular pain, 729.1	Slipping rib syndrome, 733.99

1. Musculoskeletal.
   a. Costochondritis.
      • Most often at 2nd to 5th costal cartilages.
      • Often reproducible pain with pressure at costochondral junctions.
      • Treated with nonsteroidal anti-inflammatory drugs (NSAIDs).
   b. Slipping rib syndrome.
      • Pain at lower costal margin, often associated with click.
      • Reproducible at times with anterior motion of lower rib.
      • Treated with avoidance of inciting movements.
   c. Trauma (nonaccidental or accidental).
      • Point tenderness at site of trauma.
      • Pain is worse with movement of chest, self-limited.
   d. Muscular pain.
      • History of new physical activity, pain is worse if affected muscles are used.
   e. Precordial catch.
      • Sharp pain in anterior chest, often when child is bent over.
      • Short, intermittent pain, relieved by shallow respirations.
   f. Pleural pain.
      • Infection affecting intercostal and upper abdominal muscles, intensified with coughing.
      • Tender muscles lasting 3–7 days.
      • Intense pain separated by pain-free intervals.
2. Pulmonary.
   a. Asthma, particularly exercise-induced asthma.
   b. Pneumonia.
   c. Foreign body aspiration.
   d. Pleuritis: often is remote occurrence to viral infection.

    e. Diaphragmatic irritation.

    f. Pulmonary embolus: associated with dyspnea, usually is acute episode.

    g. Pneumothorax: associated with dyspnea, usually is acute episode.

   3. Gastrointestinal: typically localized to substernal area.

    a. GER.

    b. Related to mealtimes. Exacerbated by supine positioning.

    c. Esophagitis.

    d. Biliary colic.

    e. Acute pancreatitis: pain radiates to back.

    f. Peptic ulcer disease.

   4. Psychogenic causes: often have witnessed episodes of chest pain in family members.

 G. Treatment.

   1. Musculoskeletal.

    a. Analgesics and anti-inflammatories.

    b. Avoidance of inciting movements, rest.

   2. Pulmonary.

    a. Asthma: trial of bronchodilators, particularly if exercise-induced symptoms.

    b. Immediate referral for concern of pulmonary embolus or pneumothorax.

   3. Gastrointestinal.

    a. GER: H_2 blockers, dietary modifications, weight loss if obesity contributing to symptoms.

    b. Referral to specialist if initial medical therapy does not relieve symptoms.

   4. Psychogenic.

    a. Frank discussion with patient, family about nonorganic cause of chest pain.

     • Changes in patient's life leading to stress or depression?

     • Assess for secondary gain that pain yields patient.

     • Counseling may be indicated.

    b. Refer to specialist.

   5. Cardiac causes.

    a. Refer to specialist.

    b. Coronary artery anomalies, valvular defects: medical management, surgical repair.

    c. Infectious etiologies.

     • Cardiomyopathy/myocarditis.

- Treatment of inciting infection if elucidated.
- Supportive care until recovery of function.
- Consideration for transplantation if function does not recover.

   d. Kawasaki disease (see later section).

   e. Myocardial issues.

- Obstructive cardiomyopathy.
- Activity restriction.
- Consideration of medical or surgical therapy.

   f. Dysrhythmias.

- Identification of dysrhythmia.
- Antidysrhythmic agents.
- Ablation of accessory pathways.

H. Follow up.

1. Follow up with pediatrician or specialist as indicated.
2. Support for chronic pain.
3. Assess for missed diagnosis if pain persists or worsens.
4. No cause of chest pain may have been identified. Patient, family may require ongoing support, education, particularly if pain continues.

I. Complications.

1. Misdiagnosis.
2. Sudden cardiac death rare.

J. Education.

1. Most often require assurance and education as to noncardiac nature of chest pain and resumption of normal activities.
2. If cause of chest pain found, education regarding cause and treatment plan.

II. HYPERTENSION

Adrenal disorders, 255.9	Papilledema, 377
Anorexia, 783	Papilledema with increased intracranial pressure, 377.01
Diabetes, 250	
Epistaxis, 784.7	Pheochromocytoma, 194
Headache, 784	Renal vascular diseases, 593.9
Hypertension, 401.9	Seizure, 780.39
Hypertension, family history of, V17.4	Stroke, 436

Hypertension, secondary, 405.99	Systemic lupus erythematosus, 710
Hyperthyroidism, 242.9	Tiredness, 780.79
Irritability, 799.2	Tuberous sclerosis, 759.5
Myocardial infarction, 410	Turner syndrome, 758.6
Nausea, 787.02	Vascular lesions, 459.9
Obesity, 278	Vomiting, 787.03

A. Etiology.
  1. May be early onset of essential hypertension.
  2. Etiology of adult-onset essential hypertension is unclear and thought to be multifactorial with genetic, familial, environmental factors contributing to development of essential hypertension. Becoming more clear that elevations of blood pressure in childhood are beginnings of adult essential hypertension.
  3. May be a sign of underlying pathology (secondary hypertension).
     a. Renal, cardiac, endocrine diseases.
  4. Related to systemic disease, chronic illness, or medication.
B. Occurrence.
  1. By definition, 5% of children will have hypertension.
  2. Secondary hypertension is more common in children.
C. Clinical manifestations.
  1. Definition is systolic and/or diastolic blood pressure consistently above 95th percentile for age, sex, height taken on 3 separate occasions.
     a. Stage 1 hypertension is 95th to 99th percentile +5 mmHg and should be repeated on 3 or more separate occasions to confirm.
     b. Stage 2 hypertension is greater than the 99th percentile +5 mmHg.
        • Prompt referral.
        • Immediate referral if patient is symptomatic.
     c. Prehypertension now defined as readings between the 90th and 95th percentile, and/or greater than or equal to 120/80 in adolescents.
     d. Check blood pressure in left arm and one lower extremity if hypertension present.
  2. Secondary hypertension.
     a. Hypertension secondary to another cause.
     b. Typically more severe elevation of blood pressure.
     c. Younger age.
     d. Severe elevation of blood pressure at any age should trigger an aggressive evaluation to look for an underlying cause.

3. Essential hypertension.
   a. Typically milder elevation in blood pressure, but still > 95th percentile.
   b. Often associated with obesity.
   c. Typically, family history of essential hypertension.
   d. Elevated heart rate is common.
   e. Variable blood pressure measurements on repeated evaluation.
   f. Often no additional findings on history or physical.
   g. For mild elevation of blood pressure in asymptomatic adolescent, it is more likely to be essential hypertension, particularly if positive family history and/or presence of comorbid conditions.

D. Physical findings.
   1. Essential hypertension: May be few abnormal physical findings but patient history is important adjunct to determine whether hypertension is essential or secondary.
      a. Family history of hypertension in first- or second-degree relative, myocardial infarction, stroke, renal vascular diseases, diabetes, obesity.
      b. Obesity in patient.
   2. Secondary hypertension: May be physical findings or important clues in patient's history as to possible cause of secondary hypertension.
      a. Neonatal history of invasive umbilical lines.
      b. History of urinary tract infections.
      c. Medication history: OTC, prescribed, and illicit drugs.
         • Tobacco, alcohol, diet pills, anabolic steroids, oral contraceptive pills, pseudoephedrine, phenylpropanolamine.
      d. Headaches.
      e. Weight loss (pheochromocytoma, hyperthyroidism).
      f. Overall slowing of growth parameters may indicate underlying chronic disease.
      g. Webbed neck (Turner syndrome associated with coarctation).
      h. Presence of skin lesions (tuberous sclerosis, systemic lupus erythematosus).
      i. Retinal exam: presence of vascular lesions due to chronic hypertension, papilledema with increased intracranial pressure.
      j. Dysmorphic features: Williams syndrome, Turner syndrome.
      k. Adrenal disorders.
      l. Anorexia, nausea.
      m. Tiredness, irritability.
      n. Epistaxis.
      o. Neurologic symptoms.

- Headache, nausea, vomiting, anorexia, visual complaints, seizure, papilledema.

E. Diagnostic tests.

1. Errors in blood pressure measurement are common: use correct technique, appropriately sized equipment for repeated measurement.
   a. All children 3 years of age or older: blood pressure measured at every pediatric visit.
   b. Appropriate cuff size essential for accurate measurement.
   c. Bladder width of cuff should be 40% of child's arm circumference, bladder should cover 80% or more of circumference of arm.
   d. At least 3 separate measurements to diagnose hypertension.
   e. Measurement should occur after 5 minutes of quiet; child should be seated with back supported and feet on floor.
   f. Auscultation preferred method.
   g. Right arm preferred for measurement.
   h. Ambulatory blood pressure monitoring may be utilized by specialists to more accurately delineate blood pressure readings throughout the day and night.

2. For all identified as hypertensive:
   a. Serum electrolytes, blood urea nitrogen, and creatinine.
   b. Urinalysis and urine culture.
   c. Complete blood count.
   d. Renal ultrasound.

3. If overweight and prehypertensive and for all hypertensive:
   a. Fasting lipid panel and fasting glucose.

4. Drug screen if concern for use of licit or illicit drugs.

5. Polysomnography if history elucidates snoring.

6. Evaluation for end-organ damage may be ordered by specialists.
   a. Echocardiogram.
   b. Retinal exam.
   c. Plasma renin.
   d. Renovascular imaging.
   e. Plasma and urine steroid and catecholamine levels.

F. Differential diagnosis.

Cushing's syndrome, 255	Systemic lupus erythematosus, 710
Hypertension, secondary, 405.99	Tuberous sclerosis, 759.5
Hyperthyroidism, 244.9	Turner syndrome, 758.6
Renal vascular disease, 593.9	

1. Secondary hypertension.
2. Renal vascular disease, renal parenchymal disease.
3. About 60–80% of secondary hypertension in childhood is due to renal causes.
4. Coarctation of aorta (Turner syndrome).
5. Endocrine and adrenal causes: hyperthyroidism, Cushing's syndrome.
6. Systemic diseases: systemic lupus erythematosus, tuberous sclerosis.
7. Pharmacologic effect: steroids, amphetamine or sympathomimetics, oral contraceptives, illicit drugs.
8. CNS manifestations: increased intracranial pressure, intracranial mass.

G. Treatment.
1. Treatment goal is to achieve blood pressure < 95th percentile, or < 90th percentile if concurrent conditions present.
2. Nonpharmacologic treatment first-line therapy.
   a. Weight loss if obese; prevention of obesity if normal weight.
   b. Increase physical activity.
   c. Dietary modifications.
   d. Family-based interventions.
   e. Tobacco cessation; avoid drugs of abuse, particularly cocaine.
   f. Reevaluation of blood pressure.
3. Pharmacologic treatment indicated if symptoms present, target organ damage present, type 1 or 2 diabetes present, or failure of nonpharmacologic treatment with lifestyle modifications.
4. Single drug therapy preferred. Provider preference since no studies show absolute long-term benefit of any class or drug.
   a. Angiotensin converting enzyme inhibitors (preferred if diabetes or proteinuria).
   b. Angiotensin receptor blockers (preferred if diabetes or proteinuria).
   c. Beta blockers (preferred if patient experiences migraine headaches).
   d. Calcium channel blockers (preferred if patient experiences migraine headaches).
   e. Diuretics.
5. Add second class of medication if maximum dose achieved or side effects experienced before blood pressure control achieved.
6. Consider gradual withdrawal of medication if target blood pressure achieved for long period of time.

H. Follow up.
1. Continued monitoring of blood pressure.
2. Encouragement of and follow up on lifestyle changes.
3. Refer back to pediatrician or specialist if treatment goals not achieved with lifestyle changes, current medication regime.

I. Complications.
    1. End-organ dysfunction.
    2. Hypertensive crisis.
J. Education.
    1. Essential hypertension.
        a. Chronicity of disease, likely long-term morbidity, end-organ damage if not controlled.
        b. Potential improvements with dietary, lifestyle changes and medications if necessary.
        c. Need for continuous follow up.
        d. Adherence to medication regime if prescribed.
        e. Encourage patients to return to prescriber if side effects unacceptable because many classes of medications are available for blood pressure control.
        f. Goals of therapy.
    2. Suspected or known secondary hypertension.
        a. Thorough evaluation of cause, may be extensive testing.
        b. Follow up with specialists.
        c. Adherence to treatment or medication regimen.

III. INNOCENT HEART MURMURS

Bruit, 785.9	Peripheral pulmonary arterial stenosis murmur, 747.3
Chromosomal abnormality, 758.89	
Clubbing of digits, 781.5	Pulmonary flow murmur, 424.3
Cyanosis, 782.5	Shock, 785.5
Diaphoresis, 780.8	Splenomegaly, 789.2
Easily fatigued, 780.79	Still's murmur, 782.2
Edema, 376.33	Tachycardia, 785
Hepatomegaly, 789.1	Tachypnea, 786.09
Hypotension, 458.9	Weak pulses, 785.9
Innocent heart murmurs, 785.2	

A. Etiology.
    1. Innocent murmur is abnormal heart sound caused by turbulent blood flow not associated with structural heart disease, also called functional or nonorganic murmur.

B. Occurrence.
1. Cardiac murmurs are noted in 50–70% of children who are asymptomatic.
2. Vast majority of murmurs heard in infants and children are innocent in nature.
C. Clinical manifestations.
1. Innocent murmur is typically found on routine physical exam.
2. Presence of other clinical manifestations: concern for congenital, acquired heart disease.
3. Any murmur, innocent or organic, is typically louder with fever, anemia, other high cardiac output states.
D. Physical findings.
1. Absence of physical findings other than murmur should be expected if innocent murmur is suspected. Innocent murmurs often more prominent during high cardiac output states such as fever, anemia, pregnancy.
2. Physical exam findings of congenital or acquired heart disease that follow should specifically be evaluated.
   a. Known or suspected syndrome or genetic or chromosomal abnormality.
   b. Failure to grow.
   c. Easily fatigued.
   d. Tachypnea, increased work of breathing, retractions, flaring, grunting.
   e. Diaphoresis particularly with exertion, feeding in the infant.
   f. Cyanosis, central or peripheral.
   g. Clubbing of digits.
   h. Tachycardia.
   i. Edema, particularly periorbital and facial in infant.
   j. Active precordium.
   k. Palpable thrill.
   l. Weak pulses, delayed capillary refill, hypotension, or other signs of shock.
   m. Differential between upper and lower extremity pulses or blood pressures.
   n. Hepatomegaly or splenomegaly.
   o. Murmur of grade IV (see **Box 25-1**) or higher in intensity.
   p. Diastolic murmur.
3. Careful consideration of murmur description.
   a. Location.
      • Where murmur is heard best, described by location over cardiac structures or location on chest.

Box 25-1 Grading of Cardiac Murmurs

Grade I/VI: soft, difficult to hear unless room quiet and child cooperative.
Grade II/VI: soft but heard immediately.
Grade III/VI: easily heard, moderately loud, no thrill associated.
Grade IV/VI: loud, can palpate the thrill of turbulent flow on chest wall.
Grade V/VI: loud, has thrill, able to hear murmur with stethoscope barely off chest wall.
Grade VI/VI: loud, has thrill, able to hear murmur with stethoscope off chest wall

---

- • Most common areas to auscultate innocent murmurs are left upper sternal border and left lower sternal border.
  - b. Radiation.
    - • Descriptor of where else murmur can be heard.
    - • Innocent murmurs rarely radiate to distant parts of chest.
  - c. Timing: where in the cardiac cycle the murmur is heard.
    - • Systole: between S_1 and S_2.
    - • Diastole: between S_2 and S_1.
    - • Continuous: starts in systole, continues into diastole, does not need to continue throughout cardiac cycle, but has same sound for duration of murmur.
    - • Innocent murmurs are typically systolic; venous hum is continuous murmur. Solely diastolic murmur is never innocent and should be referred.
    - • Children with innocent murmurs typically have normal first and second heart sounds (S_1 and S_2) that are audible in addition to murmur. Rapid heart rates of infants, particularly febrile infants, may make it difficult to distinguish between systole and diastole.
  - d. Pitch: sound frequency of murmur. Innocent murmurs typically low to medium in pitch.
  - e. Quality: musical or vibratory in quality.
  - f. Intensity: loudness of the murmur (Box 25-1).
    - • Innocent murmurs, typically Grade I–II/VI. Often change in intensity with change in position: sitting to lying, standing to sitting. May change in intensity from one visit to the next.
    - • No clicks or extra sounds if murmur is innocent.
  4. Types of innocent murmurs.
    - a. Still's murmur.
      - • Most common innocent murmur in children; occurs typically in 2- to 6-year olds.

- Low to medium in pitch, buzzing or vibratory in nature.
- Short murmur occurring in early systole.
- Grade I–III/VI.
- Loudest in supine position, diminished by standing.
- Heard best at left lower sternal border.
  b. Pulmonary flow murmur.
- Heard in children/adolescents.
- Harsh murmur, blowing, nonmusical.
- Systolic ejection murmur.
- Grade II–III/VI.
- Loudest in supine position, loudest on exhalation.
- Heard best in second to third intercostal space at left sternal border.
  c. Peripheral pulmonary arterial stenosis murmur.
- Heard frequently in infants and newborns.
- Medium in pitch.
- Short systolic ejection murmur.
- Grade I–II/VI.
- Often heard best in axillae and over back.
- Turbulence is due to relative smallness of peripheral pulmonary arteries in newborn and angulation of takeoff of right- and left-branch pulmonary arteries from main pulmonary artery.
  d. Supraclavicular or brachiocephalic systolic murmur or bruit.
- Heard in children, young adults.
- Low to medium in pitch, harsh.
- Is short, systolic murmur.
- Grade I–III/VI.
- Heard best above clavicles, radiates to neck.
- Heard best in supine, sitting positions; changes with change in neck position.
  e. Venous hum.
- Also known as cervical venous hum.
- Continuous murmur.
- Heard over neck, immediately below clavicles.
- Intensity varies, loudness varies with position, activity; best heard in sitting position.
- May disappear when head is turned toward side of murmur.
- Murmur results from turbulence of flow as large veins converge.

E. Diagnostic tests.
1. When murmur is detected, refer to pediatrician or cardiologist to determine significance.
2. Many innocent murmurs do not require further diagnostic tests after thorough history, physical, auscultatory exam.
3. CXR, electrocardiogram, cardiac echocardiography may determine whether murmur is truly innocent.
4. Murmurs associated with structural abnormalities (organic murmurs) may require additional diagnostic evaluation.
F. Differential diagnosis.

Cardiomyopathy, 425.4	Kawasaki disease, 446.1
Congenital heart disease, 746.9	Rheumatic heart disease, 398.9
Cyanotic or acyanotic disease, 782.5	

1. Congenital heart disease.
2. Cyanotic or acyanotic disease.
3. Acquired heart disease.
4. Cardiomyopathy.
5. Kawasaki disease.
6. Rheumatic heart disease.
G. Treatment.
1. Innocent heart murmurs have no organic cause, no structural abnormality, therefore, no treatment required.
2. Education of patient, family is most important treatment modality.
H. Follow up.
1. If innocent murmur confirmed, patients may return to usual health maintenance schedule for follow-up visits.
2. If innocent murmur suspected, but not yet confirmed as innocent, should return for reevaluation to physician.
I. Complications.
1. None, since no abnormality is present.
J. Education.
1. Crucial for patient, family.
2. Explain murmur as noise.
3. Noise is result of blood flow, no structural problem.
4. No heart disease or abnormality is present.
5. Murmur may change or disappear with time but if persists still no problem with heart.

6. No activity restrictions required.
7. No treatment required.

IV. KAWASAKI DISEASE

Abdominal pain, 789	Increased liver enzymes, 794.8
Bilateral conjunctivitis, 372.3	Irritability, 799.2
Cardiomegaly, 429.3	Jaundice, 782.4
Cervical lymphadenopathy, 785.6	Joint pain, 719.4
Coronary artery aneurysms, 414.11	Kawasaki disease, 446.1
Cough, 786.2	Murmur, gallop, 427.89
Diarrhea, 787.91	Peripheral arterial aneurysms, 442.89
Distention of gallbladder, 575.8	Polymorphous exanthem, 782.1
ECG changes, 794.31	Proteinuria, 791
Elevated white blood cell count, 288.8	Reye's syndrome, 331.81
Erythema, unspecified, 695.9	Rhinorrhea, 478.1
Erythematous rash, 782.1	Seizure, 780.39
Fever, 780.6	Strawberry tongue, 529.3
Hypoalbuminemia, 273.8	Systemic vasculitis, acute, 447.6
Ileus, 560.1	Vomiting, 787.03

A. Etiology.
   1. Syndrome of acute systemic vasculitis of unknown origin.
   2. Affects mostly small- to medium-sized arteries, particularly coronary arteries.
   3. Likely of infectious origin or infection-triggered immune disorder.
B. Occurrence.
   1. Most prominent in Japan.
   2. Children of Asian descent more susceptible than Caucasians.
   3. 50% of cases in younger than 2 years of age, 80% of cases in younger than 5 years of age. Peak incidence at 1 year. Rare after 10 years of age.
   4. Boys 1.5 times > girls.
   5. 1–2% of siblings affected.
   6. Recurrence rate: 1–3%.
   7. More common in winter and early spring.

C. Clinical manifestations.
1. Vasculitis of small- to medium-sized arteries, especially coronary arteries. May progress to aneurysm formation in coronary arteries; can lead to thrombosis or scarring, increased risk for myocardial infarction, ischemic heart disease, and sudden death.
D. Physical findings.
1. Fever.
2. Reddened, edematous, indurated palms/soles progressing to desquamation. May be unwilling to walk/use hands to grasp objects.
3. Erythematous rash; most prominent on trunk, groin.
4. Bilateral conjunctival injection; particularly bulbar conjunctiva; nonexudative.
5. Red or peeling lips, strawberry tongue, injected oral, pharyngeal mucosa.
6. Cervical lymphadenopathy.
7. Irritability: particularly in infants.
8. Evidence of vasculitis in other systems.
   a. Cardiovascular: murmur, gallop, ECG changes, cardiomegaly, peripheral arterial aneurysms.
   b. Gastrointestinal: diarrhea, vomiting, abdominal pain, ileus, jaundice, increased liver enzymes, distention of gallbladder.
   c. Hematologic: elevated WBC count, elevated platelet count.
   d. Renal: proteinuria, hypoalbuminemia.
   e. Respiratory: cough, rhinorrhea.
   f. Joint: pain, swelling.
   g. CNS: pleocytosis of cerebral spinal fluid (CSF), seizure.
E. Diagnostic tests.
1. No specific laboratory test to confirm diagnosis.
2. Diagnostic criteria to establish diagnosis.
3. Fever of greater than or equal to 5 days and 4 of the following 5 criteria:
   a. Erythematous, edematous, indurated palms/soles progressing to desquamation later in course.
   b. Polymorphous exanthem.
   c. Bilateral conjunctival injection.
   d. Red or peeling lips, strawberry tongue, injected oral, pharyngeal mucosa.
   e. Cervical lymphadenopathy.
   f. OR: Fever of greater than or equal to 5 days, less than 4 of the above 5 criteria, and coronary aneurysms documented by echocardiography or cardiac angiography.

4. Kawasaki should be considered in any young child with unexplained fever for 5 or more days, leukocytosis, elevated erythromycin sedimentation rate or C-reactive protein, and thrombocytosis.
   a. "Incomplete" Kawasaki, with symptoms inadequate to meet classic criteria is more common in younger than 1 year of age and adolescents.
   b. Echocardiography may show evidence of coronary arteritis.
F. Differential diagnosis.

Hypersensitivity reactions, 995.2	Stevens-Johnson pharyngitis, 695.1
Juvenile rheumatoid arthritis, 714.3	Streptococcal, 041
Measles, 055.9	Systemic lupus erythematosus, 710
Polyarteritis nodosa, 716.59	Toxic shock syndrome, 040.82
Rheumatic fever, 390	Viral exanthems, 057.9
Staphylococcus aureus, 041.11	

1. Infectious illnesses, particularly streptococcal and staphylococcal infections.
2. Drug reactions or hypersensitivity reactions.
3. Stevens-Johnson syndrome: erythema, swelling, peeling all advance beyond hands, feet.
4. Other vasculitic diseases.
5. Polyarteritis nodosa, systemic lupus erythematosus.
6. Juvenile rheumatoid arthritis: smaller joints, morning stiffness, fingers involved, joint deformities.
7. Rheumatic fever: positive antistreptococcal antibody.
8. Viral exanthems: do not meet all criteria for Kawasaki disease.
9. Measles: rash more prominent on face and neck.
10. Toxic shock syndrome: sandpaper rash, more toxic-appearing child, often hypotension with evidence of shock.
G. Treatment.
1. Referral to pediatrician and specialists.
2. Hospitalization.
3. Aspirin.
   a. Used for antipyretic, anti-inflammatory, and antiplatelet effects.
   b. High-dose aspirin for at least 48 hours.

    c. Low-dose aspirin to complete 6–8 weeks of therapy if no coronary artery abnormalities.

    d. Aspirin continued indefinitely if coronary artery aneurysms, second antiplatelet agent may be added.

  4. IV immunoglobulin.

    a. Decreases incidence of coronary artery aneurysms.

    b. Mechanism of protection unknown.

    c. If fever persists > 36 hours after IVIG repeat IVIG dose.

H. Follow up.

  1. Pediatric cardiology for echocardiographic evaluation of coronary artery aneurysms. Aneurysms may not develop until after acute stage of illness.

I. Complications.

Congestive heart failure, 428.0	Myocarditis, 429.0
Coronary artery aneurysms, 414.11	Pericardial effusion, 423.9
Coronary artery thrombosis, 410.9	Pericarditis, 423.9
Intrahepatic vasculitis, 447.6	Valvular heart disease, 424.0

  1. Coronary artery aneurysms: develop in < 20% of individuals, fewer if treated with immunoglobulin.

  2. If coronary artery aneurysms develop, increased risk of coronary artery thrombosis, stenosis, and resultant myocardial infarction.

  3. May also develop valvular heart disease; mitral valve is affected more frequently than aortic valve.

  4. Pericarditis, myocarditis, pericardial effusion, congestive heart failure may occur.

  5. Can have development of vascular aneurysms elsewhere in body.

  6. Can have liver dysfunction from intrahepatic vasculitis.

J. Education.

  1. Serious nature of illness.

  2. Importance of specialty care and follow up.

  3. Possibility of complications after initial phase of illness.

  4. Importance of adherence to prescribed medication: aspirin.

  5. Importance of not using aspirin to treat fever in other childhood illnesses: association with Reye's syndrome.

  6. Consider influenza vaccine due to association of Reye's syndrome with flulike illnesses and aspirin.

V. RHEUMATIC FEVER

Arthralgia, 719.4	Pericarditis, 423.9
Cardiomegaly, 429.3	Polyarthritis, 716.59
Carditis, 429.89	Pulmonary edema, 514
Chorea, 333.5	Rash, 782.1
Congestive heart failure, 428	Rheumatic fever, 390
Diffuse vasculitis, 447.6	Rheumatic heart disease, acute, 391.9
Erythema marginatum, 695	Streptococcal pharyngitis, 034
Erythrocyte sedimentation rate, 790.1	Subacute bacterial endocarditis, 421
Fever, 780.6	Subcutaneous nodules, 782.2
Group A streptococcal pharyngitis, 041.01	Tachycardia, 785
Migratory polyarthritis, 390	Valvular disease, 424.9
Myocarditis, 429	White blood cell count, 288.9

A. Etiology.
   1. Complication of Group A beta-hemolytic streptococcal (GABHS) pharyngitis.
   2. Thought to be unique host factors that make certain individuals more susceptible to rheumatic fever after GABHS pharyngitis.
   3. Rheumatic fever is classified as collagen vascular disease or connective tissue disease resulting in diffuse vasculitis.
B. Occurrence.
   1. Most common in underdeveloped countries but resurgence in United States.
   2. Occurs in 2–3% of patients with untreated GABHS.
   3. Rheumatic fever is rare in infants, toddlers. Most cases younger than 5 years of age.
C. Clinical manifestations.
   1. Inflammation of joints and heart.
   2. Rarely, inflammation of brain and skin.
D. Physical findings.
   1. Migratory polyarthritis.
      a. Occurs in 75% of initial episodes, 50% of recurrent episodes.
      b. Arthritis is typically of larger joints (knees, elbows, wrists, ankles).
      c. Each joint typically affected for < 1 week, often overlap so that more than 1 joint is affected at a time.
      d. Joints are painful to touch, red, swollen; painful with movement.

2. Carditis.
   a. Up to 50% of patients with rheumatic fever have evidence of carditis.
   b. May manifest as myocarditis with poor function, valvular disease with audible murmur, pericarditis with friction rub, or as general symptoms of tachycardia, cardiomegaly, pulmonary edema, or symptoms of congestive heart failure.
3. Subcutaneous nodule.
   a. Small, hard nodules typically found on elbows, knees, wrists; also felt in occipital area, over vertebrae. Relatively rare finding in rheumatic fever.
4. Chorea.
   a. Finding of abnormal, involuntary writhing, purposeless movements that extinguish with sleep.
   b. Patients often have uncontrollable facial grimacing.
   c. Often preceding emotional lability thought to be from CNS involvement.
   d. Chorea is often late sign with latent period of 1–6 months.
5. Rash.
   a. Erythema marginatum: typical rash of rheumatic fever; painless, does not itch. Spreads peripherally while central clearing, most common on trunk, limbs; face is usually spared.
6. Low-grade fever.
7. Painful joints without obvious joint inflammation.
E. Diagnostic tests.
   1. Evidence of previous GABHS.
   2. Modified Jones criteria to make diagnosis.
      a. Major criteria:
         • Carditis.
         • Polyarthritis.
         • Chorea.
         • Erythema marginatum.
         • Subcutaneous nodules.
      b. Minor criteria:
         • Arthralgia.
         • Fever.
         • Elevated acute-phase reactants (erythrocyte sedimentation rate, C-reactive protein, WBC count).
         • Prolonged PR interval.
      c. Diagnosis requires 2 major criteria, or 1 major and 2 minor criteria, and evidence of previous GABHS infection.
      d. Electrocardiogram and echocardiogram for confirmed diagnoses.

F. Differential diagnosis.

Congenital heart disease, 746.9	Kawasaki disease, 446.1
Infective carditis, 429.89	Myocarditis, 429
Juvenile rheumatoid arthritis, 714.3	

1. Juvenile rheumatoid arthritis: small joints involved, swelling and deformities of joints, morning stiffness, no positive antistreptococcal antibody.
2. Kawasaki disease.
3. Congenital heart disease: murmur without associated symptoms of rheumatic fever.
4. Infective carditis or myocarditis: positive viral or bacterial cultures.

G. Treatment.
1. Prevention: appropriate diagnosis and treatment of streptococcal pharyngitis.
2. Referral to pediatrician or specialist if diagnosis suspected.
3. Antibiotics to eradicate streptococcal infection (primary prevention; see **Table 25-1**).
4. Bed rest until fever, symptoms resolve. With carditis, bed rest may be indicated for longer period of time.
5. Aspirin.
    a. If no relief in arthritis with initiation of aspirin therapy, question diagnosis.
    b. Steroids may be considered if no response to aspirin therapy and/or for those with moderate to severe carditis.
6. Secondary prevention (Table 25-1).
    a. To prevent recurrence of rheumatic fever in susceptible individuals.
    b. Antibiotics until 21 years of age and minimum of 5 years if no cardiac involvement.
    c. Antibiotics until 21 years of age and minimum of 10 years if cardiac involvement but no residual cardiac disease.
    d. Antibiotics until 40 years of age and minimum of 10 years if residual valve abnormalities; consider lifelong antibiotic prophylaxis.

H. Follow up.
1. With specialist.
2. Subacute bacterial endocarditis (SBE) prophylaxis if residual valve disease.

I. Complications.

Valvular heart disease, 424.9

Table 25-1 Primary and Secondary Antibiotic Prophylaxis for Rheumatic Heart Disease

Antibiotic	Dose	Duration	Route
Primary prevention			
Benzathine penicillin G	< 27 kg: 600,000 units; > 27 kg: 1.2 million units	once	IM
Penicillin V	< 27 kg: 250 mg 2–3 times/day; > 27 kg, adolescents and adults: 500 mg 2–3 times/day	10 days	orally
Amoxicillin	50 mg/kg once daily (maximum 1 g)	10 days	orally
If penicillin allergic			
Narrow spectrum cephalosporin	variable	10 days	orally
Clindamycin	20 mg/kg/day in 3 doses (maximum 1.8 g/day)	10 days	orally
Clarithromycin	15 mg/kg/day in 2 doses (maximum 250 mg bid)	10 days	orally
Azithromycin	12 mg/kg/dose once daily (maximum 500 mg)	5 days	orally
Secondary prevention (see text for duration of therapy)			
Benzathine penicillin G	< 27 kg: 600,000 units; > 27 kg: 1.2 million units	once every 4 weeks	IM
Penicillin V	250 mg 2 times daily	daily	orally
Sulfadiazine	< 27 kg: 500 mg once daily; > 27 kg: 1000 mg once daily		orally
If allergic to penicillin and sulfadiazine: macrolide or azalide	variable		orally

Source: Adapted from: Gerber MA, Baltimore RS, Eaton CB, et al. Prevention of rheumatic fever and diagnosis and treatment of acute Streptococcal pharyngitis: a scientific statement from the American Heart Association Rheumatic Fever, Endocarditis and Kawasaki Committee of the Council on Cardiovascular Disease in the Young, the Interdisciplinary Council on Functional Genomics and Translational Biology and the Interdisciplinary Council on Quality of Care and Outcomes Research: endorsed by the American Academy of Pediatrics. *Circulation.* 2009; 119(11):1541-1551.

    1. Cardiac involvement.
       a. Valvular heart disease.
    2. Recurrence.
       a. Increased risk of recurrence in susceptible hosts.
       b. Cardiac damage is cumulative with each recurrence.
J. Education.
    1. Nature of disease.
    2. Recurrence risk.
    3. Prompt diagnosis and treatment of Group A streptococcal pharyngitis.
    4. Cumulative nature of cardiac damage with repeat episodes.
    5. Secondary prevention.
       a. Streptococcal infections do not have to be symptomatic to cause additional cardiac damage.
    6. Importance of continued pediatric subspecialty follow up and transition to adult healthcare providers when appropriate.
    7. SBE prophylaxis if indicated.

BIBLIOGRAPHY

Baker EJ. Non-rheumatic inflammatory disease of the heart. In: Anderson RH, Baker EJ, Penny DJ, et al., eds. *Paediatric cardiology.* 2nd ed. Philadelphia, PA: Churchill Livingstone; 2010.

Coelho Mota CC, Demarchi Aiello V, Anderson RH. Rheumatic fever. In: Anderson RH, Baker EJ, Penny DJ, et al., eds. *Paediatric cardiology.* 2nd ed. Philadelphia, PA: Churchill Livingstone; 2010.

Danford DA, McNamara DG. Innocent murmurs and heart sounds. In: Garson A, et al., eds., *The science and practice of pediatric cardiology.* 2nd ed. Baltimore: Williams & Wilkins; 1998.

Gerber MA, Baltimore RS, Eaton CB, et al. Prevention of rheumatic fever and diagnosis and treatment of acute Streptococcal pharyngitis: a scientific statement from the American Heart Association Rheumatic Fever, Endocarditis and Kawasaki Committee of the Council on Cardiovascular Disease in the Young, the Interdisciplinary Council on Functional Genomics and Translational Biology and the Interdisciplinary Council on Quality of Care and Outcomes Research: endorsed by the American Academy of Pediatrics. *Circulation.* 2009;119(11):1541-1551.

National High Blood Pressure Education Program Working Group on High Blood Pressure in Children and Adolescents. The fourth report on the diagnosis, evaluation and treatment of high blood pressure in children and adolescents. *Pediatrics.* 2004:555-576.

Takemoto CK, Hodding JH, Kraus DM. *Pediatric dosage handbook.* 16 th ed. Hudson, OH: Lexi-Comp; 2009.

Urbina E, Alpert B, Flynn J, et al. Ambulatory blood pressure monitoring in children and adolescents: recommendations for standard assessment: a scientific statement from the American Heart Association atherosclerosis, hypertension and obesity in youth committee of the Council on Cardiovascular Disease in the Young and the Council for High Blood Pressure Research. *Hypertension.* 2008;52: 433-451.

CHAPTER 26

Gastrointestinal Disorders

Robin Shannon

I. ABDOMINAL PAIN, ACUTE

Abdominal pain, acute, 789	Mittelschmerz, 625.2
Appendicitis, 541	Ovarian cyst, 620.2
Cholelithiasis, 574.2	Pancreatitis, 577
Colic, 789	Pharyngitis, 462
Constipation, 564	Pelvic inflammatory disease (PID), 614.9
Dysmenorrhea, 625.3	Pneumonia, 486
Ectopic pregnancy, 633.9	Testicular torsion, 608.2
Incarcerated hernia, 552.9	Urinary tract infection, 599
Intussusception, 560	Viral gastroenteritis, 008.8

A. Etiology.
   1. Pain located in abdomen with 2 weeks' duration. Symptom can originate from within or outside gastrointestinal (GI) tract.
   2. Pain from visceral (stomach, intestine), parietal (peritoneum), or referred areas.
   3. Frequently caused by viral gastroenteritis, urinary tract infection (UTI), constipation.
   4. Other possible causes vary by age:
      a. Infant: colic, intussusception, incarcerated hernia, testicular torsion.
      b. Preschool: appendicitis, intussusception, pneumonia, pharyngitis, trauma.
      c. School age: appendicitis, pneumonia, pharyngitis, pancreatitis, trauma.
      d. Adolescent: appendicitis, pancreatitis, cholelithiasis. Female: mittelschmerz, pelvic inflammatory disease (PID), dysmenorrhea, ectopic pregnancy, ovarian cyst.

B. Occurrence.
   1. Gastroenteritis, appendicitis are most common causes.
C. Clinical manifestations.
   1. Must take child's age, developmental level into consideration regarding location, duration of pain. Younger children often indicate periumbilical region.
   2. Associated symptoms: fever, vomiting, diarrhea, cough, anorexia depending on etiology.
   3. Important subjective data should include:
      a. Location, duration, frequency of pain.
      b. Stool frequency, consistency; history of hematochezia or melena.
      c. Vomiting: frequency, presence of bile or hematemesis.
      d. Symptoms outside GI tract (cough, congestion, dysuria, sore throat, fever).
      e. Medication and diet history.
      f. Sexual activity, vaginal discharge.
      g. Alleviating and aggravating factors.
D. Physical findings.
   1. Weight, temperature, vital signs.
   2. General appearance: Assess degree of discomfort and hydration.
   3. Complete physical exam with attention to following:
      a. Abdominal exam: Ask child to indicate location of pain. Observe for peristaltic waves, distention, guarding. Palpate for masses, stool, hepatosplenomegaly, tenderness. Percuss for rebound tenderness. Have child stand, jump to assess for signs of peritoneal irritation.
      b. Rectal exam: Assess for fissures, erythema.
E. Diagnostic tests.
   1. May include CBC, comprehensive metabolic panel, amylase, lipase, and urinalysis. Consider pregnancy test in postmenarchal girls.
   2. Test stool for occult blood if history dictates.
   3. Chest X-ray (CXR) if pneumonia suspected.
   4. Abdominal X-ray if intestinal obstruction or perforation suspected. Useful to rule out fecal impaction.
   5. Abdominal ultrasound if appendicitis, ovarian cyst, ectopic pregnancy suspected.
F. Differential diagnosis.

       1. Appendicitis.
          a. Vague periumbilical pain, localized to right lower/middle quadrant.
          b. Often associated with fever, vomiting; may see elevated WBC count.
          c. Guarding, rebound, signs of peritoneal irritation on abdominal exam.
       2. Constipation, gastroenteritis, intussusception, incarcerated hernia, colic, peptic ulcer.
       3. Pancreatitis.
          a. Inflammation of pancreas from infection, medications, trauma, genetic defect, or structural abnormality.
          b. Epigastric pain often with nausea, vomiting.
          c. Elevated amylase, lipase.
       4. Cholelithiasis.
          a. Epigastric or right upper quadrant pain, often radiates to back.
          b. Ultrasound shows stones in gallbladder or bile duct.

G. Treatment.
       1. Appendicitis, cholelithiasis: surgical consult.
       2. Pancreatitis: possible hospital admission for IV hydration, pain control.
       3. Intussusception: admission for diagnosis and barium enema incarcerated hernia: admission for surgery.

H. Follow up.
       1. Telephone contact for any changes/increase in symptoms.
       2. Ensure follow through with any consults that have been requested.

I. Complications.
       1. School absence.

J. Education.
       1. Reassure if physical exam consistent with nonsurgical abdomen. Parents most often concerned about appendicitis.
       2. Review hydration/nutrition needs.
       3. Treat fever as needed.
       4. Monitor for any changes in symptoms or worrisome signs such as hematochezia, hematemesis, increased or newly localized pain.
       5. Education otherwise depends on final diagnosis.

II. ABDOMINAL PAIN, CHRONIC: CHILDHOOD FUNCTIONAL ABDOMINAL PAIN (FAP)

Chronic abdominal pain syndrome (FAP), 789

A. Diagnostic criteria: Must experience *all* of the following symptoms, at least once per week for at least 2 months prior to diagnosis:
   1. Episodic or continuous abdominal pain.
   2. Insufficient criteria for other functional gastrointestinal disorders.
   3. No evidence of an inflammatory, anatomic, metabolic, or neoplastic process that explains the symptoms.
B. Functional abdominal pain syndrome (FAP-S) includes all of the above plus at least 25% of the time one or more of the following:
   1. Some loss of daily functioning.
   2. Additional somatic symptoms such as headache or difficulty sleeping.
C. Etiology.
   1. Considered to be functional disorder: defined as absence of specific structural, infectious, inflammatory, or biochemical abnormalities as cause of pain.
   2. No longer thought to be caused by psychologic stressors. However, coping skills may be different in patients with FAP. Stress may affect pain experience, perpetuate symptoms.
   3. May be greater likelihood of anxiety, somatization in parents of children with FAP.
D. Occurrence.
   1. Equal incidence among males and females until age 10 years; then female-to-male ratio is 1.5:1.0. Most common between 8–15 years of age.
E. Clinical manifestations.
   1. Periumbilical abdominal pain lasts from 1 hour to 3 hours.
   2. Occurs daily or intermittently (at least once per week) over at least 8-week period.
   3. May be associated with nausea, fatigue, headache, pallor.
   4. Patient may assume fetal position, grimace/cry during episode.
   5. Pain does not wake child from sleep.
   6. Patient may have school absence, withdraw from social/extracurricular activities.
   7. No weight loss or growth delay.
   8. Not associated with fever, vomiting, melena, or hematochezia.
   9. Important subjective data to obtain:
      a. Description of normal elimination pattern; alleviating or aggravating factors.
      b. Dietary history, medications.
      c. Psychosocial stressors, parent/caregiver usual reaction to the pain.
F. Physical findings.
   1. Weight/height: Plot on growth curve and compare with previous.

2. Perform thorough physical exam at first visit with attention to following:
   a. Abdominal exam: Ask patient to indicate location of pain. Assess for tenderness, masses, hepatosplenomegaly.
   b. Rectal exam: inspect for erythema, fissures, skin tags. Perform digital exam.
3. Tanner staging.

G. Diagnostic tests.
   1. No diagnostic test to make diagnosis of FAP.
   2. Screening laboratories to obtain:
      a. Urinalysis, urine culture.
      b. Complete blood count, erythrocyte sedimentation rate (ESR), and/or CRP, comprehensive metabolic panel, amylase, lipase.
      c. Stool for occult blood, ova and parasite, giardia antigen.
      d. Consider lactose breath hydrogen test to rule out lactose intolerance.

H. Differential diagnosis.

Abdominal tenderness, 789.6	Lactose intolerance, 271.3
Constipation, 564	Melena hematochezia, 578.1
Crohn's disease, 555.9	Rectal skin tags, 455.9
Diarrhea, 787.31	Ulcerative colitis, 556.9
Inflammatory bowel disease, 569.9	Upper respiratory infection, 465.9
Intestinal parasite, 129	Weight loss, 783.21
Irritable bowel syndrome (IBS), 564.1	

1. Irritable bowel syndrome (IBS).
2. Infection: UTI, intestinal parasite.
3. Lactose intolerance: positive lactose breath test or okay after no lactose in diet after 2-week trial.
4. Constipation.
5. Inflammatory bowel disease (Crohn's disease, ulcerative colitis): associated with melena, hematochezia, and/or diarrhea. Possible weight loss, growth delay. Physical exam may reveal abdominal tenderness, multiple anal fissures/skin tags, possible joint symptoms. Refer to pediatric gastroenterologist.

I. Treatment.
   1. Most valuable treatment is establishment of therapeutic relationship with patient and family. Discuss possibility of FAP at first visit.
   2. Can do trial of lactose-reduced diet. Eliminate caffeine.

3. Trial of fiber supplementation: may regulate intestinal motility. American Academy of Pediatrics (AAP) recommends: child's age + 5 = grams of fiber/day.
4. Counseling: self-hypnosis, biofeedback.
5. Symptom diary.

J. Follow up.
   1. Arrange for clinic visit about 1 month after diagnosis of FAP.
   2. Telephone contact for any changes in symptoms.

K. Complications.
   1. School absence or avoidance, decreased participation in extracurricular activities.
   2. Interference with peer relationships.

L. Education.
   1. If physical exam normal, reassure family that it is unlikely any specific cause will be found.
   2. Acknowledge pain is real, not fabricated.
   3. Insist on return to normal, daily activities, school participation.
   4. Educate family about reaction to the pain: may be altered reaction to pain or secondary gain if too much attention is given to symptom.
   5. Discuss prognosis: Pain may persist for months or years.

III. COLIC

Colic, 789

A. Often defined by "rule of 3": crying for 3 hours a day on 3 days a week for 3 weeks during first 3 months of life in otherwise healthy infant. Diagnostic criteria: Must include all of the following in infants from birth to 4 months of age:
   1. Paroxysms of irritability, fussing, or crying that starts and stops without obvious cause.
   2. Episodes lasting 3 or more hours/day and occurring at least 3 days/week for at least 1 week.
   3. No failure to thrive.

B. Etiology.
   1. Unknown, probably multifactorial.

C. Occurrence.
   1. Most studies estimate incidence rates of up to 25% of infants. Equal incidence among males and females, all socioeconomic levels, breastfed versus bottle-fed.

D. Clinical manifestations.
   1. Inconsolable crying for 3 or more hours per day, often clustering in after-noon or evening. Episodes seem to have a clear beginning and end.
   2. Associated symptoms may include pain facies/grimacing, clenched fists, taut/distended abdomen, drawing legs up to abdomen, flatus.
   3. Crying often described as more intense than normal crying.
   4. Ask parents to describe quality, frequency, duration, timing of crying.
   5. Ask about any other symptoms such as vomiting, regurgitation.
   6. Detailed diet history, including mother if breastfeeding.
   7. Frequency, consistency of stool, hematochezia.
   8. Alleviating or aggravating factors.
   9. Medications given to baby or that breastfeeding mother is taking.
   10. Ask about coping skills of caregivers and opportunity for respite.
E. Physical findings.
   1. Weight/length/head circumference, temperature, vital signs.
   2. Complete physical exam.
   3. Abdominal exam may reveal mild distention.
   4. Check baby for evidence of incarcerated hernia, testicular torsion, hair tourniquet.
   5. Observe caregiver and infant: assess caregiver's anxiety, coping skills.
F. Diagnostic tests.
   1. No test to diagnosis colic: made by history and physical exam.
G. Differential diagnosis.

Constipation, 564	Milk protein intolerance, 578.8
Gastroesophageal reflux, 530.81	Parental stress, 308.9
Inappropriate feeding, 783.3	Testicular torsion, 608.2
Incarcerated hernia, 552.9	

   1. Inappropriate feeding: Assess infant's intake by history.
   2. Milk protein intolerance or allergy: usually associated with vomiting/diarrhea. May have history of hematochezia.
   3. Constipation: hard or dry stools regardless of frequency.
   4. Incarcerated hernia.
   5. Parental stress tension, poor coping.
   6. Testicular torsion: testis tender, cord thickened/shortened.
   7. Gastroesophageal reflux (GER).
H. Treatment.
   1. Consider 2-week trial of hypoallergenic formula. Avoid sorbitol-containing fruit juices.

2. Encourage continued breastfeeding; trial of caffeine elimination from mother's diet.
3. Swaddling of infant, rhythmic movement, gentle massage, warm baths.
4. "White noise" such as soft music.
5. Avoid overstimulation. Avoid exposure to tobacco smoke.
6. Counsel parents: alleviate guilt about cause of colic, need for respite. Reassure them: Infant is not in pain. Acknowledge importance of problem, discuss prognosis.

I. Follow up.
   1. Frequent clinic and/or telephone follow up may be necessary to assess any formula changes, parental coping skills.
   2. Plan to see baby 2 weeks after initial diagnosis.

J. Complications.
   1. Poor parental coping skills.
   2. Disruption of maternal–infant relationship.
   3. Child abuse.

K. Education.
   1. Discuss normal crying patterns. Infants cry more in first 3 months of life than at any other time. Crying increases at 2 weeks and usually peaks in second month with gradual decline thereafter. Pattern of crying different in all babies.
   2. Explain that taut/distended abdomen and flatus are probably result of, not cause of, crying. Reassure them that infant not in pain.
   3. Alleviate parental guilt and discuss range of emotions may be experiencing.
   4. Stress need for respite: Suggest parents leave baby with reliable caregiver for few hours. Infant may sense tension in parents if do not allow themselves a break.
   5. Trial of hypoallergenic formula may be indicated, but multiple formula changes are not warranted and should be discouraged. There is minimal if any evidence that lactose intolerance plays a role.

IV. CONSTIPATION

Anal stenosis, 569.2	Hirschsprung's disease, 751.3
Anterior ectopic anus, 751.5	Hypercalcemia, 275.42
Change in diet, 269.9	Hypothyroidism, 244.9

A. Delayed or difficult defecation for 2 weeks; passage of hard and/or dry stools.
B. Etiology.
   1. Functional: most common, no underlying pathology.
      a. Diet low in fiber/fluids; sudden change in diet (e.g., formula/breast to cow's milk).
      b. Lack of exercise, obesity.
      c. Stool withholding secondary to painful defecation ("pain-retention cycle").
      d. Family history.
   2. Outlet dysfunction: Hirschsprung's disease, anterior ectopic anus, tethered spinal cord (secondary to occult spinal dysraphism), anal stenosis.
   3. Metabolic/gastrointestinal: celiac disease, hypothyroidism, hypercalcemia.
   4. Other: cystic fibrosis, malnutrition, sexual abuse, cow's milk protein intolerance (infants), medications (e.g., narcotics).
C. Occurrence.
   1. Accounts for about 3% of visits to general pediatrics, 25% to pediatric gastroenterology.
D. Clinical manifestations.
   1. Hard bowel movements (BMs), usually infrequent. May be dry, small (incomplete evacuation).
      a. Size, consistency, frequency of BMs: Ask when change in stool became apparent.
      b. Stool-withholding symptoms (hides for BM, crosses legs, dances around).
      c. Blood associated with stool.
      d. Fecal soiling in underwear of previously toilet-trained child.
      e. Did child pass meconium within first 48 hours of life?
      f. What treatments have been instituted thus far?
   2. Associated symptoms: abdominal pain/distention, poor appetite, irritability.
   3. Other important questions: Diet history, any changes? Child on any medications? Child toilet trained? Any possibility of sexual abuse?
E. Physical findings.
   1. Height/weight: Plot on growth curve.

2. Complete physical exam with attention to:
   a. Abdomen: Assess for fecal masses, particularly in lower quadrants. Assess for distention, tenderness.
   b. Anus: Assess for placement, fissures, erythema. Digital exam to assess anal tone, quality of stool present. Observe for soiling at anal opening.
   c. Lower back: Assess for tuft of hair over lumbar sacral area or deep sacral dimple above gluteal crease. Assess for deviated gluteal crease.
   d. Assess muscle tone throughout, deep tendon reflexes (DTRs).
F. Diagnostic tests.
   1. Testing not usually necessary.
   2. Abdominal flat-plate X-ray to assess fecal load if question diagnosis/to tailor disimpaction.
   3. X-ray of lumbar/sacral spine: assess for occult spinal dysraphism if abnormality on L/S spine area and/or history of lower extremity weakness. If abnormal: MRI.
   4. Labs only if red flags in history/physical exam: serum electrolytes, calcium, lead level, thyroid function (TSH, free T4). Celiac screen (total serum IgA and tissue transglutaminase IgA) and sweat test if poor growth.
   5. Unprepped barium enema: if history of delayed passage of meconium, to assess for transition zone associated with Hirschsprung's disease.
G. Differential diagnosis.

Anal stenosis, 569.2	Hirschsprung's disease, 751.3
Anterior ectopic anus, 751.5	Infant dyschezia, 564
Constipation, 564	Sexual abuse, 995.53
Cow's milk protein intolerance, 579.8	Side effect of narcotics, 564.09
Encopresis, 787.6	

1. Vast majority have functional constipation, diagnosis by history and physical exam.
2. Infant dyschezia: at least 10 minutes of crying and straining before passage of soft stools in healthy infant younger than 6 months of age. Reassure, self-limited.
3. Encopresis: constipation with fecal soiling.
4. Hirschsprung's disease: absence of ganglion nerve cells in colon to varying degrees. Usually have history of delayed passage of meconium. May have thin caliber stools, abdominal distention, failure to thrive. No stool in rectal vault on digital exam.
5. Structural: anterior ectopic anus, anal stenosis.

6. Sexual abuse.
7. Side effect of drugs such as narcotics.
8. Cow's milk protein intolerance: anal irritation/fissures, subsequent stool retention.

H. Treatment.
1. Stool softeners: Most children will benefit from stool softener as first-line treatment. May be needed for longer than 2 weeks
   a. Lactulose/sorbitol: 1 mL/kg/dose bid, maximum 30 mL bid. Must be ingested quickly. May mix in beverage. Good choice for infants who don't respond to dietary management.
   b. Polyethylene glycol/PEG 3350 (Miralax, Glycolax): for children older than 1 year of age and younger than 3 years start with 2 teaspoons in 4 ounces of any noncarbonated beverage/day; older than 5 years can increase to 17 g (1 heaping tablespoon) in 8 ounces beverage/day. Stir powder well to dissolve; excellent palatability and acceptance. Titrate dose to achieve soft stools.
   c. Mineral oil: Never give to infants younger than 1 year or patients at risk for aspiration (e.g., neurologically impaired). Difficult to regulate dose, start with 1–3 mL/kg/day. Rarely used.
   d. Milk of magnesia: 1–3 mL/kg/day (400 mg/5mL). Avoid in infants.
2. Laxatives/cathartics: used for disimpaction only, usually over period of 1–3 days.
   a. Magnesium citrate: older than 2 years: 1–3 mL/kg/day in single or divided doses.
   b. Senna: 2–6 years: 2.5–7.5 mL/day; 6–12 years: 5–15 mL/day.
   c. Bisacodyl: younger than 2 years: 1–2 tablets/dose.
3. Enemas/suppositories: for disimpaction only, over 1–3 days.
   a. Glycerin suppository: for children younger than 2 years.
   b. Bisacodyl suppository: older than 2 years: 0.5–1 suppository/day.
   c. Pediatric Fleet enema: older than 2 years: 1–2 times/day for 1–3 days.
4. High-fiber diet: AAP recommends age + 5 g fiber/day. Infants: prune or pear juice good choice for stool softening.
5. Toilet training, not yet trained: Delay until constipation resolved. Trained: Encourage scheduled time on toilet bid following meal, for 5–10 minutes. Provide footstool.
6. Positive reinforcement for toilet sitting, successful passage of stool.

I. Follow up.
1. Close telephone contact after disimpaction, to monitor response to stool softeners.

    2. Refer to pediatric gastroenterology if patient unresponsive to treatment, red flags in history, or abnormal test results.

    3. Refer to pediatric surgery if Hirschsprung's disease/anal abnormalities concerns.

J. Complications.

Anal fissure, 565

Encopresis, 787.6

---

    1. Encopresis.

    2. Anal fissure (treat with stool-softening agents, diet, topical cream, e.g., Anusol).

    3. Delayed toilet training.

K. Education.

    1. Reassure family if history and physical consistent with functional constipation. Explain pain-retention cycle.

    2. Reassure that stool softeners are not habit forming and are necessary part of breaking pain-retention cycle. Stool softeners are often given daily for a minimum of several weeks.

    3. Parents may report child unable to have BM despite effort; explain that what appears to be straining may be child's attempt to withhold stool to avoid pain.

    4. Avoid chronic use of laxatives, enemas, suppositories.

    5. School-age children frequently avoid using bathroom at school for BM.

    6. Explain normal defecation patterns: not necessary to have BM every day; goal is passage of soft, comfortable stools in good quantities.

    7. Instruct family to call if soiling occurs or if child not responding to treatment.

V. DIARRHEA, ACUTE

Diarrhea, acute, 787.91

A. Noticeable or sudden increase in frequency and fluid content of stools; usually infectious, self-limited lasting for 2 weeks. Diarrhea is a symptom, can result from disorders involving digestive, absorptive, secretory functions of intestine.

B. Etiology.

    1. Infectious: intestinal.

      a. Viral: rotavirus, adenovirus, Norwalk.

       b. Bacterial: salmonella, shigella, *Clostridium difficile, Escherichia coli* 0157:H7.

       c. Parasite: giardia, cryptosporidium.

   2. Infectious: outside GI tract: may be concurrent symptom of systemic illness.

   3. Dietary, medications, toxic ingestion.

   4. Other: intussusception, HUS, appendicitis, UTI.

C. Occurrence.

   1. Common symptom in children.

   2. Most commonly caused by infection in older infants/children.

   3. Dietary changes or indiscretions common in early infancy.

D. Clinical manifestations.

   1. Increased frequency, fluid content of stools.

       a. Frequency, consistency of diarrhea?

       b. Hematochezia, melena, mucus, or pus in stool.

       c. Any fecal incontinence in toilet-trained child?

       d. Anyone else in family/school or daycare have diarrhea?

   2. Possible associated symptoms: abdominal pain or cramping, fever, vomiting.

   3. Systemic illness: Are there signs of illness outside the GI tract?

   4. Medication history: recent antibiotics? OTC diarrhea remedies? others?

   5. Travel history.

   6. Toxic ingestions?

   7. Complete diet history: type, quantity of fluids; appetite; new/contaminated foods.

   8. Urine output.

E. Physical findings.

   1. Height, weight, temperature, vital signs.

   2. Complete physical exam with attention to following:

       a. Abdomen: assess bowel sounds, tenderness, organomegaly, masses, distention.

       b. Rectal: Observe for stool around anus, erythema, fissures.

   3. Assess hydration: activity level, irritability; degree of thirst; degree of dehydration (**Table 26-1**) and signs/symptoms of dehydration (**Table 26-2**).

F. Diagnostic tests.

   1. If patient appears nontoxic, mild/no dehydration: none; most episodes isonatremic.

   2. Moderate to severe dehydration: serum electrolytes.

   3. Test stool for occult blood (**Table 26-3**).

Table 26-1 Assessment of Degree of Dehydration

	Mild	Moderate	Severe
Infant	5	10	15
Adolescent	3	6	9
Infant/young children	Thirsty, alert, possibly restless	Thirsty, restless, or lethargic	Drowsy, limp, cold, sweaty
Older child	Thirsty, alert, restless	Thirsty, usually alert	Usually apprehensive, cold, sweaty

Table 26-2 Signs and Symptoms of Dehydration

	Mild	Moderate	Severe
Tachycardia	–	+	+
Palpable pulses	Normal	Weak	Decreased
Blood pressure	Normal	Orthostatic hypotension	Hypotension
Skin turgor	Normal	Slight decrease	Decreased
Mucous membranes	Moist	Dry	Dry
Fontanel	Normal	Normal to slightly depressed	Sunken
Urine output	Normal	Decreased	Oliguria, anuria
Tears	+	+/–	Absent

4. When testing for *C. difficile*, ask for toxins A and B.
5. Not usually necessary to check for parasites unless diarrhea becomes chronic.
6. Test for rotavirus in stool if infant has moderate to severe symptoms.
7. Stool for *E. coli* 0157:H7 is ordered separately.
8. Stool culture in febrile children with bloody diarrhea, check for *C. difficile* if recent antibiotic use.

Table 26-3 Diagnostic Testing for Diarrhea

	Stool	Stool	Stool	Serum	CBC
	Symptom	C&S	*C. difficile*	O&P/giardia electrolytes	w/diff
Well appearance	−	−	−	−	−
Toxic, 323.7	+	−	−	+	+
Blood in stool, 578.1	+	+	−	−	+
Blood in stool, history of antibiotics	+	+	−	−	+
Weight loss, 783.20	−	−	−	+	+

G. Differential diagnosis.

Adenovirus, 008.62	Giardia, 007.1
Allergic gastroenteritis, 558.3	Norwalk, 008.63
Antibiotic induced, 960.9	Rotavirus, 008.61
Bacterial, 008.5	Salmonella, 003.9
Clostridium difficile, 008.45	Shigella, 004.9
Cryptosporidium, 007.4	Toxic ingestions, 558.2
Diarrhea, 787.91	Viral, 008.8
Escherichia coli, 008	

1. Viral: most common GI infectious cause: rotavirus, adenovirus, Norwalk.
2. Bacterial.
    a. Salmonella: foodborne. Most resolve in 5–7 days without treatment. Fever, diarrhea +/− blood, abdominal cramping for 4–7 days.
    b. Shigella: foodborne, usually during warmer months. Sudden high fever, abdominal cramps, nausea, vomiting, diarrhea with blood, mucus, pus. Usually self-limited. Dehydration common.

    c. *E. coli* 0157:H7: strain that produces toxin. Bloody diarrhea. Most common form of traveler's diarrhea, cause of most cases of hemolytic uremic syndrome (HUS).

    d. *C. difficile*: found frequently in stool of children with antibiotic-associated diarrhea and in healthy infants, role as etiologic agent in these cases controversial. In pathologic cases, diarrhea can occur within days or up to 8 weeks after antibiotic use or any drugs that alter GI flora. Watery diarrhea, +/– blood. Fecal–oral route. Common in hospitals.

3. Parasitic.

    a. Giardia: waterborne, foodborne. Diarrhea, bloating, abdominal cramping, nausea. Temporary lactase deficiency. Often self-limited. Outbreaks can occur in daycare and long-term care facilities.

    b. Cryptosporidium: mild diarrhea, usually self-limited.

4. Dietary.

    a. Increase in fluids with high osmotic load: fruit juices, sports drinks, or any sugared beverages can cause temporary osmotic diarrhea in otherwise healthy infant/child.

    b. Introduction of new food: possible allergic response.

5. Antibiotic induced.

6. Toxic ingestions.

7. Systemic illness: may have history of upper respiratory infection (URI) or other illness.

H. Treatment.

1. Viral: self-limited, supportive care (see rehydration guidelines on p. 345).

2. Bacterial.

    a. Salmonella: supportive.

    b. Shigella: supportive, can be self-limited. Antimicrobial treatment for children in hospitals, daycare centers, institutions, and those with severe symptoms. Antibiotic resistance increasing: consult health department or MD for selection of appropriate antibiotic in your community.

    c. *E. coli* 0157:H7: supportive.

    d. *C. difficile*: metronidazole (20–30 mg/kg/day divided tid for 10–14 days) oral.

3. Parasite.

    a. Giardia: metronidazole (5–10 mg/kg/dose tid for 7–10 days) or nitazoxanide (Alinia) for children 1–11 years; 12–47 months: 5 mL (100 mg) bid for 3 days; 4–11years: 10 mL bid for 3 days; 12 and older 500 mg (1 tab) bid for 3 days, oral.

b. Cryptosporidium: supportive in immunocompetent patients; if therapy required: nitazoxanide.

4. Rehydration.
   a. Mild dehydration: oral replacement solution 50 mL/kg (5 teaspoons/pound) over 4 hours. Once repletion completed, ORS continued for ongoing diarrhea losses.
   b. Moderate dehydration: oral replacement solution 100 mL/kg + replacement of stool losses over 4 hours, reassess hourly.
   c. Severe dehydration: IV fluid: normal saline (0.9% saline); consult MD; transfer to tertiary care facility.
   d. No dehydration: Continue to feed age-appropriate diet including milk.
5. Dietary.
   a. Remove possible offending/allergenic foods.
   b. No fruit juice, sports drinks, other sugared beverages.
   c. Feed full diet: Restricting food deprives gut of nutrients needed for healing.
   d. Continue to breast/formula feed, can alternate with oral replacement solution (ORS).
   e. Eliminate dairy only if known giardia infection or if symptoms severe.
   f. With dehydrated patient: refeed age-appropriate diet as soon as rehydrated.
6. Antidiarrheal medication/bismuth: avoid; not advised for children.

I. Follow up.
   1. Telephone: Instruct parent to call and arrange for immediate clinic visit if not improving, new symptoms develop, signs of dehydration.
   2. Return to clinic next day with mild–moderate dehydration.
   3. Referral to MD or local ED for moderate–severe dehydration or lack of response to treatment.
   4. Repeat stool studies after treatment for *C. difficile*, giardia if symptoms persist.
J. Complications.

Dehydration, 276.5	Hemolytic uremic syndrome (HUS), 283.11
Diarrhea, chronic, 787.91	Malnutrition, 263.9
Escherichia coli, 008	Shigella, 004.9

1. Dehydration, malnutrition.
2. Chronic diarrhea may develop, especially if restricted diet/inappropriate fluids.
3. Hemolytic uremic syndrome (*E. coli*), bacteremia (shigella).

K. Education.
1. Reassure: most cases viral, self-limited.
2. Review proper hygiene, handwashing techniques, handling of soiled objects. Alcohol-based hand sanitizers are not effective for *C. difficile*.
3. Review dehydration signs/symptoms: Instruct parent when to call.
4. Review dietary instructions: Explain restricting diet may prolong diarrhea. Appropriate beverage selection essential.
5. Skin care: Prevent diaper rash with effective barrier ointment.

VI. ENCOPRESIS

Abdominal distention, 787.3	History of urinary tract infection, V13
Abdominal pain, 789	Poor appetite, 783
Encopresis, 787.6	Sexual abuse, 995.53
History of enuresis, V13	

A. Fecal incontinence in clothing usually after toilet training completed. Vast majority caused by chronic, functional constipation (retentive encopresis).
B. Etiology.
1. Chronic, functional constipation. Stool accumulates in rectum, which subsequently leaks out through anus. Soiling is not volitional/intentional.
2. Underlying pathology is rare: tethered spinal cord (secondary to occult spinal dysraphism), prior anal–rectal surgery, Hirschsprung's disease, ectopic anus.
C. Occurrence.
1. Stool incontinence, usually during day, of varying quantities.
2. Soiling often has soft consistency and parents misinterpret this as diarrhea, child "can't make it to the bathroom in time."
3. Parents commonly believe this is volitional or result of laziness.
4. Important questions to ask:
   a. Age of toilet training? Was process difficult?
   b. Frequency, consistency, size/amount of BM on toilet. Any blood? What time of day does it usually occur?
   c. Does child hide soiled clothing?
   d. How has family dealt with problem?
5. Associated symptoms may include abdominal pain, abdominal distention, poor appetite, school avoidance.

     6.   Ask about history of UTI and enuresis.

     7.   Any possibility of sexual abuse?

D. Clinical manifestations.

     1.   Common pediatric problem: boys affected more than girls.

E. Physical findings.

     1.   Abdomen may appear distended or full. Dull on percussion. Stool may be palpable in lower quadrants (smooth, movable mass).

     2.   Anus may appear erythematous with stool around exterior. Observe for fissures. Digital exam may reveal decreased tone, copious stool in vault of varying consistency. Check for position of anus, anal wink.

     3.   Assess back for signs of occult spinal dysraphism: sacral dimple or hair tuft above gluteal crease, deviated gluteal crease.

     4.   Assess muscle tone throughout, DTRs.

F. Diagnostic tests.

     1.   Rarely necessary.

     2.   Abdominal flat-plate X-ray can be useful to assess fecal load, tailor disimpaction. However, good physical exam and history often eliminates need for X-ray.

     3.   MRI of lumbosacral spine if concern for tethered spinal cord.

G. Differential diagnosis.

Constipation, 564	Tethered spinal cord, 724.9
Fecal incontinence, 787.6	Urinary incontinence, 788.3

     1.   Majority of cases are from functional constipation.

     2.   Tethered spinal cord: can result in fecal/urinary incontinence.

H. Treatment.

     1.   All children with encopresis must first start with disimpaction ("clean out"). Soiling will not resolve without this. Depending on amount of stool on X-ray exam, can give oral cathartics at bedtime for 1–3 nights in row and up to 1 Fleet enema bid for 1–3 days in row.

     2.   After clean out, child immediately starts daily stool softening.

     3.   Keep track of BMs, soiling episodes on calendar.

     4.   High-fiber diet.

     5.   Toilet retraining: child to sit on toilet after meals 2–3 times/day, work up to 5–10 minutes. Provide footstool. Ask child to "try" to have BM, to "practice," not expected to produce BM each time.

     6.   Positive reinforcement only. No punishment for soiling. Soiling should be cleaned up swiftly with child's assistance and little attention paid to it.

I. Follow up.
   1. Encourage telephone contact. If continues to soil, may need further clean out.
   2. Follow up in clinic about 1 month after diagnosis.
   3. May need follow-up abdominal X-ray if results of clean out are in doubt.
   4. Referral if patient not responding to treatment once compliance has been assured.
J. Complications.

Enuresis, 788.3

Urinary tract infection, 599

---

   1. Low self-esteem/shame.
   2. Child abuse.
   3. School avoidance.
   4. UTI (due to proximity of stool in clothing to urinary tract).
   5. Enuresis.
K. Education.
   1. Stress to parents that child has not had control over soiling episodes.
   2. Relieve parental guilt over prior negative reinforcement.
   3. Explain to parent and child why soiling occurs, discuss normal defecation.
   4. Treatment will take at least 6 months. Parents are advised to be diligent about daily stool softening, toilet training during this time.
   5. Reassure about functional nature of chronic constipation.
   6. Advise parent to speak with school about problem so child will have better access to restroom at school, may need to provide written request.

VII. GASTROESOPHAGEAL REFLUX DISEASE (GERD)

Gastroesophageal reflux, 530.81

A. Passage of stomach contents into esophagus. Gastroesophageal reflux (GER) is normal, physiologic process, can occur in healthy individuals. GERD refers to pathologic degree of GER, causing symptoms.
B. Etiology.
   1. Infants (up to 18 months).
      a. Very common in infants, may be result of immaturity of lower esophageal sphincter (LES).

      b. Position of LES and feeding techniques may induce GER.

      c. GERD probably multifactorial.

  2. Children/adolescents.

      a. Probably multifactorial, exact cause not known.

      b. May be malfunctioning LES: inappropriate relaxation.

      c. Environmental/dietary influences may induce GER.

C. Occurrence.

  1. About 50% of infants have recurrent vomiting in first 3 months, 67% of 4-month olds, 5% of 10- to 12-month olds.

  2. Increased incidence among premature babies, neurologically impaired children.

D. Clinical manifestations.

  1. Infants: recurrent vomiting, regurgitation ("spit up"); usually effortless.

  2. Important questions to ask for affected infants:

      a. Type, quantity, frequency of feedings? How positioned during, after feeding?

      b. Quality, quantity, timing of emesis? Does baby cry/grimace with emesis?

      c. History of apnea?

  3. Children: regurgitation (reswallowed/spit up), possible vomiting, nausea, epigastric abdominal pain. Pain may be poorly localized. Can have any/all of these symptoms.

  4. Important questions to ask for affected children:

      a. Frequency, timing of symptoms including regurgitation with/without emesis.

      b. Abdominal pain: location, timing, frequency, quality.

      c. Any specific foods that provoke symptoms?

      d. Complete diet history including type and amount of beverages.

      e. Any dysphagia, food lodging, chronic throat clearing, dental decay?

  5. For all age groups:

      a. History of hematemesis, melena, asthma, recurrent pneumonia, otitis media, sinusitis?

      b. Any decrease in appetite, poor weight gain, weight loss?

E. Physical findings.

  1. Height, weight: plot on growth curve.

  2. Full physical exam with attention to following:

      a. Abdomen: assess for tenderness, particularly over epigastrium.

      b. Rectal exam: obtain stool to test for occult blood.

      c. Mouth: assess for dental caries, enamel erosion.

F. Diagnostic tests.
1. Upper GI series: only to rule out anatomic abnormalities. Not used to make diagnosis of GERD. Presence of GER on upper GI is common in all people. Must order in infants if forceful vomiting; in older children with frank vomiting, dysphagia.
2. Stool for occult blood: if positive, may indicate esophagitis.
3. Other tests by pediatric GI specialist if referral necessary (endoscopy, pH probe).
G. Differential diagnosis.

Gastritis, 535.5	Overfeeding, 783.6
Gastroesophageal reflux, 530.81	Pyloric stenosis, 537

1. GER: normal physiologic event. Infants with regurgitation who are otherwise well, growing normally, without pain.
2. GERD: Infants who in addition to emesis have irritability during feeds, poor feeding/growth, recurrent lung problems. May be related to apnea. May have one or all of these symptoms. Recurrent GER symptoms in children older than 18 months is almost always considered pathologic (GERD).
3. Overfeeding; cow's milk protein allergy.
4. Pyloric stenosis.
5. Gastritis.
H. Treatment.
1. Conservative management, infants: for GER, as adjunct to medical therapy in GERD:
    a. Smaller, more frequent feedings. Increase burping opportunities.
    b. Hold upright after feeds; do not place infant in car seat after feedings.
    c. Consider change to commercially available prethickened formula (Enfamil AR). Consider 2-week trial of extensively hydrolyzed infant formula (hypoallergenic)
    d. Can add 1 teaspoon/ounce of cereal to bottle. Cross-cut nipple for easier flow.
    e. Elevate head of crib mattress. No extra bedding in crib. No prone positioning.
2. Conservative management, children: essential component along with medications.
    a. Smaller, more frequent meals. No skipping meals.
    b. Avoid caffeine, carbonated drinks; fatty, fried foods; citrus; chocolate; peppermint.

         c. Avoid or correct obesity.

         d. Avoid tobacco and alcohol.

         e. Elevate head of bed; no eating within 2 hours of bedtime.

    3. Medical management.

         a. Histamine-2 blockers (H2 blockers): ranitidine (Zantac), famotidine (Pepcid).

         b. Proton pump inhibitors (PPI): can try after 2-week trial of H2 blockers if no response. Must give about 30 minutes before breakfast, do not skip meal.

            • Lansoprazole (Prevacid): approved for use in children.

            • Omeprazole (Prilosec).

            • OTC antacids: not for long-term use. Only for temporary relief.

    4. Surgery: fundoplication. Reserved for severe GERD that failed medical management.

I. Follow up.

    1. Telephone contact after 2 weeks on H2 blocker or proton pump inhibitor.

    2. Return to clinic for increased symptoms, new symptoms.

    3. Refer to pediatric GI specialist if symptoms severe/no response to initial treatments, lifestyle changes.

J. Complications.

Esophagitis, 530.1	Otitis media, 382.9
Failure to thrive, 783.41	Pneumonia, aspiration, 507
Nutritional deficits, 269.9	Sinusitis, 473.9

    1. Esophagitis, stricture formation.

    2. Failure to thrive, nutritional deficits.

    3. Recurrent aspiration pneumonia.

    4. May be related to recurrent otitis media, sinusitis.

K. Education.

    1. In otherwise healthy infant with normal growth, reassure parent: GER is common, most outgrow by first birthday.

    2. Children: prognosis usually very good but unlikely to "outgrow."

    3. Take medication exactly as prescribed. If helpful, medicate minimum of 2 months before discontinuing or stepping down therapy from PPI to H2 blocker.

    4. Nutritional guidance: Avoid overfeeding, review all dietary restrictions/history at each visit.

VIII. HERNIA, INGUINAL

Abdominal distention, 787.3	Hernia, inguinal, 550.9
Abdominal masses, 789.3	Vomiting, 787.03
Abdominal tenderness, 789.6	

A. Protrusion of abdominal organ, usually bowel, into inguinal canal.

B. Etiology.
 1. Indirect: Bowel protrudes through deep inguinal ring through inguinal canal lateral to inferior epigastric artery.
 2. Direct: Bowel protrudes between interior epigastric artery and edge of rectus muscle.
 3. Incarcerated: hernia that cannot be returned or reduced by manipulation. Can become strangulated.

C. Occurrence.
 1. Most common surgical condition in children.
 2. 60% are on right side.
 3. Most common type is indirect (approximately 99%).
 4. Approximately 50% present before 1 year of age, most seen in first 6 months.
 5. Ratio of boys to girls, 4:1. Incidence approximate 10–20 in 1000 live births.
 6. Higher incidence in premature babies, positive family history, cystic fibrosis, undescended testes, hypospadias, congenital dislocation of hip, and congenital abdominal wall defects.

D. Clinical manifestations.
 1. Bulge in inguinal region may extend to scrotum. Especially noticeable during crying/straining.
 2. History of intermittent groin, labial/scrotal swelling.
 3. Parents are usually first to notice.
 4. Hernia reduces spontaneously when relaxed/sleeping.
 5. Important questions to ask:
   a. When was swelling/bulge first noticed? How often/when does it occur?
   b. Does infant/child appear uncomfortable with it?
   c. Any signs of intestinal obstruction such as vomiting, abdominal distention?

E. Physical findings.
 1. Bulge at level of internal/external ring.
 2. Scrotal/labial swelling.
 3. Do not place finger in inguinal canal, done only for adult hernia exam.

4. In supine position, with legs and arms extended over head: wait for cry, which will increase intra-abdominal pressure. Should demonstrate bulge over external ring/scrotal swelling.
5. Have older children stand.
6. Palpate testes before palpation of inguinal bulge (retractile testes are common in infants and young children, can be mistaken for hernia).
7. Abdominal exam: Assess for distention, masses, tenderness.
8. If swelling not apparent during exam, check for thickening of spermatic cord (silk sign) by palpating spermatic cord over pubic tubercle. Rubbing together area feels like silk.

F. Diagnostic tests.
   1. All girls with inguinal hernia should have rectal exam by experienced examiner; may need to order pelvic ultrasound.
   2. Diagnosis otherwise made by history and physical exam.
G. Differential diagnosis.

Hernia, incarcerated inguinal, 550.1
Hydrocele, 603.9

   1. Inguinal hernia: Scrotal swelling varies during day, increase in size with crying/straining.
   2. Incarcerated inguinal hernia: usually associated with discomfort, positive/negative abdominal distention. Bulge persists.
   3. Hydrocele: circumscribed fluid collection in scrotum; swelling does not change in size throughout day, gradually disappears over first year of life. Transillumination of scrotum cannot distinguish between hydrocele, inguinal hernia.
H. Treatment.
   1. Surgery: Inguinal hernia does not resolve spontaneously, surgery usually elective shortly after diagnosis.
   2. Supports/trusses are not indicated, may be hazardous.
I. Follow up.
   1. Referral to pediatric surgeon when diagnosis of inguinal hernia made.
J. Complications.

Hernia, incarcerated inguinal, 550.1	Ischemia/infarction of testis, 608.83
Hernia, strangulated incarcerated, 552.9	Ovary/fallopian tube infarction, 620.8

   1. Incarcerated hernia: immediate referral for reduction under sedation.
   2. Strangulated incarcerated hernia: blood supply compromised: surgical emergency.

3. Ischemia/infarction of testis: can occur in boys with undescended testicles, inguinal hernia.
4. Ovary/fallopian tube infarction.

K. Education.
1. Uncomplicated indirect inguinal hernia: review signs, symptoms of incarcerated/strangulated hernia with family: abdominal distention, vomiting, pain, persistent bulge that does not reduce.
2. Family understands importance of following through with surgical appointments.
3. Operative repair necessary within first year of life due to increased incidence of incarceration after that time.

IX. HERNIA, UMBILICAL

> Abdominal distention, 787.3
>
> Abdominal pain, 789
>
> Hernia, umbilical, 553.1

A. Protrusion of part of intestine at umbilicus; defect is at abdominal wall, protruding bowel covered with skin, subcutaneous tissue.
B. Etiology.
1. Due to weakness/incomplete closure of umbilical ring.
C. Occurrence.
1. Increased incidence among African American infants, low-birth-weight infants, females.
D. Clinical manifestations.
1. Soft mass covered by skin that protrudes from umbilicus, usually with increased intra-abdominal pressure (crying/straining) or may be more persistent (ask parent about fluctuations in mass size/presence).
2. Size of defect varies from 1 cm in diameter to 5 cm.
3. Usually disappears spontaneously by 1 year of age. Larger hernias may resolve spontaneously by 5–6 years of age unless defect 2 cm.
E. Physical findings.
1. Examine infant in supine position.
2. Abdomen will reveal soft protrusion through umbilicus, usually easy to reduce through fibrous umbilical ring. Assess for abdominal distention.
3. Increased size may be visible with crying. Observe for signs of pain.

F. Diagnostic tests.
   1. None.
G. Differential diagnosis.

Hernia, strangulated umbilical, 552.1

1. Strangulated umbilical hernia (very rare): may show signs of intestinal obstruction such as pain, vomiting, persistent umbilical bulge that will not reduce.
H. Treatment.
   1. Most resolve spontaneously.
   2. Surgery reserved for hernias after 3–4 years of age, those causing symptoms (become strangulated), those becoming progressively larger after 1–2 years of age.
I. Follow up.
   1. Assess hernia routinely at all visits. Immediate return if signs of incarceration.
J. Complications.

Incarceration umbilical hernia, 552.1

1. Incarceration: very rare.
K. Education.
   1. Instruct parent not to tape or bind umbilicus and on signs, symptoms of incarceration.
   2. Reassure most resolve spontaneously.

X. INTUSSUSCEPTION

Abdominal pain, 789	Lethargy, 780.79
Bilious vomiting, 787.1	Shock, 785.5
Blood in stools, 578.1	Vomiting, 787.03
Intussusception, 560	

A. Prolapse or "telescoping" of one part of intestine into lumen of adjoining intestine.
B. Etiology.
   1. Can follow infections such as gastroenteritis, otitis media, URI, adenovirus.

    2. About 10% have "lead point" such as Meckel's diverticulum, polyp, duplication.

    3. May be alteration in intestinal peristalsis that provokes condition.

C. Occurrence.

    1. Most common cause of intestinal obstruction 3 months to 6 years of age.

    2. 60% occur in infants younger than 1 year, 80% by 2 years. Rare in neonates.

    3. Incidence 1–4 in 1000 live births.

    4. Male-to-female ratio is 4:1.

    5. Peaks in spring and fall.

D. Clinical manifestations.

    1. Sudden onset severe abdominal pain, usually periumbilical/lower abdomen, in previously well child.

    2. Pain colicky, paroxysmal occurring at frequent intervals.

    3. Child may appear well between episodes of pain at first.

    4. During pain, child flexes legs, pulls knees toward abdomen, cries.

    5. Vomiting common.

    6. Stools may appear normal in first few hours, after which little or no stool.

    7. Blood per rectum can occur within first 12 hours or up to 2 days after symptoms start. May be mixed with mucus described as "currant jelly stool."

    8. If symptoms unrecognized, may progress to lethargy, bilious vomiting, shock.

E. Physical findings.

    1. Weight, temperature, vital signs.

    2. Assess overall affect and activity level, observe during pain episode.

    3. Abdomen may be distended. Guarding during exam if having pain. About 70% may have palpable, ill-defined ("sausage-shaped") mass, may be mildly tender.

    4. Rectal exam may reveal bloody mucus.

F. Diagnostic tests.

    1. Diagnosis usually made by history and physical exam.

    2. Barium enema: may show filling defect.

    3. Abdominal ultrasound can also detect intussusception.

G. Differential diagnosis.

Gastroenteritis, 558.9

Henoch-Schönlein purpura, 287

Meckel's diverticulum, 751

1. Gastroenteritis.
2. Meckel's diverticulum: painless, rectal bleeding from congenital append-age of ileum.
3. Henoch-Schönlein purpura: associated with joint symptoms, purpura rash.

H. Treatment.
   1. Barium enema: hydrostatic/"air contrast" used to diagnose, treat intus-susception.
   2. Untreated, condition almost always fatal.
   3. 10% recurrence rate after reduction by barium enema.
   4. Intussusception secondary to "lead point" from Meckel's diverticulum or polyp requires surgery.

I. Follow up.
   1. Immediate referral to tertiary care facility.
   2. Telephone or clinic follow up after reduction.

J. Complications.

Dehydration, 276.5

   1. Dehydration, bowel necrosis, death.

K. Education.
   1. Reassure parent that vast majority of cases have no specific lead point and are successfully treated with barium enema.
   2. Counsel family to call immediately if any signs of abdominal pain, rectal bleeding following reduction.

XI. IRRITABLE BOWEL SYNDROME (IBS)

Abdominal distention, 787.3	Loose stools, 787.91
Abdominal pain, 789	Nausea, 787.02
Constipation, 564	Rectal fissures, 565
Hepatosplenomegaly, 571.8	Rectal fistula, 565.1
Irritable bowel syndrome (IBS), 564.1	Rectal skin tags, 455.9

A. Functional bowel disorder characterized by abdominal pain and changes in bowel function. Diagnostic criteria (fulfilled at least once/week for at least 2 months prior to diagnosis): Must include both of the following:

1. Abdominal discomfort or pain associated with 2 or more of the following at least 25% of the time:
   a. Improvement with defecation.
   b. Onset associated with change in frequency of stool.
   c. Onset associated with change in appearance of stool.
2. No evidence of an inflammatory, anatomic, metabolic, or neoplastic process that explains the patient's symptoms.

B. Etiology.
   1. Thought to be combination of visceral hypersensitivity and possibly altered gut motility. May be due to alterations in enteric nervous system (ENS) and relationship to central nervous system (CNS).
   2. Stress/anxiety may induce/worsen symptoms but probably not root cause.
   3. May be preceded by episode of viral gastroenteritis or past history of constipation.

C. Occurrence.
   1. Common cause of recurrent abdominal pain in older children and adolescents.
   2. Estimated that about 6% of middle school students and 14% of high school students may fit criteria.

D. Clinical manifestations.
   1. Abdominal pain/discomfort, usually lower abdomen or periumbilical; relieved by defecation/onset associated with change in frequency/appearance of stool.
   2. Otherwise well, without evidence of underlying structural/metabolic abnormalities.
   3. BMs may be predominantly loose, constipated, or fluctuate between the two.
   4. May pass mucus with stool.
   5. Stool urgency, especially in morning; occasional feeling of incomplete defecation.
   6. Abdominal bloating/distention, especially later in day.
   7. Important questions to ask:
      a. Location, timing, frequency, duration, quality of pain.
      b. BM frequency, consistency, size. Straining? Mucus or blood? Stool urgency?
      c. Does BM relieve abdominal pain? Anything that helps or aggravates symptoms?
      d. Is patient on medications? Any OTC remedies?
      e. Sensation of abdominal bloating? What time of day?
   8. Complete diet history including beverages. Any weight loss?

9. May have functional dyspepsia symptoms such as nausea. No vomiting.
10. Red flags in history indicating diagnosis other than IBS include growth failure, weight loss, joint symptoms, vomiting, blood in stool, fever, family history of inflammatory bowel disease (Crohn's or ulcerative colitis), dysphagia.

E. Physical findings.
   1. Height, weight, temperature, vital signs.
   2. Complete physical exam with attention to:
      a. Abdomen: Assess for tenderness, masses, stool, hepatosplenomegaly.
      b. Rectal: Assess for fissures, skin tags, fistula.

F. Diagnostic tests.
   1. No test to diagnose IBS.
   2. Screening studies usually necessary to be sure no underlying pathology.
      a. Stool for occult blood, ova and parasite, giardia antigen.
      b. CBC, ESR.
      c. Consider lactose breath hydrogen test to rule out lactose intolerance.

G. Differential diagnosis.

Constipation, 564	Inflammatory bowel disease, 558.9
Crohn's disease, 555.9	Recurrent abdominal pain syndrome, 789
Gastroesophageal reflux, 530.81	Ulcerative colitis, 556.9

   1. Constipation, GER.
   2. Lactose intolerance: Decreased lactase enzyme in small intestine causes malabsorption, subsequent diarrhea, abdominal pain, gas if excessive lactose ingested.
   3. Recurrent abdominal pain syndrome.
   4. Inflammatory bowel disease: Crohn's disease, ulcerative colitis: usually associated with growth delay/weight loss, anemia, diarrhea with/without blood, possibly joint pain, mouth ulcerations. Physical exam may reveal abnormal appearance to anus, abdominal tenderness.

H. Treatment.
   1. There is currently a lack of high-quality evidence on the effectiveness of dietary interventions.
   2. High-fiber diet, consider starting fiber supplement (OTC). AAP recommends: child's age +5 grams of fiber/day.
   3. Regular meals, avoid caffeine.
   4. Ensure adequate rest and exercise.
   5. Bloating/loose stools: Reduce sorbitol and fructose in diet.

6. Predominantly constipation: Add stool softener such as MiraLax, milk of magnesia.
7. Cognitive–behavioral therapy, such as relaxation and biofeedback.
8. Pharmacologic treatment reserved for continuing symptoms usually monitored by MD. Low-dose tricyclic antidepressants used with some success, probably due to effect on ENS. Antispasmodics used but little data at this time to support their use. Studies using probiotics inconclusive and ongoing at this time.

I. Follow up.
1. Return to clinic for any change/worsening of symptoms.
2. Refer to counselor as needed for relaxation therapy or biofeedback.
3. Refer to pediatric GI specialist if red flags or if treatment not successful.

J. Complications.
1. School absence/avoidance.

K. Education.
1. Discuss IBS at first visit. Explain that although diagnosis of exclusion, real diagnosis.
2. Reassure if history consistent with IBS and physical exam and screening studies are negative, further testing not necessary.
3. Discuss enteric nervous system and possible reasons for symptoms of IBS.
4. Explain importance of regular meals and exercise; both can help control symptoms.
5. Fiber supplementation may take 8 weeks to make difference.
6. Identify psychologic triggers such as family upset/school difficulties.
7. Insist on regular school attendance.

XII. PYLORIC STENOSIS (PS)

Dehydration, 276.5	Pyloric stenosis, 537
Electrolyte imbalance, 276.9	Vomiting, 787.03
Peristalsis, 787.4	Weight loss, 783.21

A. Gastric obstruction at pylorus muscle.
B. Etiology.
1. Unknown.
C. Occurrence.
1. Most common form of nonbilious vomiting in infants.
2. Usually in infants after 2–3 weeks of age, up to 5 months of age.

3. About 3 per 1000 live births in United States.
4. Male-to-female ratio = 4:1, especially firstborn males.
5. Caucasians > African Americans.
6. Increased incidence if mother had PS as infant (20% of her male offspring, 10% of female offspring will develop PS).
7. Can be associated with other congenital defects (e.g., tracheoesophageal fistula).

D. Clinical manifestations.
1. Nonbilious vomiting. Vomiting progressively projectile, immediately after feeding.
2. Can occur intermittently or with every feeding.
3. Infant hungry after emesis.
4. As condition worsens, increased fluid losses, electrolyte imbalance, weight loss.

E. Physical findings.
1. Length, weight, temperature, vital signs.
2. Assess overall hydration, activity level, signs of hunger.
3. Abdomen: may palpate firm mass, approximately 2 cm in length, olive shaped. Usually to right of umbilicus in upper abdomen, toward midepigastrium. Easier to palpate after vomiting. Mass may not be palpable in early PS.
4. Visible peristalsis may occur after feeding.

F. Diagnostic tests.
1. Abdominal ultrasound confirms majority of cases.

G. Differential diagnosis.

Gastroenteritis, 558.9	Inborn errors of metabolism, 277.9
Gastroesophageal reflux, 530.81	Overfeeding, 783.6

1. GERD.
2. Gastroenteritis.
3. Inborn errors of metabolism.
4. Overfeeding.

H. Treatment.
1. Admit patient for rehydration/electrolyte management with referral to pediatric surgery (pyloromyotomy).

I. Follow up.
1. Post-hospitalization office visit to ensure infant regaining weight, tolerating feeds.
2. Follow up with surgical team.

J. Complications.

Dehydration, 276.5
Failure to thrive, 783.41
Weight loss, 783.21

1. Dehydration.
2. Failure to thrive.
3. Weight loss.

K. Education.
1. Reassure that infants do very well after surgical correction.
2. Infant may resume normal feeding within 1–2 days postoperatively.

XIII. PEPTIC ULCER DISEASE (PUD)

Anemia, chronic iron deficiency, 280.9	Irritability, 799.2
Family history of PUD, V12.71	Melena, 578.1
Gastrointestinal hemorrhage, 578.9	Peptic ulcer disease, 533.9
Hematemesis, 578	Periumbilical pain, 789
Hematochezia, 578.1	Vomiting, 787.03

A. Erosion or ulceration of gastroduodenal mucosa.
B. Etiology.
1. Imbalance between cytotoxic and cytoprotective factors.
   a. Cytotoxic: acid, pepsin, medications, infection.
   b. Cytoprotective: Gastric mucous layer provides mechanical barrier.
2. Primary PUD: mainly caused by *Helicobacter pylori* infection in adults.
   a. Route of transmission unknown, may be fecal–oral, acquired early in life.
   b. Can cause gastritis positive/negative peptic ulcer, usually in older than 10 years of age.
3. Secondary PUD: physiologic stress (burns, trauma), medications (NSAIDs, aspirin, corticosteroids), caustic ingestion (including alcohol), viral infections, Zollinger-Ellison syndrome, eosinophilic gastroenteritis (allergic inflammation), Crohn's disease.
C. Occurrence.
1. *H. pylori.*
   a. Increased risk for acquiring infection in developing countries, poor socioeconomic conditions, overcrowding.

  b. Possible ethnic/genetic predisposition: higher rate among Asians, African Americans, Hispanics.

  c. Less common in children, but may acquire infection in childhood that is asymptomatic until later.

  d. Among most common bacterial infections in humans.

D. Clinical manifestations.

 1. Neonates (up to 1 month): usually present with GI hemorrhage/perforation.

 2. Infants to 2 years: vomiting, irritability, poor growth, GI hemorrhage.

 3. Preschool: periumbilical pain, often postprandial, vomiting, GI hemorrhage.

 4. School age and older: epigastric abdominal pain that may awaken child from sleep. Acute/chronic GI blood loss (hematemesis, hematochezia, melena) may occur along with iron-deficiency anemia.

 5. Family history of PUD.

 6. Difficult to distinguish from other GI disorders such as GERD.

 7. Obtain full diet and medication history.

 8. Location, frequency, quality, duration, timing of pain. Does it wake child from sleep?

 9. Any regurgitation or vomiting? Hematemesis, coffee ground–like emesis?

 10. Frequency, consistency of stools. Any melena or hematochezia?

E. Physical findings.

 1. Height, weight: Plot on growth curve and compare with previous.

 2. Temperature, vital signs.

 3. Full physical exam with attention to following:

  a. HEENT: Assess for dental caries, enamel erosion.

  b. Abdomen: Assess for tenderness, masses, hepatosplenomegaly.

  c. Rectal: Perform digital exam. Assess for fissures.

F. Diagnostic tests.

 1. Physical exam: CBC (anemia); comprehensive metabolic panel, amylase, lipase; urinalysis and urine culture.

 2. Test stool for occult blood.

 3. Upper GI series: to assess anatomy in child with vomiting. Little value in diagnosing ulcers or gastritis in children.

 4. *H. pylori* serology: unreliable in children, not recommended. *H. pylori* stool antigen: fairly reliable for diagnosis of current infection.

 5. Endoscopy with biopsies (test of choice) to diagnose *H. pylori* and PUD.

G. Differential diagnosis.

Crohn's disease, 555.9

Secondary peptic ulcer disease, 533.9

Helicobacter pylori infections, 041.86

1. *H. pylori* infections: reliable diagnosis in children by upper endoscopy.
2. Secondary PUD:
   a. Medication: history of NSAID, aspirin, corticosteroid use, and others.
   b. Trauma/stress PUD: history of burns, trauma, surgery.
   c. Caustic ingestion/ETOH.
   d. Crohn's disease: History may include growth problems, diarrhea, blood in stool.
H. Treatment.
1. *H. pylori*: 14 days of amoxicillin and Biaxin (Clarithromycin) and at least 1 month of proton pump inhibitor (e.g., Prevacid [Lansoprazole]).
2. Secondary PUD.
   a. Discontinue offending medication/caustic substance. If on corticosteroids to treat another disease, may wean or give acid-reducing medicine until therapy complete.
   b. Gastritis/PUD can be treated first with H2 blocker (Zantac [Rantadine], Pepcid [Farnotidine]). If no response in 7–14 days, can increase therapy to PPI.
   c. History of upper GI bleed, melena, hematochezia requires referral to tertiary care facility/consultation of MD before therapy.
   d. Treat iron-deficiency anemia.
I. Follow up.
1. *H. pylori*: follow-up testing (repeat endoscopy) for patients symptomatic after treatment. Other methods can be unreliable or not approved for children.
2. Return to clinic 1 month after treatment started for nonspecific/suspected PUD.
3. Immediate return for any worsening symptoms.
J. Complications.

Anemia, chronic iron deficiency, 280.9	Massive gastrointestinal bleed, 578.9
Gastric cancer, 151.9	Perforation, 531.6
Helicobacter pylori, 041.86	

---

1. *H. pylori* (chronic colonization carries theoretical risk of developing gastric cancer).
2. Massive GI bleed/perforation.
3. Chronic iron-deficiency anemia.
K. Education.
1. *H. pylori* not common in children, communicability low. Increased risk among household contacts of others with this infection.

2. Explain that because differentiating between GERD and PUD is difficult, if no response to treatment with acid-reducing medication, possible endoscopy may be necessary.
3. Employ conservative management for symptoms, such as dietary restrictions.

XIV. PINWORMS (ENTEROBIASIS)

Perianal erythema, 695.9	Pinworms (enterobiasis), 127.4
Perianal irritation, 569.49	Sleeplessness, 780.52

A. Etiology.
1. Humans only known hosts for this obligate parasite; ingest embryonated eggs, which hatch in stomach. Larvae migrate to cecum area where mature into adult worms.
2. Adult worms are about 1 cm in length. Females migrate by night to perianal region to deposit eggs.
3. Ova mature after approximately 6 hours. Larvae viable for about 20 days.
4. Eggs carried under fingernails, transmitted directly to another human or deposited in environment (dust, bed clothes) where others come in contact. Autoinfection/reinfection common; highly communicable.
B. Occurrence.
1. Highest prevalence in children 5–14 years of age.
2. Increased incidence in crowded living conditions, among family members of infected patients, in institutions.
C. Clinical manifestations.
1. Anal pruritus, especially nocturnal (most likely from female pinworm depositing eggs).
2. Sleeplessness.
3. Perianal irritation/erythema may occur (most likely from scratching).
D. Physical findings.
1. Child should appear well. Physical exam normal or nonspecific perianal irritation.
E. Diagnostic tests.
1. Cellophane tape test.
    a. Adult worms sometimes visualized in evening around anus using flashlight: white, thread-like moving worm.
    b. Essentially diagnostic, specimen rarely required.

F. Differential diagnosis.

Erythema, unspecified, 695.9

Perianal streptococcal infection, 041
---

1. Perianal streptococcal infection: anal erythema, pain. No pruritus.
G. Treatment.
    1. Vermox: children older than 2 years, adults: 100 mg (chew, crush, swallow). Repeat in 2 weeks.
    2. Consider simultaneous treatment for household contacts (except pregnant women and children younger than 2 years).
H. Follow up.
    1. As needed, not usually necessary.
    2. Consult with MD for patients younger than 2 years.
I. Complications.

Perianal irritation, 569.49
---

1. Perianal irritation/discomfort; secondary bacterial infection from scratching.
2. Rarely affects ectopic sites (i.e., female genital tract, appendix, peritoneal cavity, liver, spleen).
J. Education.
    1. Teach parent proper technique for obtaining specimen if needed.
        a. Use only clear cellophane tape. Spread buttocks early in morning, before toileting, or at night and apply tape sticky side down to perianal area.
        b. Place tape sticky side down on clear glass slide.
        c. Teach proper precautions for handling communicable specimen.
    2. Infection highly contagious and reinfection is common.
    3. Discuss strategies to avoid reinfection.
        a. Keep fingernails very short. Frequent handwashing, especially with toileting.
        b. Wash bedclothes, underwear daily; handle with precaution. Bathe daily.
        c. Discourage child from scratching anus and from placing fingers in mouth.
    4. Infections are spread only human to human. Cannot be spread by pets.
    5. Eggs are viable in environment for several days or longer.
    6. Discuss importance of second dose of medication at 2 weeks.
    7. Reassure about benign nature of the infection.
    8. Treatment side effects include abdominal pain, diarrhea.

XV. VIRAL GASTROENTERITIS

Abdominal cramps, 789	Headache, 784
Dehydration, 276.5	Muscle aches, 729.1
Diarrhea, 787.9	Viral gastroenteritis, 008.8
Fever, 780.6	Vomiting, 787.03

A. Viral infection of GI tract.
B. Etiology.
  1. Caused by several viruses, mainly:
     a. Rotavirus: highly contagious, incubation period 1–3 days. Spread by fecal–oral route. Most common viral cause.
     b. Adenovirus: second most common cause, mainly children younger than 2 years. Incubation period: 8–10 days.
     c. Norwalk group: mainly older children, adults. Main cause of viral gastroenteritis epidemics. Highly contagious, fecal–oral route. From contaminated food, water, or person to person.
  2. Osmotic diarrhea usually results from carbohydrate malabsorption, increased fluid/salts in intestines.
C. Occurrence.
  1. Rotavirus most common cause of severe, dehydrating diarrhea in infants/young children. Occurs mainly during winter months.
  2. Adenovirus can occur year-round, slight increase in summer months.
  3. Norwalk can occur year-round.
D. Clinical manifestations.
  1. Watery diarrhea most common symptom. Vomiting and fever common.
  2. Rotavirus may cause severe, watery diarrhea for 5–7 days.
  3. Adenovirus diarrhea may last for 1–2 weeks with/without vomiting at onset. May be associated with low-grade fever.
  4. Norwalk may cause acute-onset vomiting, abdominal cramps, diarrhea for 1–2 days. Vomiting main symptom in children; can have fever, headache, muscle aches.
  5. Pertinent history to obtain:
     a. Onset of symptoms, sudden? Any sick contacts? Fever history?
     b. Stools: consistency, frequency, quantity, history of melena/hematochezia.
     c. Vomiting: frequency, quantity, quality. Contain bile or blood?
     d. Abdominal pain, cramping: frequency, duration, relation to stools.
     e. Complete diet and medication history.

E. Physical findings.
1. Weight, temperature, vital signs.
2. Assess hydration status and level of activity.
3. Complete physical exam with attention to abdomen (tenderness, guarding, masses) and rectal (perianal irritation, diaper rash from diarrhea).
F. Diagnostic tests.
1. Not usually necessary.
2. Rotavirus/adenovirus diagnosed using commercially available kit.
3. If dehydrated: serum electrolytes.
G. Differential diagnosis.

| Bacterial infection, 041.9 |
| Giardia, 007.1 |

1. Parasite infection (giardia, campylobacter).
2. Bacterial infection.
H. Treatment.
1. Supportive care: prevent/correct dehydration.
I. Follow up.
1. Return to clinic if any increased symptoms or signs of dehydration.
J. Complications.

| Dehydration, 276.5 |
| Diaper rash, 691 |

1. Dehydration.
2. Diaper rash.
K. Education.
1. Reassure family about self-limited nature of viral gastroenteritis.
2. Review signs/symptoms of dehydration with family.
3. Discuss communicability, precautions (handwashing, handling of soiled objects).

XVI. VOMITING, ACUTE

Abdominal pain, 789	Hematochezia, 578.1
Diarrhea, 787.91	Joint pain, 719.4
Dysuria, 788.1	Melena, 578.1
Headache, 784	Vomiting, acute, 787.03

A. Forceful expulsion of stomach contents through mouth. Highly coordinated reflex; can be symptom of disease within or outside GI tract.

B. Etiology.
   1. Common symptom of infection such as gastroenteritis. Can also be from infection outside GI tract such as UTI, otitis media, other systemic infections.
   2. Different from regurgitation-type emesis (nonforceful), common sign of GERD.
   3. Additional etiologies vary by age:
      a. Infant: overfeeding, mechanical obstruction (pyloric stenosis, malrotation, volvulus), necrotizing enterocolitis, Hirschsprung's disease, intussusception, cow's milk protein allergy.
      b. Child: appendicitis, sinusitis, toxic ingestions, gastritis, mechanical obstruction (foreign body, malrotation).
      c. Adolescent: appendicitis, sinusitis, toxic ingestion, inflammatory bowel disease (IBD), migraine, pregnancy, bulimia.

C. Occurrence.
   1. Common pediatric symptom.
   2. Infection is one of most common medical causes of nonbilious vomiting in first year of life, usually acute gastroenteritis.

D. Clinical manifestations.
   1. Usually forceful, may be preceded by nausea, increased salivation, retching.
      a. Describe vomiting and symptoms preceding it.
      b. How often is child vomiting? When did it first begin?
      c. Any bile staining or hematemesis?
      d. How soon after oral intake does vomiting occur?
   2. Ask about possible associated symptoms:
      a. Fever? How is it treated? Any headache, body aches, joint pain?
      b. Describe stools; any diarrhea? Any melena or hematochezia?
      c. Is child continuing to urinate? Any dysuria or frequency?
      d. Any URI symptoms, cough, ear, throat pain? Abdominal pain?
   3. Diet history:
      a. Type, quantity of fluids, foods.
      b. History of ingestion of contaminated food?
      c. Medications/drugs or toxic ingestion history?
      d. Exposure to others with similar symptoms?

E. Physical findings.
   1. Weight, compare with previous measurements.
   2. Temperature, vital signs.

3. Assess level of activity; does child appear ill?
4. Complete physical exam with attention to:
    a. Abdomen: Assess for distention, guarding, tenderness, masses.
    b. Hydration status.
    c. Rectal exam: Observe for any abnormalities, digital exam may be necessary to check for occult blood.
    d. CNS: Assess fontanel. Assess for irritability, nuchal rigidity, Brudzinski and Kernig's signs, funduscopic exam.
F. Diagnostic tests.
    1. If child appears ill, dehydrated: serum electrolytes, CBC.
    2. If bilious vomiting, consider upper GI series to rule out mechanical obstruction.
    3. Projectile vomiting in infant younger than 5 months: abdominal ultrasound to rule out pyloric stenosis.
    4. Abdominal flat-plate X-ray: if ingested radiopaque foreign body/bezoar suspected.
    5. Urinalysis with specific gravity.
    6. Other tests to be determined by history, physical exam.
G. Differential diagnosis.

Bulimia, 783.6	Pneumonia, 486
Hirschsprung's disease, 751.3	Pregnancy, 643.9
Inflammatory bowel disease, 558.9	Pyloric stenosis, 537
Medication overdose, 977.9	Upper respiratory tract infection, 456.9
Metabolic, 277.9	Urinary tract infection, 599
Migraine, 346.9	Viral gastroenteritis, 008.8
Overfeeding, 783.6	

1. Infection: usually associated with fever/all ages: viral gastroenteritis, UTI, pneumonia, upper respiratory tract infections (otitis media, sinusitis, pharyngitis).
2. Mechanical: pyloric stenosis, infants, malrotation/volvulus (infants, children: bilious vomiting, abdominal pain, anorexia), foreign body ingestion or bezoar (children), Hirschsprung's disease (infants: delayed passage of meconium, constipation).
3. Metabolic: inborn errors of metabolism (infants, rare).
4. CNS: migraine (children, adolescents: headache, photophobia, family history common), brain tumor (rare), labyrinthitis.
5. Medication overdose, reaction, toxic ingestion (including lead).
6. Overfeeding (infants): normal physical exam, review feeding techniques.

7. Pregnancy: consider in postmenarchal girls.
8. Bulimia.
9. Inflammatory bowel disease (child, adolescent): Crohn's disease, ulcerative colitis. Hematochezia, melena, abdominal pain, diarrhea, weight loss, anemia.

H. Treatment.
1. Treat, prevent dehydration.
   a. Mild–moderate dehydration: oral rehydrate solution 5 mL every 1–5 minutes plus replacement of estimated volume of emesis. Mild dehydration: goal 50 mL/kg + losses over 4 hours. Moderate: 100 mL/kg + losses over 4 hours, reassess hourly.
   b. Severe dehydration: emergency department or admission for IV fluids. Start with normal saline or lactated Ringer's solution at 10–20 mL/kg over 1 hour.
2. As vomiting decreases, offer larger amounts of ORS at less frequent intervals.
3. After rehydration, other fluids including milk, food may be reintroduced.
4. Antiemetic medications are generally not warranted/recommended.

I. Follow up.
1. No/mild dehydration: Telephone next day.
2. Moderate dehydration: See patient next day.
3. Immediate return if increased symptoms, signs of dehydration.
4. Severe dehydration requires visit following discharge from emergency department/hospital.

J. Complications.

Dehydration, 276.5

Mallory-Weiss tear, 530.7

---

1. Dehydration.
2. Mallory-Weiss tear (linear tear at gastroesophageal junction from repeated vomiting): fresh red blood in emesis after multiple episodes of vomiting.
3. Other complications depend on etiology.

K. Education.
1. Most cases of acute vomiting are from viral gastroenteritis.
2. Can be successfully treated at home if no signs of or mild dehydration.
3. Review dehydration signs/symptoms with family, reassure most cases self-limited.
4. Repeated vomiting can induce reflux of bile into stomach resulting in bile staining.

BIBLIOGRAPHY

Aiken JJ. Inguinal hernias. In: Kleigman, RM, Behrman RE, Jensen HB, et al., eds. *Nelson textbook of pediatrics.* 18th ed. Philadelphia, PA: Saunders Elsevier; 2007.

Baker SS, et al. Evaluation and treatment of constipation in infants and children: recommendations of the North American Society for Pediatric Gastroenterology, Hepatology and Nutrition. *J Pediatr Gastroenterol Nutr.* 2006;43:e1–e13.

Bhutta, ZA. Gastroenteritis. In: Kleigman RM, Behrman RE, Jensen HB, et al., eds. *Nelson textbook of pediatrics.* 18th ed. Philadelphia, PA: Saunders Elsevier; 2007.

Blanchard, SS, et al. Peptic ulcer disease in children. In: Kliegman RM, Behrman RE, Senson HB, et al., eds. *Nelson textbook of pediatrics.* 18th ed. Philadelphia, PA: Saunders Elsevier; 2007.

Ellett, M. What is known about infant colic? *Gastroenterology Nursing.* 2003;26(2):60–67.

Gold BD, et al. Helicobacter pylori infection in children: recommendations for diagnosis and treatment. *J Pediatr Gastroenterol Nutr.* 2000;31:490–497.

Hyman, P, et al. Childhood functional gastrointestinal disorders: neonate/toddler. *Gastroenterology.* 2006;130(5):1519–1526.

Ishimine P. Abdominal pain, acute. In: Zorc JJ, ed. *Schwartz's clinical handbook of pediatrics,* 4th ed. Philadelphia: Lippincott, Williams & Wilkins; 2009.

King C, et al. Managing acute gastroenteritis among children: oral rehydration, maintenance, and nutritional therapy. *Morb Mortal Weekly Rep.* 2003;52(16):1–16.

Liacouras CA. Vomiting. In: Zorc JJ, ed. *Schwartz's clinical handbook of pediatrics,* 4th ed. Philadelphia, PA: Lippincott, Williams & Wilkins; 2009.

Rasquin A, DiLorenzo C, et al. Childhood functional gastrointestinal disorders: child/adolescent. *Gastroenterology.* 2006;130(5):1527–1537.

Scholl J, Jackson-Allen P. A primary care approach to functional abdominal pain. *Pediatr Nursing.* 2007;33(3):247–259.

Vandenplas Y, Rudolph C, et al. Pediatric gastroesophageal reflux clinical practice guidelines: joint recommendations of the North Amercian Society for Pediatric Gastroenterology, Hepatology and Nutrition (NASPGHAN) and the Euorpean Society for Pediatric Gastroenterology, Hepatology and Nutrition (ESPGHAN). *Journal of Pediatric Gastroenterology and Nutrition.* 2009;49(4):498–547.

Vernacchio L, et al. Characteristics of persistent diarrhea in a community-based cohort of young US children. *Journal of Pediatric Gastroenterology and Nutrition.* 2006;43(1):52–58.

Wiley CC. Diarrhea, acute. In: Zorc JJ, ed. *Schwartz's clinical handbook of pediatrics,* 4th ed. Philadelphia, PA: Lippincott, Williams & Wilkins; 2009.

Wyllie R: Pyloric stenosis and congenital anomalies of the stomach. In: Kliegman RM, Behrman RE, Senson HB, et al., eds. *Nelson textbook of pediatrics.* 18th ed. Philadelphia, PA: Saunders Elsevier; 2007.

Young RJ, Philichi L, eds. *Clinical handbook of pediatric gastroenterology.* St. Louis, MO: Quality Medical Publishing; 2008.

Genitourinary Disorders

Shelly J. King

I. MALE GENITALIA DISORDERS

Absent testicle, 752.59	Hypospadias, 752.61
Congenital adrenal hyperplasia, 255.2	Intersexuality, 752.7
Cryptorchidism, 785.51	Retractile testicles, 752.52
Disorders of male genitalia, 608.9	

A. Cryptorchidism.
B. Etiology/incidence.
   1. Cryptorchid testes can be absent, undescended, ectopic.
   2. Can be result of chromosomal, hormonal, anatomic factors.
   3. Majority (about 80%): palpable, are undescended or ectopic testes. Retractile testes: also palpable, sometimes misdiagnosed as undescended. Nonpalpable (20%) can be intra-abdominal, inguinal, absent testes.
C. Occurrence.
   1. Most common male congenital anomaly, affects nearly 1% of term infants.
D. Clinical manifestations.
   1. Risk of cryptorchidism increases in premature infant.
   2. Bilateral nonpalpable testes or cryptorchid testes associated with hypospadias should be evaluated at birth for life-threatening intersex conditions such as congenital adrenal hyperplasia.
   3. Parents may note retractile testicles in scrotum intermittently, especially after warm bath. Retractile testes are associated with an overactive cremasteric reflex. When examined they can be placed in the scrotum and will remain there for a short time after released. If they retract immediately they should be considered undescended.
   4. In case of absent testicle, contralateral testicle may be larger than expected.

E. Physical findings.
1. Often helpful to have child in cross-legged sitting position for exam.
2. Retractile testes can be placed into scrotum, remain there for short period.
3. Nonpalpable testes maybe ectopic, found in femoral or perineal regions.
4. Scrotum may be flat/underdeveloped on affected side.
5. Larger than expected testicle may represent absent or nonfunctioning testicle on contralateral side.
F. Diagnostic tests.
1. Unilateral or bilateral palpable testes: No diagnostic testing indicated.
2. Bilateral nonpalpable testes or unilateral nonpalpable testes associated with phallic abnormality: Evaluate with karyotype, endocrine testing, appropriate radiographic studies.
   a. Human chorionic gonadotropin (hCG) stimulation test differentiates between anorchia and undescended testicles.
   b. hCG can stimulate testosterone production in functioning testes and can also result in testicular descent.
G. Differential diagnosis.

Intersex conditions, 752.7

Retractile testes, 752.52
---

1. Retractile testes.
2. Intersex conditions.
H. Treatment.
1. If at 6 months of age testes remain undescended, intervention is necessary.
   a. Type of treatment depends on testes' location, patient's age, association with other anomalies.
   b. Reasons for treatment: reduced fertility, risk of tumor formation, trauma, torsion, repair of commonly associated defects such as inguinal hernia, psychological factors related to body image.
2. Placing testes into scrotum does not decrease risk of testicular cancer but does provide easy exam for early detection. Risk of testes cancer in cryptorchid male is 1 in 2000.
3. Orchiopexy or open surgery fixes testicle in scrotum and repairs hernia if needed. Laparoscopy can be used to locate nonpalpable testes or blind-ending vessels. There is also laparoscopic approach to orchiopexy.
4. Hormone administration is not as successful as surgical approach but good option in high-risk patients and/or patients who have testes found in high scrotum or at external inguinal ring.

I. Follow up.
    1. After surgery, examine incisions at 2–4 weeks, 4–6 months postop.
    2. Hormonal therapy: Examine at 1 month, 6 months post-treatment (higher risk of reascension).
    3. Yearly exam important; patient should be taught self-exam at puberty. Can be performed by local medical provider or pediatric urologist.
       a. Asymmetry of testes needs further evaluation.
    4. Retractile testes should be evaluated annually for possible ascension.
J. Complications.

Testicular atrophy, 608.3
---

    1. Testicular atrophy is rated most serious complication of orchiopexy.
K. Education.
    1. All males need to be taught self-scrotal exam at puberty. Especially important with history of undescended testicle due to increased risk of cancer.
    2. Prior to puberty, annual exam should be done. Scrotal pain needs to be evaluated immediately to rule out risk of testicular torsion, trauma, epididymitis, torsed testicular appendage.

II. HYDROCELE

Hernia, 553.9	Scrotal swelling, 608.86
Hydrocele, 603.9	Processus vaginalis, 616.1
Intersexuality, 752.7	

A. Etiology.
    1. Occurs when processus vaginalis (channel that allows testicle to move from abdomen to scrotum during development) remains patent.
    2. Difference between hernia and hydrocele is size of patent processus vaginalis and its contents.
       a. Narrow channel only allows fluid from peritoneal cavity to pass, resulting in hydrocele.
       b. Inguinal hernia: much wider, can allow both fluid and intestinal contents to pass.
B. Occurrence.
    1. About 80% of infants are born with patent processus vaginalis; by end of first month of life, decreases to about 60%.

2. By 18–24 months of age, only 20–30% remain.
3. Rare in females: 6 males to 1 female.
C. Clinical manifestations.
  1. Females: rare, usually presents with soft bulge in labia or inguinal canal.
    a. Bulge can represent ovary or hernia.
    b. Intersex conditions (especially testicular feminization): evaluate in female.
  2. Males: parents complain of scrotal swelling in one or both sides. Can be continuous or intermittent; size can fluctuate.
    a. Parent may describe bluish hue to scrotum, often small in size in morning and growing larger during day as fluid accumulates.
    b. History is very important because may not be present at time of exam.
D. Physical findings.
  1. Hydroceles typically transilluminate with penlight to scrotum.
  2. Palpate testicle; if testicle cannot be palpated, can be seen by transillumination. If testes not seen or palpated, need scrotal ultrasound to differentiate.
  3. Classified as communicating (patent processus vaginalis) or noncommunicating. Almost all congenital hydroceles are communicating. Noncommunicating hydroceles do not fluctuate in size.
  4. Condition rarely painful unless associated with hernia that becomes incarcerated.
E. Diagnostic tests.
  1. If any concern regarding testes, ultrasound imaging is indicated.
F. Differential diagnosis.

Ectopic testes, 752.51	Inguinal hernia, 550.9
Epididymitis, 604.9	Retractile testes, 752.52

  1. Inguinal hernia.
  2. Epididymitis.
  3. Retractile testes.
  4. Ectopic testes.
  5. Absent testes.
G. Treatment.
  1. Generally safe to watch hydroceles until 18–24 months. After that age spontaneous resolution is uncommon.
  2. Earlier surgical intervention is indicated if hydrocele is large or associated with hernia secondary to increased risk of incarceration. Any abnormality of testes requires evaluation by scrotal ultrasound and could lead to earlier surgical intervention.

H. Follow up.
1. Child younger than 18 months of age should be examined every 6 months. If no change, no intervention indicated until 18–24 months.
2. If hydrocelectomy is performed, see patient 4 weeks postop to evaluate incision and scrotum. If exam is normal, can return to routine annual exam with healthcare provider.
I. Complications.

Hydrocele, 603.9	Testicular atrophy, 608.3
Incarcerated hernia, 552.9	Processus vaginalis, 616.1

1. Complications from hydroceles are rare.
2. Risk of incarcerated hernia in patients with wide patent processus vaginalis.
3. Postoperative complications are rare; include recurrent hydrocele, testicular atrophy, lysis of vas deferens.
J. Education.
1. Although hydroceles and hernias are not really associated with increased risk of testicular cancer, discuss importance of self-scrotal exam.
2. Teach parents importance of regular exam during observation period.
3. If any scrotal pain, child needs to be seen immediately.

III. EPIDIDYMITIS

Chlamydia, 079.98	Neisseria gonorrhea, 098
Disorders of male genitalia, 608.9	Neurogenic bladder, 596.54
Dysuria, 788.1	Orchitis, 604.9
Epididymitis, 604.9	Testicular torsion, 608.2
Exstrophy, 753.5	Urethral discharge, 788.7
Imperforate anus, 751.2	Torsed appendix testes, 608.2

A. Etiology.
1. Epididymitis refers to edema, irritation of epididymis or lining of testicle.
2. Can occur from infectious/inflammatory cause.
3. Can be difficult to distinguish epididymitis from testicular torsion because both can be quite painful.
4. Can be sexually acquired; Neisseria gonorrhoeae and Chlamydia are common pathogens.
5. Can be related to genitourinary abnormalities or urethra manipulation.

      6.   Rarely associated with heavy lifting or straining that result in efflux of urine into vas deferens. If urine is infectious, then bacterial epididymitis can occur; if not, chemical inflammation develops.

B. Occurrence.
    1.   Rare in children before puberty unless child has genitourinary abnormality.
    2.   More commonly occurs in sexually active adolescents.

C. Clinical manifestations.
    1.   Most likely to occur in postpubertal male and very young males.
    2.   Those with imperforate anus, exstrophy, neurogenic bladder, any conditions requiring intermittent catheterization are more prone to this type of infection.

D. Physical findings.
    1.   Include sexual history in postpubertal male.
    2.   Urethral discharge may be present.
    3.   Often slow onset of pain that continues to become more severe.
    4.   May have dysuria and see blood or discharge in urine.
    5.   Physical exam yields swollen and inflamed scrotum.
    6.   May complain of tenderness along epididymis.
    7.   If testicle is tender and swollen, may also have orchitis.
    8.   Up to 33% may be febrile.

E. Diagnostic tests.
    1.   Urine culture and urinalysis may be positive or negative for bacteria. If positive then X-ray evaluation by voiding cystourethrogram (VCUG) and renal-bladder ultrasound is indicated.
    2.   Scrotal ultrasound with Doppler flow is useful in differentiating epididymitis from testicular torsion. Ultrasound will show enlarged epididymis with increased blood flow unless edema is so severe it results in ischemia. May also show enlarged testicle with increased low flow in orchitis.

F. Differential diagnosis.

Bacterial epididymitis, 604.9	Torsion of testicular appendage, 608.2
Chemical epididymitis, 604.9	Urinary tract infections, 599
Testicular torsion, 608.2	Orchitis 604.9
Henoch-Schönlein purpura inflammatory vasculitis, 287	

    1.   Testicular torsion.
    2.   Chemical epididymitis.

3. Bacterial epididymitis.
4. Torsion of testicular appendage.
5. Urinary tract infection (UTI).

G. Treatment.
1. Start 2 weeks of appropriate broad-spectrum antibiotic while cultures are pending. If necessary, change appropriately when cultures are final.
   a. Children not sexually active: cephalexin: 40 mg/kg/day in 2 divided doses. Can also use:
      - Ampicillin: 50 mg/kg bid.
      - Trimethoprim-sulfamethoxazole (TMP-SMX): older than 2 months of age: 4 mg/kg and 20 mg/kg bid.
      - Ciprofloxacin: 15 mg/kg bid postpuberty. Quinolone clinical trials are evaluating the safety and efficacy of use in children. Some clinical situations may warrant off-label use.
2. Ibuprofen for several days will help decrease inflammation, pain.
3. Scrotal support and elevating scrotum will help resolve edema.
4. Limited activity for 2–3 days.
5. Application of heat/cold compresses help reduce pain and edema.
6. If pain and edema are severe or not responding to treatment, consider IV antibiotics. Prolonged infection can result in damage to epididymis.
7. Identified STD should be treated with appropriate antibiotic regimen.

H. Follow up.
1. If pain increases, see patient immediately.
2. If condition is resolving, follow up in 2 weeks with repeat ultrasonography.
3. If positive urine cultures, a VCUG and renal–bladder ultrasound should be done. Increased likelihood of genitourinary abnormalities in males with positive urine cultures. Prophylactic antibiotics should be given until radiographic evaluation is complete (see UTI section).

I. Complications.
1. Possible damage to vas deferens, epididymis with recurrent or untreated infection.

J. Education.
1. Preventive education especially when epididymitis is associated with sexually transmitted infections (STIs).
2. Signs/symptoms of testicular torsion and acute scrotum indicate need for immediate attention by medical professional.
3. Genitourinary abnormalities can be associated with urinary infections so follow up with necessary testing.

IV. HYPOSPADIAS/CHORDEE

Disorders of male genitalia, 608.9

Hypospadias, 752.61

Chordee, 607.89

A. Etiology/incidence.
 1. Cause of hypospadias is unknown; genetic link is suspected (many families with multiple occurrences).
 2. Hypospadias is a congenital anomaly in which urethral meatus is ectopic; it is located on the undersurface of the penis any place between the glans and the scrotum.
 3. Spectrum defect ranging from mild to severe, depending on degree of chordee (bend of penis), location of urethral opening. Mild forms can be found during newborn circumcision; stop circumcision—foreskin used to repair defect.
B. Occurrence.
 1. Occurs in 1/250 of males in United States, 1/100 if immediate family history.
C. Clinical manifestations.
 1. Difficult for older child to stand to urinate.
 2. If associated with chordee, future intercourse may be difficult.
 3. Parental anxiety/guilt common with genital malformation.
D. Physical findings.
 1. Urethral opening lies on undersurface of penis.
 2. Degrees of hypospadias: distal shaft refers to opening being closest to natural location.
    a. As opening gets closer to scrotum, condition becomes more severe.
    b. Referred to as midshaft, penoscrotal (located at penoscrotal junction), and perineal (located just beneath scrotum).
 3. Chordee or bend of penis is often present.
 4. Foreskin typically seen only on dorsal side of penis, gives "hooded" appearance.
 5. Penile glans has spade-like appearance and cleft/blind-ending pit may be seen at location where meatus would normally reside.
 6. Cryptorchidism may be associated.
E. Diagnostic tests.
 1. Rarely necessary with hypospadias.
 2. Early referral to experienced pediatric urologist important: Allay fears about child's masculinity, opportunity to assess for intersex disorders

(uncommon but considered with severe hypospadias and hypospadias associated with cryptorchidism).

3. In some of more extensive cases, urinary tract will need to be evaluated.

F. Differential diagnosis.

Intersexuality, 752.7
---

1. Intersex disorders.

G. Treatment.
1. Referral to pediatric urologist as soon after birth as possible (reassure parents after surgical intervention child's potency/fertility no longer affected; makes it easier to discuss problem with other family members).
2. More than 200 surgical techniques described for hypospadias repair.
   a. Goals same in each repair; cosmetically normal-appearing penis, straight with urethral meatus at tip. Repairs are performed in healthy males as early as 6 months of age.
   b. Patient should be able to stand to void.
   c. Selected cases may require preadministration of testosterone to enhance blood supply to genitalia.
   d. Most surgery is done on outpatient basis.
   e. Many approaches to postoperative dressing. Absorbable sutures are used in repairs, will not need to be removed.
   f. Stent may be left through urethra to drain bladder while urethra heals. Nonabsorbable suture may be used to hold stent in place, will need to be removed about 1 week postop.

H. Follow up.
1. See in 1 week to inspect incision, remove any dressings, stent if necessary.
2. See again 2–3 months later, after majority of edema is resolved, to ensure penis is straight, meatus is widely open.
3. Some surgeons schedule visit after toilet training to visualize normal voiding stream; others see child after puberty to discuss surgery, alleviate fears.
4. If ever difficulty voiding or UTI, patient should be seen immediately by pediatric urologist.

I. Complications.

GU hematoma, 863.8	Urethral stricture, 598.9
Meatal stenosis residual chordee, 607.89	Urethrocutaneous fistula, 599.1
Urethral diverticulum, 599.2	Wound infection, 958.3

    1. Experienced hypospadiac surgeon is important to minimize complications.
    2. Rate of complication varies according to severity of defect.
       a. Early postoperative complications: uncommon but include wound infection, urethrocutaneous fistula, hematoma.
       b. Late complications: urethral stricture, meatal stenosis residual chordee, urethral diverticulum.
       c. If secondary procedure necessary, not performed until tissues well healed—approximately 6 months after initial repair.
J. Education.
    1. Important to educate newborn-care providers not to circumcise if any penile defects: Foreskin is used for repair.
    2. Understanding defect and its correction can alleviate parental fears. Reassure them child's masculinity not affected; structural problem that can be corrected surgically.
    3. Patient must understand potential for complications. Any difficulty voiding or urinary tract infection need follow up with pediatric urologist.

V. FEMALE GENITALIA DISORDERS

Disorders of female genitalia, 629.9	Incontinence, 788.31
Dysuria, 788.1	Labial adhesions, 752.49

A. Etiology.
    1. Labial adhesions are fusion of labia minora, occur as result of vulvar irritation, lack of estrogen.
    2. Possible causes: chronic inflammation, irritation secondary to infection, trauma, incontinence.
B. Occurrence.
    1. Primarily in girls 3 months to 6 years of age.
C. Clinical manifestations.
    1. Dysuria and incontinence are common complaints when efflux of urine is blocked and urine is trapped behind adhesions.
    2. Toilet-trained girls may complain of postvoid dribbling. Maternal estrogens seem to prevent adhesions in newborns.
D. Physical findings.
    1. Labial adhesions appear as thin film that begins posteriorly and advance anteriorly.
    2. In more severe cases, cannot see vaginal introitus or urethral meatus.

      3.   Presence of scarring that deviates from midline or more dense adhesions should raise question of repeat trauma/sexual abuse.

E. Diagnostic tests.

      1.   None.

F. Differential diagnosis.

Intersexuality, 752.7

Sexual abuse, 995.53

---

      1.   Intersex conditions.

      2.   Sexual abuse.

G. Treatment.

      1.   Majority requires no treatment, resolve spontaneously.

          a.   Keep child clean and dry to prevent irritation and superficial infection.

      2.   More significant adhesions that present with dysuria and postvoid dribbling can be treated with hormone cream or lysis of adhesions.

          a.   Premarin cream: 0.625 mg applied with gentle pressure to the translucent midline twice a day for 10–14 days.

          b.   Betamethasone cream 0.05% bid can be used up to 4 weeks.

      3.   Lysis of thinned adhesions can be done in office after EMLA cream application.

      4.   More dense-appearing adhesions or those that have been broken down previously may be done more effectively and with less trauma in operating room. Critical to prevent readherence by applying barrier cream to previously attached tissues twice a day for 8–12 weeks.

H. Follow up.

      1.   No treatment: Follow up with each well-child check, may become more severe with time (best obtained by urethral catheterization).

      2.   If complaints of dysuria: Careful collection of urine specimen is important; it is difficult to collect valid specimen by voiding when adhesions are present (catheterization preferred).

      3.   Post-treatment: See patient 4–6 weeks later to ensure no reoccurrence.

I. Complications.

Urinary tract infections (UTI), 599

---

      1.   Biggest risk is reoccurrence due to poor parental compliance with barrier cream placement after adhesions have been lysed.

      2.   If painful voiding, child may delay voiding, empty more poorly resulting in true UTIs.

3. Prolonged use of estrogen can result in development of secondary sex characteristics.

J. Education.

1. Importance of post-treatment management must be stressed to parents; most important in preventing further problems with adhesions. Sometimes difficult for parents, especially if child complains of discomfort when medication is applied.
2. Child should learn to void with legs widely separated to facilitate good bladder emptying and to keep labia separated during voiding.
3. If urine specimen necessary, take care to avoid contamination; done best by catheterization.
4. Parents understand length of Premarin treatment; possible side effects of prolonged or repeated use.

VI. PEDIATRIC URINARY TRACT INFECTIONS

Constipation, 564	Nausea, 787.02
Diarrhea, 787.91	Poor feeding, 783.3
Dysuria, 788.1	Suprapubic/urethral pain, 788
Fever, 780.6	Urinary frequency, 788.41
Flank pain, 789	Urinary tract infections, 599
Incontinence, 788.31	Vomiting, 787.03
Irritability, 799.2	

A. Etiology.
1. Periurethral bacteria infect bladder, ureter, kidney. *Escherichia coli* most frequently identified pathogen.

B. Occurrence.
1. Fairly common: 2.4% of children yearly, majority are ascending.
2. Up to 6 months of age, more common in males than females, incidence of 2 cases per 100 live births. Uncircumcised males less than 6 months old have a tenfold increased risk for UTI development.
3. After 1 year of age, much more common in females.
4. Approximately 3% of toilet-trained females will develop infection.
   a. Of children who develop infection, 17% will develop infection-related renal scarring.
   b. Of those, 10–20% will have hypertension.

C. Clinical manifestations.
  1. Symptoms of UTI in infants often difficult to recognize.
  2. Usually generalized illness with fever, irritability, poor feeding, vomiting, diarrhea. Suspect when no other source for illness.
  3. Older children complain of dysuria, suprapubic/urethral pain, urinary frequency, incontinence. Can also have fever, flank pain, nausea, vomiting if kidney is involved.
  4. Foul-smelling urine, constipation (commonly associated, obtain stool history).
D. Physical findings.
  1. Perform thorough exam.
  2. May detect renal mass in infants with gross anatomic abnormalities such as obstruction or mass.
  3. Costal-vertebral angle (CVA) tenderness seen while palpating flank of older children.
  4. If dysuria is primary concern, perineal exam may show external irritation related to incontinence, vaginal voiding, labial adhesions.
  5. Sometimes treated as UTIs: vaginitis and pinworms sometimes mistaken (because often present with dysuria).
  6. Vaginal discharge: culture if present; may have suprapubic tenderness.
  7. Males: scrotal exam to rule out epididymitis, especially in older males who may be sexually active.
      a. Look for urethral discharge; culture if present.
      b. UTIs younger than 6 months of age are very uncommon, need evaluation.
      c. Abdominal exam may also yield large stool burden; constipation very common in children with UTIs.
E. Diagnostic tests.
  1. Collecting urine specimen is very important in documenting infection. Four techniques for obtaining a specimen are listed in **Table 27-1**.
  2. X-ray evaluation: infants, febrile UTIs, males, recurrent UTIs, children who are not toilet trained. Important that true infection is documented by catheterized culture when deciding what additional evaluation is necessary.
  3. If criteria met, then VCUG and renal–bladder ultrasound are ordered to evaluate urinary tract.
      a. Obstructions of urinary tract seen in 5–10%; 21–57% have vesicoureteral reflux.
          • If tests are negative, no additional evaluation necessary unless further problems arise.

Table 27-1 Techniques for Obtaining a Specimen

Techniques	Use for specimen	Drawbacks
Bagged specimen (baggy attached to perineum)	Helpful in ruling out UTI	If positive, catheter specimen needs to be obtained (false positives: 90%, especially if left on for 20 minutes)
Clean-catch midstream	Better collection; provides results of multiple organisms of small colony counts that are suggestive of contamination	Difficult for children (parents have a hard time cleaning, separating labia in girls); urine often hits perineum before reaching the cup
Catheterized specimen	Most widely accepted technique for determining true UTIs	Some offices not set up to catheterize children
Urinalysis	Provides information on leukocytes and nitrates (positive nitrates is highly predictive of infection), urine culture should be sent to assess colony count, pathogens present, appropriate antibiotic treatment	
Suprapubic aspirate	Most reliable	Rarely utilized because of anxiety associated with placing needle through abdominal wall and into bladder; can be threatening to child, parent/care provider

- If tests are positive, refer to pediatric urologist for evaluation, consultation, possibly treatment.
4. In case of febrile child, serum chemistries can identify elevation in creatinine or BUN, may implicate urinary tract. CBC with elevated WBC count can indicate bacterial infection.
F. Differential diagnosis (see **Table 27-2**).
G. Treatment.
   1. Goals: Prevent renal damage, urosepsis, future infections.
      a. How goals are accomplished varies according to severity and age of patient.

Table 27-2 Urinary Tract Infections

Febrile UTIs	Afebrile UTIs
Obstruction of urinary tract, 599.6	Perineal irritation, 709.9/chemical irritation
Renal mass, 593.9	Labial adhesions, 752.49/vaginal voiding
Urosepsis, 599	Pinworms, 127.4
Pelvic inflammatory disease, 614.9	Abuse (rare)
Sexually transmitted infections	Hematuria, 599.7/hypercalciuria, 275.4

2. Infants who appear systemically ill or are less than 3 months of age should be hospitalized.
   a. Parenteral broad-spectrum antibiotics, usually aminoglycoside (e.g. gentamicin), ampicillin. Third-generation cephalosporins can also be used.
   b. Some situations can be managed with outpatient therapy:
      • Parenteral ceftriaxone if child is taking fluids well, parents are reliable enough to contact provider if condition changes.
      • Some older children can be managed as outpatients with cephalosporins, penicillins, sulfonamides. Antibiotic treatment is 7–10 days.
      • Parent involvement is very important when managing patients outside hospital; provider must have confidence in family.
   c. Continue parenteral treatment until culture, sensitivity returns and clinical picture is improving, then place child on appropriate oral antimicrobial.
   d. Quinolones are not yet approved for pediatric UTI management but clinical trials are evaluating the safety and efficacy in children. Some clinical situations may warrant limited off-label use.
   e. Nitrofurantoin is not a good antimicrobial in a systemically ill patient, does not attain high serum concentrations.
3. Lower tract or bladder infections are referred to as uncomplicated UTI.
   a. Children: 3- to 5-day course of oral antimicrobials.
   b. Nitrofurantoin: good option, provides high urinary concentration (other agents used: sulfonamides, cephalosporins, penicillins).
   c. Antibiotic prophylaxis: maintained after infection is treated to prevent infection from reoccurring before completion of X-ray evaluation. May need to be continued after X-ray evaluation: vesicoureteral

reflux, urinary tract obstruction, immunosuppression, recurrent UTIs, or less than 6 monthss of age.
- Nitrofurantoin: 1.2–2.4 mg/kg or TMP-SMX 2 mg/kg of trimethoprim once a day are common choices.
- Cephalosporins (such as cephalexin) or ampicillin: 25% treatment dose daily.
- Nitrofurantoin: Do not use until older than 1 month of age.
- TMP-SMX: Do not use until older than 2 months of age.
- Both Keflex and ampicillin can be used in newborn.
  d. Treatment must also include good oral intake of fluids, encouraging toilet-trained patient to void more frequently.
  e. If associated constipation, this must also be addressed.
- Prevents good urinary evacuation.
- Provides good medium for microbial growth.
- Dysfunctional elimination syndrome (poor emptying of bowel and bladder) is hallmark of UTIs in toilet-trained patients.
  f. Educate parent in treatment of problem.
- Urination on timed schedule usually every 2 hours with techniques for relaxation of external urinary sphincter.
- Voiding to completion with each attempt is vital to preventing further infections. Have child sit comfortably on the toilet with legs widely separated and feet supported on a footstool if they don't reach the floor. Some children sit backward on the toilet.
- Stool softeners are often necessary while working on dietary measures to prevent constipation.
  g. Perineal irritation.
- Scented soaps, bubble baths may irritate urethra, cause burning that results in disrupted urinary stream, poor emptying of bladder; discontinue in patients with recurrent UTIs.
- Covering perineum with barrier cream helps prevent burning caused from irritation especially with incontinence associated with infection.
- Vulvovaginitis can be treated with baking soda sitz bath (3 tablespoons) in a shallow tub bath daily for 1 week.

H. Follow up.
1. Follow-up culture to prove infection has resolved.
2. If X-ray evaluation is positive or if infections are recurrent: urology consult preferably with pediatric urology group. Specialist can do postvoid ultrasound/other treatments to help patient learn to empty more effectively, correct any structural abnormalities if necessary.

3. More thorough education of problems associated with infection will help family and provider.

I. Complications.

Chronic cystitis, 595.2	Incontinence, 788.31
Hypertension, 401.9	Loss of renal function, 593.9

1. Serious risks, warrants effective management.
   a. Renal scarring, loss of renal function are most serious complications.
   b. Hypertension can result from renal scaring.
   c. Chronic cystitis can result in poor functional use of bladder, sometimes incontinence.

J. Education.
   1. Understand signs/symptoms of UTIs and need for treatment/evaluation.
   2. Importance of daily antibiotic and/or stool softener (if prescribed); easy to forget to take medication.
   3. Understand dysfunctional elimination and its treatment, primarily need to empty bladder frequently to completion, to avoid constipation.
   4. Follow up critical in management of UTIs due to risk of renal sequelae.

VII. HEMATURIA

Alport syndrome, 759.89	Hemolytic uremic syndrome, 283.11
Anatomic abnormalities, 759.9	Hypercalciuria, 275.4
Benign familial hematuria, 599.7	Lupus erythematosus, 710
Calculi, 592.9	Purpura, 287
Disorders of renal parenchyma, 588.9	Sickle cell nephropathy, 583.81
Glomerulonephritis, 583.9	Urethralgia, 788.9
Hematuria, 599.7	Urinary tract infection, 599

A. Etiology/incidence.
   1. Gross hematuria (blood visible to naked eye) can originate from upper/lower urinary tract.
   2. Causes: variable; include trauma, UTI, calculi, disorders of renal parenchyma, glomerulonephritis, Alport syndrome, hypercalciuria, benign exercise-induced hematuria, anatomic abnormalities, hemolytic uremic syndrome, sickle cell nephropathy, Henoch-Schönlein purpura, Goodpasture disease, lupus erythematosus, medication toxicity/chemotherapy, urethralgia, viral bladder infections, STDs (in postpubertal child).

B. Occurrence.
   1. Common in children (unlike adults): rarely associated with neoplasm (1%).
   2. Microscopic hematuria found on routine health exam by dipstick urinalysis in 0.5–2% of school-aged children.
C. Clinical manifestations.
   1. History important in determining diagnosis.
      a. Urinary frequency, fever, dysuria may indicate infection, most common cause of blood in school-aged child's urine.
      b. May describe recent trauma.
      c. Blood in other sites (i.e., sputum/stools) may indicate blood dyscrasia.
   2. Family history: familial diseases such as hypercalciuria, Alport syndrome, calculi, structural anomalies.
   3. Hemolytic uremic syndrome, one of most common causes of acute renal failure in children: preceded by gastroenteritis, bloody diarrhea.
      a. Question child regarding any joint pain, edema, tenderness.
      b. Any recent cold, upper respiratory symptoms? Sore throat/skin infection present?
   4. Acute nephritic syndrome: associated with gross hematuria, edema, hypertension, renal insufficiency.
      a. Post-streptococcal glomerulonephritis occurs 7–14 days after onset of strep infection.
      b. Winter months: commonly associated with strep pharyngitis.
      c. Summer months: more likely to be skin infections.
   5. When bleeding occurs, urine color is important.
      a. Brown/cola-colored urine: more likely from kidney.
      b. Red/pink urine: more likely from bladder.
      c. Red blood spotting at end of urinary stream/in underwear: most likely from urethra.
D. Physical findings.
   1. Full-body exam to look for:
      a. Abdominal or renal mass.
      b. Presence of abdominal, CVA tenderness.
   2. Check child's underwear for blood, perineum for signs of trauma.
   3. Assess joints for edema, inflammation, tenderness.
   4. Edema of face, hands, or feet.
   5. Assess for signs of upper respiratory infection, pharyngitis, or other illness.

E. Diagnostic tests.
   1. Urinalysis may reveal infection or proteinuria.
   2. Laboratory analysis: formal urinalysis, culture if thought to be infection; urine calcium/creatinine ratio; urine protein/creatinine ratio.
   3. Serum studies: CBC with differential and platelet count, complete metabolic panel, anti-streptolysin enzyme (ASO) or streptozyme, antinuclear antibody (ANA) and C3.
   4. Skin or throat cultures when appropriate.
   5. Sickle cell screen in all African American patients.
   6. Coagulation studies with history of bleeding from other sites.
   7. Cystoscopy: only if persistent gross hematuria.
F. Differential diagnosis.

Hematuria (benign, essential, idiopathic), 599.7

Idiopathic hypercalcemia, 275.42

---

   1. Pseudohematuria.
   2. Idiopathic hypercalcemia.
   3. Extrarenal hematuria.
   4. Exercise-induced hematuria.
G. Treatment.
   1. Systemically ill child with gross hematuria: Admit while being evaluated.
   2. If elevated ASO and low C3 (hypocomplementemia), refer to nephrologist to rule out/treat nephritis.
   3. If abnormal ultrasound, referral to urologist to determine presence of structural anomalies.
   4. With UTIs, refer to urologist and consider VCUG.
   5. Abnormal ANA results, elevated ANA: consult rheumatology, nephrology; commonly associated positive crithidia may indicate lupus erythematosus.
   6. Other blood dyscrasias: consult hematology.
   7. Elevated serum creatinine, hypertension, peripheral edema, abnormal calcium/creatinine ratio, protein/creatinine ratio: refer to nephrologist. Renal biopsy/cystoscopy may be necessary to diagnose.
   8. Urethralgia: hallmarked by blood at end of urinary stream or in underwear, can persist without negative consequence in child for years. Treatment is controversial: Some use antibiotics, but have not been proven effective.

9. If child develops hypertension or proteinuria, refer to nephrologist. Renal biopsy may be indicated.

10. If chlamydia or gonorrhea is suspected:

   a. Younger than 9 years of age: erythromycin 50 mg/kg/day qid (max 2 g/day).

   b. 9–15 years of age: ceftriaxone 250 mg IM single dose followed by 7 days of doxycycline 200 mg/day bid.

   c. Older than 15 years of age: azithromycin 1 g in 1 dose.

H. Follow up.

1. Determined by disease, usually done by appropriate specialist.

2. Urethralgia without significant symptoms and benign familial hematuria without proteinuria and hypertension: Monitor by checking urine and blood pressure every 6–12 months.

I. Complications.

Electrolyte imbalance, 276.9
Renal failure, 586

1. Renal failure.

2. Significant electrolyte imbalance.

3. Follow up with specialist very important for children with these complications.

J. Education.

1. Parents must understand importance of having studies done and follow up with specialists.

2. If medications prescribed, how and when to give and possible side effects.

3. Know signs/symptoms of progressive renal disease: edema, hypertension, increasing blood in urine, proteinuria, UTI, lethargy, pallor.

VIII. PROTEINURIA

Cold exposure, 991.9	Hypertension, 401.9
Congestive heart disease, 428	Obstructive uropathy, 599.9
Edema, 782.3	Polycystic kidney disease, 753.12
Febrile illness, 780.6	Proteinuria, 791
Glomerulonephritis, 583.9	Pyelonephritis, chronic, 590.8
Hematuria, 599.7	Tubular necrosis, acute, 584.5

A. Etiology.
1. Renal insufficiency often associated with proteinuria.
2. Diagnosed by random urinalysis on well-child checkup or associated with serious illness.
3. Common causes of proteinuria include chronic pyelonephritis, renal scarring, febrile illness, glomerulonephritis, exercise induced, idiopathic, orthostatic, polycystic kidney disease, acute tubular necrosis, cold exposure, congestive heart disease, obstructive uropathy, pregnancy, drug induced, trauma.

B. Occurrence.
1. Positive screening by dipstick: approximately 10% of 8- to 15-year olds.
   a. Dipstick finding considered positive if it is 1+ (30 mg/dL). False positives can occur with concentrated urine specimens; if specific gravity is 1.015, dipstick finding for protein needs to be higher than 2+.
2. If in doubt, look for other symptoms: hypertension, edema, hematuria.
3. Always best to confirm lower range and asymptomatic results by rechecking/confirming by protein-to-calcium ratio.

C. Clinical manifestations.
1. Varies with diagnosis.
2. Glomerulonephritis presents with hematuria and proteinuria.
   a. Decreased glomerular filtration rate can result in sodium and water retention, oliguria, circulatory overload, edema, hypertension.
   b. Chronic glomerulonephritis results in failure to thrive, slow growth, fatigue.
3. Postural or orthostatic proteinuria: usually discovered on well-child check.
   a. Usually older than 8 years of age and totally asymptomatic.
   b. Exercise-induced proteinuria is seen after vigorous exercise, resolves with 48 hours rest.
   c. Febrile proteinuria resolves as temperature returns to normal.
4. Henoch-Schönlein purpura nephritis (a systemic vasculitis) presents with abdominal cramping, purpuric rash, joint pain.
   a. Bloody diarrhea occurs in 50% of patients.
   b. Hemolytic uremic syndrome, systemic lupus erythematosus can also present with purpura, inflammatory bowel.
   c. Known history of renal disease or strong family history of renal compromise.

D. Physical findings.
1. Urinalysis shows proteinuria ranging from trace to 4+, microscopic/gross hematuria.

2. May be associated infection indicated by elevated urine WBC, nitrites.
3. Blood pressure may be elevated.
4. Edema (especially periorbital) may be present.
5. Patient complains of joint pain, stiffness. Joints swollen, inflamed on exam.
6. Complaints of dysuria or frequency: signs of infection, CVA tenderness, flank pain may indicate obstruction or pyelonephritis.

E. Diagnostic tests.
1. In nonacute setting: obtain protein-to-creatinine ratio.
   a. If > 0.2, repeat; if still elevated, obtain 12- or 24-hour urine.
   b. Supine and upright collection obtained to rule out orthostatic proteinuria. Nonpathologic proteinuria associated with posture, fever, or exercise usually yields results < 1 g/24 hours.
   c. Renal ultrasound is normal.
2. Pathologic proteinuria results from glomerular, tubular disorders of kidney.
   a. Protein-to-creatinine ratio is > 0.2, 24-hour urine results are = 3 g of protein in 24 hours.
   b. Renal ultrasound can show infectious or obstructive nephropathy.
   c. Complete metabolic panel, CBC with differential and platelets, ASO, C3, ANA help sort out the immunologic from the nephrologic causes.
   d. Throat and/or skin cultures can identify post-streptococcal glomerulonephritis.

F. Differential diagnosis.
1. See Etiology.

G. Treatment.
1. Treatment is dependent on type and severity of proteinuria, obstructive uropathy can be repaired surgically.
2. Infectious uropathy: Treat with antibiotics.
3. Associated hypertension: may need short- or long-term treatment.
4. Urgent nephrology referral with edema and hypertension.
5. Systemically ill patients require hospitalization to determine cause.
6. If creatinine-to-protein ratio is > 0.2, refer to nephrology for further evaluation.

H. Follow up.
1. Follow up may be lifelong depending on cause.
2. Recheck asymptomatic proteinuria annually by dipstick analysis and blood pressure: If either is abnormal, referral or additional evaluation needed.

I.   Complications.

> Failure to thrive, 783.41
> Hypertension, 401.9
> Renal failure, 584.9

   1.   Failure to thrive, renal failure, hypertension.
J.   Education.
   1.   Know signs/symptoms of progressive disease process.
   2.   Ensure routine urinalysis remains part of well-child check so early evaluation and treatment can be done.
   3.   Follow nonpathologic proteinuria annually.
   4.   Close observation for pathologic proteinuria.

BIBLIOGRAPHY

Behrman RE, et al. *Textbook of pediatrics*. 17th ed. Philadelphia, PA: W.B. Saunders; 2004.
Gearhart JP, Rink RC, Mouriquand PD. *Pediatric urology*. Philadelphia, PA: WB Saunders; 2010.
Johnson KB, Oski FA. *Oski's essential pediatrics*. Philadelphia, PA: Lippincott-Raven; 1997.
Oneil JA, Jr., et al. *Principles of pediatric surgery*. 2nd ed. St. Louis, MO: Mosby; 2004.
Wein AJ, Kavoussi LR, Novick AC, et al. *Campbell-Walsh urology*. Philadelphia, PA: Elsevier; 2010.

CHAPTER 28

Gynecologic Disorders

Mary Lou C. Rosenblatt and Meg Moorman

I. AMENORRHEA

A. Primary: No episodes of spontaneous uterine bleeding by 16.5 years. Evaluate for delayed puberty if no secondary sex characteristics by 14 years.

B. Secondary: After onset of menarche, absence of uterine bleeding for 6 months or time equal to 3 previous menstrual cycles. Regular monthly cycles not often seen until 1–2 years after menarche. Because evaluation of amenorrhea applies to all amenorrhea, not necessary to categorize workup as primary or secondary.

C. Etiology.
1. External genital anomaly: androgen insensitivity (46,XY).
2. Internal genital anomaly:
   a. Vaginal agenesis.
   b. Imperforate hymen.
   c. Transverse vaginal septum.
   d. Agenesis of the cervix.
   e. Agenesis of the uterus.
   f. Gonadal dysgenesis.
3. Hypogonadotropic hypogonadism:
   a. Stress.
   b. Weight loss or gain.
      • Obesity.
      • Eating disorders.

- Competitive athletics.
- Familial (ask ages of menarche for mother, sisters).
- Drugs (phenothiazines, oral contraceptives, medroxyprogesterone acetate (Depo Provera), illicit drugs).
- Environmental changes (such as going away to college).
4. Pregnancy.
5. CNS tumor.
6. Pituitary gland infarct, irradiation, surgery.
7. Adrenal gland tumor, disease.
8. Chronic diseases.
9. Hypo- or hyperthyroidism.
10. Autoimmune oophoritis.
11. Ovarian failure, tumor, irradiation, or surgery.
12. Polycystic ovary syndrome (PCOS).
13. Asherman's syndrome (history of uterine surgery).
D. Occurrence.
1. Primary: 3 out of 1000 girls have menarche after 15.5 years.
2. Secondary: Most common reason is pregnancy. Also consider stress, weight changes, eating disorders.
    a. 8–10% of 14–18-year olds report missing 3 consecutive menses in past year.
E. Clinical manifestations.
1. May have no signs or, depending on cause, may be specific signs, such as wide-spaced nipples, web neck, short stature of Turner syndrome, obesity, acanthosis nigricans of PCOS, or wasting of anorexia.
2. Evaluate galactorrhea/amenorrhea for prolactinoma and empty sella syndrome.
F. Physical findings.
1. Physical exam to rule out nonreproductive system problems.
2. Plot height and weight looking for Turner syndrome, obesity, anorexia; explain need for genital exam.
3. On external exam check for patent hymen.
4. A cotton Q-tip can determine the length of the vagina.
5. A one-finger, vaginal–abdominal or rectal–abdominal exam may determine the presence of a cervix and uterus.
6. Estrogenized vaginal mucosa is pink.
7. A pelvic exam for sexually active teens to identify normal organ structure. Clitoromegaly is seen in the presence of excess androgens.
G. Diagnostic tests.
1. Testing indicated in stepwise progression based on history and physical exam.

   2. If any concern about sexual activity, obtain pregnancy test. Keep in mind admitting sexual activity may be difficult for some teens.
      a. Negative pregnancy test: Follow stepwise progression again, starting with thyroid-stimulating hormone (TSH) and prolactin.
      b. Pelvic ultrasound to look at pelvic structures may be needed.
      c. Vaginal maturation index can be obtained to evaluate estrogenization of vagina.
      d. Progestational challenge checks endogenous estrogen levels and competency of outflow tract.
H. Differential diagnosis.
   1. See Etiology.
I. Treatment.
   1. Cause of amenorrhea determines treatment.
J. Follow up.
   1. Determined by the cause and treatment.
   2. Referral may be needed in cases of anatomic or chromosomal abnormality, CNS tumor, eating disorder, or specialized management.
K. Complications.

Infertility, 628.9
---

   1. Infertility may result from some causes of amenorrhea, making it important to listen to patient's questions and concerns and to offer emotional support.
L. Education.
   1. Offer information relevant to the cause and treatment of the individual's diagnosis.

II. CHLAMYDIAL INFECTION

Abdominal tenderness, 789.6	Penile discharge, 788.7
Cervicitis, 616	Salpingitis, 614.2
Chlamydial infection, 079.98	Urethritis, 597.8
Epididymitis, 604.9	Vaginal discharge, 623.5
Hypertrophic cervical ectopy, 622.6	

A. Etiology.
   1. An obligate intracellular bacterial agent with at least 18 serologic variants.

B. Occurrence.
   1. Most common sexually transmitted infection (STI) in United States with high rates among sexually active adolescents.
C. Clinical manifestations.
   1. Causes urethritis, cervicitis, epididymitis, salpingitis, perihepatitis, endometritis, reactive arthritis.
   2. Can lead to acute and chronic pelvic inflammatory disease (PID).
   3. Incubation varies; about 1 week.
D. Physical findings.
   1. May be no symptoms for males or females.
   2. Females: mucopurulent vaginal discharge, hypertrophic cervical ectopy, abdominal tenderness.
   3. Males: penile discharge, abdominal tenderness, testicular tenderness.
E. Diagnostic tests.
   1. Tissue culture.
   2. Nucleic acid amplification: highly sensitive from cervical, urethral, rectal, vaginal swabs, or urine.
F. Differential diagnosis.

Gonorrhea, 098

   1. Other STIs, such as gonorrhea.
G. Treatment.
   1. Recommended regimens:
      a. Azithromycin 1 g one dose PO, OR
      b. Doxycycline 100 mg PO bid for 7 days.
      c. See Centers for Disease Control and Prevention (CDC) guidelines (see Bibliography) for alternative regimens or treatment guidelines for PID.
H. Follow up.
   1. Rescreen 3–4 months after treatment in high-risk population.
I. Complications.

Chronic pelvic pain, 625.9	Infertility, 628.9
Ectopic pregnancy, 633.9	Pelvic inflammatory disease, 614.9

   1. PID.
   2. Ectopic pregnancy.
   3. Infertility.
   4. Chronic pelvic pain.

J. Education.
   1. Abstain from sexual intercourse until 7 days after single-dose treatment or completion of 7-day regimen.
   2. Sex partner(s) need treatment.
   3. Inform about risks associated with untreated infection to motivate completion of treatment.
   4. Avoid multiple partners.
   5. Educate about safer sex: Use condoms during all intercourse, limit number of sexual partners, carefully screen any potential partner.

III. DYSMENORRHEA

Abdominal pain, 789	Headache, 784
Diarrhea, 787.91	Nausea, 787.02
Dizziness, 780.4	Nervousness, 799.2
Dysmenorrhea, 625.3	Pain with menses, 625.3
Fatigue, 780.79	Vomiting, 787.03

A. Primary: pain associated with menstrual cycle without organic source.
B. Secondary: menstrual pain due to organic disease.
C. Etiology.
   1. Primary: elevated prostaglandins, prostaglandin levels are higher in women with ovulatory cycles.
   2. Secondary: due to pelvic pathology such as infection, structural abnormalities, endometriosis.
D. Occurrence.
   1. 60% of teens report pain with menses; 10–14% of those miss school days due to pain.
E. Clinical manifestations.
   1. Primary: may begin 6–36 months after menarche.
      a. Lower abdominal pain; may radiate to thighs or back.
      b. Nausea, vomiting, diarrhea, dizziness, nervousness, headache, fatigue may accompany.
      c. Commonly pain starts within 1–4 hours of onset of menses, lasts 1–2 days. Pain may begin before menses and last 2–4 days.
   2. Secondary: pain with menses and associated symptoms. History should include sexual history, gastrointestinal and genitourinary systems history.

F. Physical findings.
1. Primary: normal physical exam.
2. Patients with STIs may have purulent cervical discharge, cervical motion tenderness, uterine tenderness, adnexal tenderness. Mass in adnexa could be cyst, ectopic pregnancy, tubo-ovarian abscess. Tender/nodular cul-de-sac may be found with endometriosis.
G. Diagnostic tests.
1. For sexually active teens: pelvic exam to rule out STIs, gonorrhea and chlamydia tests, pregnancy test (if menses are irregular/missed).
2. Urinalysis if urinary symptoms.
H. Differential diagnosis.

Cervicitis inflammatory disease, 616	Inflammatory bowel disease, 558.9
Chlamydia, 079.98	Ovarian cysts, 620.2
Constipation, 564	Pelvic inflammatory disease, 614.9
Cystitis, 595.9	Postsurgical adhesions, 614
Dyspareunia, 625	Pyelonephritis, 590.8
Endometriosis, 617.9	Uterine malformation, 752.3
Gonorrhea, 098	

1. Cervicitis or PID caused by agents such as gonorrhea, chlamydia.
2. Cystitis, pyelonephritis.
3. Inflammatory bowel disease.
4. Constipation.
5. Endometriosis: not common in adolescents but may be significant in adolescents with chronic pelvic pain. Pain may occur before and after menses, may include dyspareunia, pain on defecation, abnormal uterine bleeding.
6. Uterine malformation.
7. Ovarian cysts.
8. Postsurgical adhesions.
I. Treatment.
1. Primary: nonsteroidal anti-inflammatory drugs (NSAIDs), oral contraceptives.
2. Secondary: treat identified cause.
J. Follow up.
1. If standard treatments such as NSAIDs or oral contraceptives do not relieve pain or if etiology is complex, refer to gynecologist.
2. When infections are the cause, treat and follow up per protocol.
   a. PID: inpatient or outpatient therapy, monitor for medication compliance.

       b. Gonorrhea or chlamydia: rescreen every 3–4 months.

K. Complications.

Dysmenorrhea, 625.3
---

1. Primary dysmenorrhea should improve with either NSAID or oral contraceptive therapy. If not, consider other causes.
2. Secondary dysmenorrhea: may have complications based on diagnosis (e.g., teens with PID may suffer from infertility, adhesions, or ectopic pregnancy).

L. Education.

1. Take anti-inflammatory agents with food; start as soon as symptoms occur.
2. Hormonal contraception is useful when contraception is needed. Teach sexually active teens about safer sex.
3. When infection is cause, partners need to be treated.

IV. GENITAL HERPES

Genital herpes, 054.1
Genitalia lesion, 625.8

A. Etiology.

1. Recurrent lifelong infection, 2 types: herpes simplex virus type 1 (HSV-1) and herpes simplex virus type 2 (HSV-2).
2. HSV-2 causes most genital HSV infection but increasing numbers of genital HSV are caused by HSV-1.

B. Occurrence.

1. 50 million persons in United States have genital HSV infection.

C. Clinical manifestations.

1. Vesicular or ulcerative lesions of male or female genitalia.
2. Infection can be more severe in immunocompromised individuals.
3. Infections caused by direct contact.
4. Incubation period: 2 days to 2 weeks. Virus persists for life in latent form.
5. Recurrent infections shed virus for 3–4 days rather than 1–2 weeks in primary infection.

D. Physical findings.

1. Vesicular or ulcerative lesions of male or female genitalia.

E. Diagnostic tests.

1. HSV culture provides best sensitivity when lesions are cultured before they begin to heal.

2. Type-specific and nonspecific antibodies to HSV develop in weeks after infection and persist indefinitely, but do not differentiate between genital and orolabial infections. Serologic type-specific glycoprotein G (gG)–based assays can be requested by providers to distinguish HSV-1 and HSV-2.

F. Differential diagnosis.

Candidal inflammation, 112.9	Syphilis, 091
Excoriation, 919.8	Warts, 078.1
Folliculitis, 704.8	

1. Folliculitis.
2. Chancre of syphilis, warts, candidal inflammation, excoriation.

G. Treatment.

1. Primary infection: Oral acyclovir therapy begun within 6 days of onset of infection can decrease viral shedding by 3–5 days. Subsequent severity/frequency of recurrences not affected by treatment. Topical antiviral drugs not recommended.

   a. Recommended regimens:
      • Acyclovir 400 mg PO tid for 7–10 days, OR
      • Acyclovir 200 mg PO 5 times per day for 7–10 days, OR
      • Famciclovir 250 mg PO tid for 7–10 days, OR
      • Valacyclovir 1 g PO bid for 7–10 days.

2. Recurrent infections: Acyclovir therapy started within 2 days of onset of recurrence may shorten clinical course by 1 day. Provide prescription so immediate therapy can begin in case of recurrence.

   a. Recommended regimens:
      • Acyclovir 400 mg PO tid for 5 days, OR
      • Acyclovir 800 mg PO bid for 5 days, OR
      • Acyclovir 800 mg PO tid for 2 days, OR
      • Famciclovir 125 mg PO bid for 5 days, OR
      • Valacyclovir 500 mg PO bid for 3 days, OR
      • Valacyclovir 1 g PO once a day for 5 days.

3. Suppressive therapy for recurrent infections (6 episodes per year): can benefit from daily therapy. Acyclovir: safety and effectiveness for 6 years; valacyclovir or famciclovir for 1 year. Because outbreaks diminish in frequency over time, periodic discontinuation of therapy (i.e., yearly) may be helpful in reassessing need for therapy.

   a. Recommended regimens:
      • Acyclovir 400 mg PO bid, OR

- Famciclovir 250 mg PO bid, OR
- Valacyclovir 500 mg PO daily, OR
- Valacyclovir 1 g PO daily.

H. Follow up.
   1. Follow patient's emotional adjustment to having HSV.
   2. Test for other STIs.
I. Complications.

> Genital HSV, 054.1
>
> Skin-colored lesions, 709.8
>
> Warts, 078.1

   1. Daily medication may not suppress recurrent outbreaks.
   2. Immune-suppressed patients may have prolonged/severe outbreaks requiring IV therapy.
   3. Transmission to neonate from infected mother is highest among women who acquire genital HSV near time of delivery.
J. Education.
   1. Psychologic burden may be great. Counseling includes supportive groups, CDC website, written materials. If depression is identified, refer to mental health provider.
   2. Latex condoms may reduce transmission if used correctly.
   3. Patients should refrain from sexual contact if lesions are present.
   4. Sexual partners should be notified by patient.
   5. Sexual transmission may occur with asymptomatic viral shedding.
   6. Explain risk of neonatal infection to male and female patients; they should inform provider during pregnancy.

V. GENITAL WARTS

> Genital warts, 078.19

A. Etiology.
   1. Human papilloma viruses (HPVs) are DNA viruses and include 100 types; 30 types can infect genital tract.
   2. Types 16, 18, and 45 are associated with cervical cancer.
B. Occurrence.
   1. Anogenital HPV occurs in 40% of sexually experienced adolescent females.
   2. HPV is etiology of 90% of cervical cancers.

C. Clinical manifestations.
  1. May have no symptoms.
  2. When present, warts are epithelial tumors of skin/mucous membrane.
  3. Immunocompromised individuals may have larger quantity of warts.
  4. Incubation unknown; likely ranges from 3 months to several years.
  5. May regress spontaneously or may persist for years.
D. Physical findings.
  1. Skin-colored lesions with cauliflower-like surface may be several millimeters to several centimeters wide; may be painless or itch, burn, bleed; can be found on vagina, cervix, vulva, penis, anus, perianal area, scrotum.
E. Diagnostic tests.
  1. For women younger than 30 years but older than age 20, HPV tests are available to detect (DNA or RNA) viral nucleic acid or capsid protein.
  2. Four Food and Drug Administration (FDA)–approved tests are available for use in the United States: Hybrid Capture (HC) II High-Risk HPV test (Qiagen), HC II Low-Risk HPV test (Qiagen), Cervista HPV 16/18 test, and Cervista HPV HR (high risk) test (Hologic).
F. Differential diagnosis.

Condyloma lata, 091.3

Molluscum contagiosum, 078

---

  1. Molluscum contagiosum.
  2. Condyloma lata (syphilis).
  3. Pink, pearly, penile papules.
G. Treatment.
  1. Recommended regimens.
    a. Patient applied:
      • Podofilox 0.5% solution or gel, OR
      • Imiquimod 5% cream, OR
      • Sinecatechins 15% ointment.
    b. Provider administered:
      • Cryotherapy with liquid nitrogen or cryoprobe.
      • Podophyllin resin 10–25%.
      • Trichloroacetic acid or bichloroacetic acid 80–90%.
      • Surgery.
H. Follow up.
  1. Females: regular Pap smears to assess for cellular damage.

I. Complications.
1. Recurrences common due to reactivation of virus. May persist for life. Duration of contagiousness unknown.
2. Local treatment can damage normal surrounding skin.
J. Education.
1. Females: regular Pap smears to assess for cellular damage from HPV.
2. Screen for other STIs.
3. Partners should be informed.
4. Teach safer sex.
K. Vaccinations.
1. Cervarix (bivalent) vaccine contains HPV types 16 and 18.
2. Gardasil (quadrivalent) vaccine contains HPV types 6, 11, 16, and 18.
3. Both vaccines protect against 70% of cervical cancers and Gardasil offers protection against 90% of genital warts.
4. Either vaccine can be administered to girls aged 11–12 years and as young as age 9. They can also be administered to women ages 12–26 who have not started or completed the vaccine. It is most beneficial if given before onset of sexual activity. Gardasil can be used in males aged 9–26 to prevent genital warts. Both vaccines are administered in a 3-series injection schedule over a 6-month period. After injection 1 is given, the second is given 1–2 months later, then at 6 months after the first injection for a total of 3 injections. Women should still receive routine cervical cancer screening after receiving the vaccine.

VI. GONORRHEA

Gonorrhea, 098

A. Etiology.
1. Neisseria gonorrhoeae is Gram-negative, oxidase-positive diplococcus.
B. Occurrence.
1. 650,000 new cases of gonorrhea per year in the United States.
2. 15- to 19-year olds have highest incidence of infection.
3. Co-infection with chlamydia is common.
C. Clinical manifestations.
1. Males tend to have symptomatic infections of urethra.
2. Females may have cervicitis, PID, perihepatitis, bartholinitis.

     3. Rectal and pharyngeal infections may be asymptomatic.

     4. Disseminated infections occur in up to 3% of untreated persons.

        a. Bacteremia causes arthritis-dermatitis syndrome.

        b. More common in females infected within 1 week of menstrual period.

     5. Incubation is 2–7 days.

D. Physical findings.

     1. May be no symptoms.

     2. Males may experience penile discharge, dysuria.

     3. Females may have vaginal discharge, abdominal pain.

E. Diagnostic tests.

     1. Culture is excellent but may require special handling.

     2. Nucleic acid amplification is highly sensitive; may be used with mucosal discharge/urine.

     3. Gram stain showing Gram-negative intracellular diplococci are most useful in acutely ill patients.

F. Differential diagnosis.

Abdominal pain, 789	Penile discharge, 788.7
Chlamydia, 079.98	Vaginal discharge, 623.5
Dysuria, 788.1	

     1. Chlamydia may cause similar symptoms.

     2. Non-gonococcal urethritis (NGU): 40% of cases caused by chlamydia; 20–30% caused by *Ureaplasma urealyticum*; and 30–40% uncertain but may include HSV, *Trichomonas vaginalis*, *Escherichia coli*, and others.

G. Treatment.

     1. Dual treatment for chlamydia should be considered in populations where chlamydia is found with 10–30% of gonococcal infections.

     2. Recommended regimens for uncomplicated gonococcal infections of cervix, urethra, rectum:

        a. Cefixime 400 mg one dose PO, OR

        b. Ceftriaxone 125 mg one dose IM, OR

        c. Ciprofloxacin 500 mg one dose PO, OR

        d. Ofloxacin 400 mg one dose PO, OR

        e. Levofloxacin 250 mg one dose PO.

        f. PLUS, if chlamydial infection is not ruled out: azithromycin 1 g PO one dose, OR doxycycline 100 mg PO bid for 7 days.

H. Follow up.

     1. Test of cure for uncomplicated gonococcal infection not indicated.

     2. Persistent infection may be due to reinfected or untreated co-infection with chlamydia.

I. Complications.

Ectopic pregnancy, 633.9	Pelvic inflammatory disease, 614.9
Infertility, 628.9	Tubal scarring, 478.9

1. PID.
2. Tubal scarring.
3. Infertility.
4. Ectopic pregnancy.
5. Hematogenous spread causing skin and joint syndrome.

J. Education.
1. Partners need to be evaluated and treated.
2. Encourage use of condom.
3. Screen for other STIs (chlamydia, HIV, syphilis, hepatitis B).

VII. SYPHILIS

Fever, 780.6	Papular lesions, 709.9
Headache, 784	Rash, 781.2
Lymphadenopathy, 785.6	Syphilis, 097.9
Malaise, 780.79	Ulcers (chancres), 091

A. Etiology.
1. Person-to-person transmission of spirochete, *Treponema pallidum*.
2. Incubation is 10–90 days.
B. Occurrence.
1. Rare in much of industrialized world but problem in large U.S. urban areas and the rural South.
C. Clinical manifestations.
1. Primary: painless, indurated ulcers (chancres) at site of inoculation, within 3 weeks of exposure.
2. Secondary: 1–2 months later, generalized maculopapular rash (includes palms and soles), fever, malaise, headache, lymphadenopathy.
3. Hypertrophic, papular lesions (condyloma lata) in moist areas of vulva or anus.
4. Latent: seroreactivity but no clinical manifestations of syphilis, may last years.
   a. Early latent: acquired in last year.
   b. Late latent: acquired more than 1 year ago or unknown duration.

5. Tertiary: may be many years after acquiring infection; features major organ damage.
6. Neurosyphilis: central nervous system (CNS) disease can occur during any stage of syphilis; examine cerebrospinal fluid in patients with neurologic involvement.

D. Physical findings.
1. Primary: chancre at site of inoculation, painless ulcer.
2. Secondary: maculopapular rash, generalized, including palms/soles, condyloma lata.
3. Neurosyphilis: abnormal neurologic exam.

E. Diagnostic tests.
1. Positive dark-field exam is definitive for syphilis but may not be readily available.
2. Nontreponemal tests (VDRL, RPR) are quantitative, testing activity, treatment response. Same lab should measure subsequent tests to ensure reliability. Tests may become negative 2 years after treatment.
3. Treponemal tests (FTA-ABS, TP-PA) must confirm nontreponemal test.
4. Tests usually positive for life. Other spirochetal disease causes positive test (yaws, pinta, leptospirosis, rat-bite fever, Lyme disease).

F. Differential diagnosis.

Pityriasis rosea, 696.3

1. Rash of secondary syphilis can be confused with pityriasis rosea, making blood evaluation important for sexually active adolescents diagnosed with pityriasis.

G. Treatment.
1. Recommended regimen for adults.
a. Primary, secondary, and early latent:
- Penicillin G benzathine, 2.4 million units IM single dose (preferred), OR
- If penicillin allergic, not pregnant: doxycycline 100 mg PO bid for 14 days, OR tetracycline 500 mg PO qid for 14 days.
b. Late latent, latent of unknown duration, tertiary or neurosyphilis, HIV-positive and pregnant patients refer to CDC guidelines for treatment. Note: Patients allergic to penicillin should be desensitized.

H. Follow up.
1. Evaluate blood tests for early-acquired syphilis at 3, 6, and 12 months.
2. Add 24-month test for persons with syphilis of 1 year duration.

I. Complications.

HIV, V08	Stillbirth, 779.9
Hydrops fetalis, 752.3	Syphilis, 097.9
Prematurity, 765.1	

1. Untreated syphilis causes damage to most body organs over time, infects partners.
2. Co-infection with HIV, other STIs.
3. Infected pregnant women pass along syphilis to fetus, resulting in stillbirth, hydrops fetalis, or prematurity. Infants may suffer numerous complications.
4. Jarisch-Herxheimer reaction (acute, febrile reaction with headache myalgia) may occur in first 24 hours after treatment (occurs most with patients being treated for early syphilis). Antipyretics may be used but may not prevent this reaction.

J. Education.
1. Sexual partners must be treated. Public health department finds contacts anonymously.
2. HIV status should be checked. If negative, recheck in 3 months.
3. Safer sex counseling.

VIII. TRICHOMONIASIS

Trichomoniasis, 131.01
Vaginal discharge, 623.5

A. Etiology.
1. *Trichomonas vaginalis* is a flagellated protozoan.
B. Occurrence.
1. Primarily sexually transmitted, may coexist with other STIs.
C. Clinical manifestations.
1. Most males have no symptoms.
2. Females may have profuse, pruritic, malodorous, yellow-green vaginal discharge or no symptoms at all.
3. Incubation period: 4–28 days.

D. Physical findings.
    1. Females: frothy white, yellow-green vaginal discharge with erythematous vaginal mucosa and friable "strawberry cervix."
E. Diagnostic tests.
    1. On wet mount, trichomonad has jerky motion and lashing flagella.
F. Differential diagnosis.

Chlamydia, 079.98	Monilia, 112.9
Gonorrhea, 098	Pruritus, 698.9

    1. Other STIs such as gonorrhea and chlamydia could be cause of discharge.
    2. Monilia could be cause of pruritus.
G. Treatment.
    1. Recommended regimen: metronidazole 2 g dose PO, OR
    2. Tinidazole 2 g orally in a single dose, OR
    3. Alternative regimen: metronidazole 500 mg PO bid for 7 days.
H. Follow up.
    1. None needed unless discharge persists.
I. Complications.
    1. If no response to initial treatment, may repeat metronidazole 1 g bid for 7 days OR 2 g daily for 3–5 days. If treatment failure occurs twice with metronidazole 2 g single dose, treat with metronidazole 500 PO bid for 7 days OR or tinidazole 2 g PO for 5 days.
    2. In rare cases where infection persists despite treatment of patient and partner, CDC may be helpful in looking at resistance of organism.
J. Education.
    1. Treat partners even if no symptoms.
    2. Patients should abstain from sex until they and any partners are treated and asymptomatic.
    3. Safer sex counseling.
    4. Screen for other STIs.
    5. No alcohol consumption for 48 hours due to disulfiram-like effects of metronidazole (flushing, pulsating headache, violent vomiting, restlessness).

IX. VULVOVAGINITIS

Vaginal discharge, 623.5
Vulvovaginitis, 616.1

A. Etiology.
   1. Bacterial vaginosis is syndrome found in sexually active females caused by changes in vaginal flora. Normal vaginal ecosystem is disrupted by increases in *Gardnerella vaginalis, Mycoplasma hominis, Ureaplasma* species, anaerobic bacteria, and marked decrease in lactobacillus species.
   2. Incubation is unknown.
B. Occurrence.
   1. Common, may occur with other infections.
   2. Although not proven to be sexually transmitted, it is uncommon in sexually inexperienced females.
C. Clinical manifestations.
   1. May have no symptoms.
   2. White, homogenous, adherent vaginal discharge with fishy odor.
D. Physical findings.
   1. White, malodorous vaginal discharge.
   2. Not associated with abdominal pain or pruritus.
E. Diagnostic tests.
   1. Three of following four criteria establish diagnosis:
      a. Homogenous, white, adherent vaginal discharge.
      b. Vaginal fluid pH 4.5.
      c. Fishy odor before or after adding 10% KOH (whiff test).
      d. Clue cells (squamous vaginal epithelial cells covered with bacteria, causing granular appearance) on microscopic exam.
F. Differential diagnosis.

Edema, 782.3
Erythema, 695.9
Vaginal discharge, 623.5

   1. Characterized by white, thick, pruritic discharge with pH 4.5; pseudohyphae are seen under microscope when 10% KOH is added. Candida also causes erythema and edema of vulva-vagina.
   2. Rule out other STIs.
G. Treatment.
   1. Not necessary in asymptomatic women.
   2. Recommended regimens:
      a. Metronidazole 500 mg PO bid for 7 days, OR
      b. Metronidazole gel 0.75%, one full applicator (5 g) intravaginally, once a day for 5 days, OR

      c. Clindamycin cream 2%, one applicator intravaginally at bedtime for 7 days.
H. Follow up.
    1. Recurrence is common.
I. Complications.

HIV, V08	Postpartum endometritis, 314.9
Pelvic inflammatory disease, 614.9	Preterm labor, 644.2

    1. May be risk factor for PID, HIV, preterm labor, postpartum endometritis.
J. Education.
    1. Not clearly sexually transmitted.
    2. Partner treatment does not affect recurrence.

BIBLIOGRAPHY

Centers for Disease Control and Prevention. Sexually transmitted diseases treatment guidelines 2010. *MMWR.* 2010; 59(No. RR-12):1–116.

Joffe A. Amenorrhea. In: Hoekelman RA, ed. *Primary pediatric care.* 4th ed. St. Louis, MO: Mosby; 2001: 975–977.

Neinstein SN. *Adolescent health care, a practical guide.* 4th ed. Baltimore, MD: Lippincott Williams & Wilkins; 2002.

Peipert, JF. Genital chlamydial infections. *NEJM.* 2003; 349:2424–2430.

Pickering LK, ed. *Red book: 2003 report of the Committee on Infectious Disease.* 26th ed. Elk Grove Village, IL: American Academy of Pediatrics; 2003.

Sanfillippo JS et al. *Pediatric and adolescent gynecology.* Philadelphia, PA: W.B. Saunders; 2001.

Speroff L, Glass RH, Kase NG. *Clinical gynecologic endocrinology and infertility.* 6th ed. Philadelphia, PA: Lippincott Williams & Wilkins; 1999:421–485.

Endocrine Disorders

Linda S. Gilman

I. HYPERTHYROIDISM

Agranulocytosis, 288	Irritability, 799.2
Amenorrhea, 626	Leukopenia, 288
Blurred vision, 368.8	Lid lag, 374.41
Breathlessness, 786.05	Lid retraction, 374.41
Cardiac enlargement, 429.3	Loss of visual acuity, 369.9
Chills, 780.99	Nervousness, 799.2
Cough, 786.2	Palmer erythema, 695
Diaphoresing, 780.8	Palpations, 785.1
Diffuse enlarged goiter, 240.9	Pedal edema, 782.3
Emotional liability, 301.3	Periorbital edema, 376.33
Enlarged thyroid, 240.9	Proptosis, 242
Euthyroid, 244.9	Rash, 782.1
Exophthalmia, 376.3	Skin reactions, 782.1
Fast heart rate, 785	Sweating, 780.8
Fatigue, 729.89	Tachycardia, 785
Fever, 780.6	Thyroid bruits, 240.9
Flushed moist skin, 782.62	Thyroiditis, 245.2
Graves' disease, 242	Trembling hands, 780.1
Heat intolerance, 992.6	Tremors, 781
Hyperthyroidism, 242.9	Weight loss, 783.21
Insomnia, 780.52	Widening pulse pressure, 785.9

A. Clinical syndrome resulting from excessive exposure of body tissues to action of thyroid hormone.

B. Etiology.
    1. Hyperthyroidism in childhood with few exceptions is due to autoimmune response to thyroid-stimulating hormone (TSH) receptors. This tissue response causes a condition known as Hashimoto thyroiditis. Graves' disease is a common cause of hyperthyroidism in children.
    2. Increases as adolescence approaches.
    3. No specific etiology known.
C. Occurrence.
    1. About 5% of all patients are younger than 15 years old.
        a. Peak incidence in adolescence at 11–15 years of age.
        b. Five times higher in girls than boys.
        c. May be present at birth if mother thyrotoxic during pregnancy.
    2. Symptoms develop gradually; time between onset and diagnosis may be 6–12 months and longer in prepubertal children compared with adolescents.
D. Clinical manifestations.
    1. Insomnia.
    2. Heat intolerance followed by diaphoresing.
    3. Weight loss, voracious appetite without weight gain.
    4. Increased sweating, palpitations, tachycardia.
    5. Muscle weakness and fatigue.
    6. Light menses or amenorrhea.
    7. Hyperactive GI tract with vomiting or frequent stooling.
    8. Tremors, nervousness, irritability, hyperactivity, emotional lability.
    9. Schoolwork suffers.
    10. Breathlessness.
    11. Blurred vision.
E. Physical findings.
    1. Enlarged thyroid, thyroid bruits, thrills.
    2. Thinning of hair.
    3. Proptosis, exophthalmia, noticeable lid lag, lid retraction, periorbital edema.
    4. Diffuse enlarged goiter.
    5. Fast heart rate, cardiac enlargement, widening pulse pressure.
    6. Trembling hands, tremor of finger with extended arm.
    7. Staring gaze, loss of visual acuity.
    8. Flushed moist skin.
    9. Pedal edema.
    10. Palmer erythema.

     11.   Increased deep tendon reflexes.

     12.   Hypercalcemia osteoporosis.

F. Diagnostic tests.

     1.   TSH produced by pituitary gland.

     2.   Thyroid hormones (T3, T4).

     3.   Iodine thyroid scan.

     4.   Antithyroid antibodies test.

G. Differential diagnosis.

Pituitary tumor, 227.3

     1.   Pituitary tumor.

H. Treatment/management.

     1.   Refer to endocrinologist.

     2.   Antithyroid agents:

         a.   Methimazole (Tapazole): to induce remission.

         b.   Propylthiouracil (PTU): to induce remission.

         c.   Propranolol (Inderal): to decrease adrenergic hyperresponsiveness symptoms.

     3.   Subtotal thyroidectomy.

     4.   Radioactive iodine (131-iodine).

I. Follow up.

     1.   Monitor for adverse side effects of antithyroid drugs such as skin reactions, leukopenia, agranulocytosis.

     2.   Most serious side effect: agranulocytosis, usually occurs in first 3 months of therapy.

     3.   Report rash, fever, chills, cough that does not resolve in 1 week.

     4.   When patient is euthyroid as determined by lab tests of TSH and T4, a 6-month follow up should be instituted to assess for risk of relapse.

J. Complications.

Agranulocytosis, 288	Hypersensitivity, 782
Glomerulonephritis, 583.9	Lupus-like syndrome, 710
Hepatic failure, 572.8	Thyrotoxicosis, 242.91
Hepatitis, 573.3	Vasculitis, 447.6

     1.   Toxic reaction with drug therapy, most severe: hypersensitivity, agranulocytosis, hepatitis, hepatic failure, lupus-like syndrome, glomerulonephritis, vasculitis of skin, thyroid storm, or thyrotoxicosis.

K. Education.
  1. Initial adjustment to therapy: Stress need to report side effects of therapy.
  2. Compliance to treatment: Do not miss doses; if dose is missed, take missed dose as soon as possible.
  3. Side effects of medication.
  4. If after several weeks of therapy symptoms continue, may need increased dose of antithyroid medication.

II. HYPOTHYROIDISM

Abdominal distention, 787.3	Hypothyroidism, 244.9
Ankle swelling, 719.07	Hypothyroidism, congenital, 243
Asymptomatic goiter, 240.9	Hypotonia, 781.3
Autoimmune destruction	Large for gestation infant, 766.1
Coarse sparse hair, 704.2	Lethargy, 780.79
Cold intolerance, 780.99	Mental retardation, 319
Constipation, 564	Mild weight gain, 783.1
Delayed dentition, 520.6	Noisy respirations, 784.49
Delayed puberty, 259	Poor feeding, 783.3
Depression, 311	Precocious puberty, 259.1
Dry skin, 701.1	Prolonged jaundice, 782.4
Dysphagia, 787.2	Sexual pseudoprecocity, 259.1
Feeding difficulties, 783.3	Short stature, 783.43
Feet swelling, 729.81	Sleep apnea, 780.57
Hashimoto thyroiditis, 245.2	Sleep disturbance, 780.5
Headaches, 784	Slow fetal growth, 764.9
Hoarseness, 784.49	Slowed pulse, 427.89
Hypoglycemia, 241.2	Visual problems, 368.8
Hypothermia, 991.6	

A. Condition resulting from deficient production of thyroid hormone or defect in hormonal receptor activity.
B. Etiology.

1. Hypothyroidism may be congenital or acquired.
   a. Congenital hypothyroidism.
      - Most commonly from inadequate production of thyroid hormone due to agenesis, dysplasia, ectopy of thyroid, or autosomal recessive defects in thyroid hormone synthesis and defects in other enzymatic steps in T4 synthesis and release.
      - Most common preventable cause of mental retardation.
   b. Acquired hypothyroidism most commonly caused by autoimmune destruction (Hashimoto thyroiditis).
C. Occurrence.
   1. One case per 3500 persons for congenital hypothyroidism.
   2. Acquired hypothyroidism: 6% of age 12–19-year olds have evidence of autoimmune disease.
      a. Depending on diagnostic criteria, may be as high as 10% in young females. Higher incidence in females (2:1).
      b. Congenital if untreated condition results in profound growth failure, developmental cognitive delay (cretinism).
      c. When untreated in older children: growth failure, slow metabolism, impaired memory.
D. Clinical manifestations.
   1. Congenital.
      a. Constipation.
      b. Hypotonia.
      c. Hypoglycemia.
      d. Hypothermia.
      e. Poor feeding.
      f. Hoarse cry, noisy respirations.
      g. Large for gestation.
   2. Acquired.
      a. Asymptomatic goiter.
      b. Hoarseness, dysphagia.
      c. Mild weight gain.
      d. Slow growth/delayed osseous maturation.
      e. Lethargy, sleep disturbance/sleep apnea.
      f. Cold intolerance.
      g. Constipation.
      h. Sexual pseudoprecocity.
      i. Headaches.
      j. Depression.

E. Physical findings.
  1. Congenital.
     a. Large for gestation infant.
     b. Hypotonia, puffy face.
     c. Wide anterior, posterior fontanel.
     d. Prolonged jaundice.
     e. Abdominal distention.
     f. Feeding difficulties/slowed gastric motility.
  2. Acquired.
     a. Visual problems.
     b. Precocious puberty (young children).
     c. Dry skin.
     d. Slowed pulse.
     e. Delayed puberty.
     f. Coarse, sparse hair.
     g. Delayed dentition.
     h. Ankle and feet swelling.
     i. Short stature.
F. Diagnostic tests.
  1. Newborn screen for T4: if low, then TSH drawn for definitive testing.
  2. Serum thyrotropin concentration/TSH.
  3. T4 and T3.
  4. Serum antithyroid globulin antibodies.
  5. Antithyroid peroxidase.
  6. Radionucleotide studies.
  7. Radioisotope-based thyroid scanning.
G. Differential diagnosis.

Bowel syndrome, chronic, 564.1	Iodine deficiency, 269.3
Cortisol excess, 255.8	Malnutrition, 263.9
Diabetes mellitus, 250	Precocious puberty, 259.1
Familial short stature, 783.43	Renal disease, 593.9
Growth hormone deficiency, 253.3	Turner syndrome, 758.6

  1. Endemic goiter/nutritional iodine deficiency.
  2. Chromosomal abnormalities such as Turner syndrome.
  3. Precocious puberty in young child.
  4. Familial short stature.
  5. Constitutional growth delay.

6. Growth hormone deficiency.
7. Chronic bowel syndrome.
8. Renal disease.
9. Malnutrition/gluten-induced enteropathy.
10. Cortisol excess.
11. Diabetes mellitus.
H. Treatment.
1. Levothyroxine (Levothroid, Levoxyl, Synthroid), a synthetic drug identical to human T4, is preferred thyroid hormone replacement.
2. Neonates: initial doses 10–15 mcg/kg PO every morning before meals. Dosage titrated on basis of thyroid function tests every 3 months until 2 years of age. Desired T4 range: 10–15 mcg/dL.
3. Children: 2–6 years of age: 5 mcg/kg PO every morning before meals; 6–12 years of age: 4–5 mcg/kg PO every morning before meals.
4. Adolescents: 100–150 mcg PO every morning before meals.
5. With age, levothyroxine dose decreases on weight basis.
I. Follow up.
1. Monitor for behavior change, school performance.
2. Monitor serum TSH 2–3 months after change in dosage.
3. Monitor for symptoms of hypothyroidism, hyperthyroidism.
J. Complications.
1. Noncompliance with treatment protocol.
K. Education.
1. Educate parents on signs/symptoms of hypothyroidism and hyperthyroidism.
2. Allow child to take responsibility for own care as soon as old enough (9–10 years of age).

III. SHORT STATURE

Constitutional growth delay, 253.3	Growth hormone deficiency, 253.3
Familial short stature, 783.43	Turner syndrome, 758.6

A. Generally accepted definition is stature below third percentile, or two standard deviations (SD) below mean, for age.
B. Etiology.
1. Familial short stature.
2. Constitutional growth delay.

3. Growth hormone deficiency.

4. Chromosomal disorder/Turner syndrome.

C. Occurrence.

1. Growth hormone deficiency estimated 10,000 to 15,000 children in United States.

2. Turner syndrome: 1 in 2500 female births.

3. About 1 million children in United States have height more than 2 SD below mean for age.

D. Clinical manifestations.

1. Familial short stature.

   a. Growth pattern remains in its centile channel for height and weight.

   b. Family history of short stature, normal birth length/weight, normal growth rate with predicted adult height of third percentile.

2. Constitutional growth delay.

   a. Bone age lower than chronological age.

   b. Family history reveals short stature in childhood, delayed puberty, eventual normal stature.

3. Growth hormone deficiency.

   a. Small child with immature face, chubby body build.

   b. Rate of growth of all body parts is slow.

4. Chromosomal disorder/Turner syndrome:

   a. Short stature.

   b. Pubertal delay.

E. Physical findings.

1. Familial short stature.

   a. Clinical/laboratory evidence of systemic disease or endocrine insufficiency.

   b. Annual growth rate within normal limits, growth at or below but progressing parallel to third percentile.

2. Constitutional growth delay.

   a. Child growing at normal or near normal rate, annual growth rate of 5 cm/year, small for age.

   b. Delayed skeletal maturity.

   c. Normal thyroid and growth hormone levels.

3. Growth hormone deficiency.

   a. Typical child with growth hormone deficiency is short, slightly overweight.

   b. When present at birth, infant may have hypoglycemia, prolonged unexplained jaundice.

4. Chromosomal disorder/Turner syndrome.
    a. Short stature, short neck, webbing of neck, low posterior hairline, shield chest, wide carrying angle, short 4th and 5th metacarpals, narrow high arched palate, epicanthal folds, nail dysplasia, clinodactyly.
F. Diagnostic tests.
    1. Detailed history, physical, and depending on findings, the following tests:
        a. X-ray of left hand and wrist to assess skeletal maturity.
        b. Urinalysis to assess ability to acidify and concentrate urine.
        c. Blood tests to include:
            - Urea nitrogen.
            - Creatinine.
            - CO_2.
            - Electrolytes.
            - Calcium.
            - Phosphorus.
            - Alkaline phosphatase.
            - T3, T4.
            - TSH.
            - Erythrocyte sedimentation rate (ESR).
            - Somatomedin C/1GF-1.
            - Complete blood count (CBC).
        d. Female patients: karyotype for abnormalities of X chromosome.
        e. X-ray of skull: sella turcica size, abnormality of sella area.
G. Differential diagnosis.

Cardiac disease, 429.9	Nutritional deficiencies, 269.9
Celiac disease, 579	Pituitary dwarfism, 253.3
Cortisol excess, 255.8	Psychosocial dwarfism, 259.4
Diabetes mellitus, 250	Renal disease, 583.9
Endocrine short stature, 783.43	Second-generation anorexia, 783
Inflammatory bowel disease, 569.9	Skeletal dysplasia, 756
Intrauterine growth retardation, 764.9	

1. Intrauterine growth retardation.
2. Skeletal dysplasia.
3. Nutritional deficiencies/second-generation anorexia.
4. Intestinal/gluten-induced enteropathy (celiac disease).
5. Chronic inflammatory bowel disease.

      6.   Renal disease.

      7.   Cardiac disease.

      8.   Diabetes mellitus.

      9.   Psychosocial dwarfism, endocrine short stature, pituitary dwarfism.

     10.   Cortisol excess.

H. Treatment.

      1.   Refer to pediatric endocrinologist for diagnosis and treatment.

      2.   Growth hormone is continued as long as potential for growth exists and child is responding to therapy; can expect to reach normal adult height.

I. Follow up.

      1.   Monitor growth patterns in response to medications.

      2.   Awareness of therapy including expected response and possible adverse reactions.

J. Complications.

Hyperglycemia, 790.6

Slipped capital femoral epiphysis, 732.9

---

      1.   Growth hormone administration: hyperglycemia, increased incidence of slipped capital femoral epiphysis.

K. Education.

      1.   Provide guidance for physical, psychologic, social development.

      2.   Assist short children and their families with ways to cope with living in bigger world.

IV. DIABETES MELLITUS

Blurred vision, 368.8	Incontinence, 788.3
Cerebral edema, 348.5	Increasing blood pressure, 401.9
Decrease in activity, 780.99	Ketonuria, 791.6
Decreasing heart rate, 427.89	Lethargy, 780.79
Dehydration, 276.5	Mental confusion, 289.9
Diabetes mellitus, 250	Monilial vaginitis, 112.1
Diabetic ketoacidosis, 250.1	Nocturia, 788.43
Enuresis, 788.3	Polydipsia, 783.5
Fatigue, 780.79	Polyphagia, 783.6
Flushed face and cheeks, 782.62	Polyuria, 788.42

Fruity odor to breath, 784.9	Seizures, 780.39
Glucosuria, 791.5	Slow, labored breathing, 786.09
Headache, 784	Vomiting 787.03
High blood glucose levels, 790.29	Weight loss, 783.21

A. Type 1 diabetes: metabolic syndrome (autoimmune disease) characterized by glucose intolerance, causing hypoglycemia/lack of pancreatic hormone (insulin). Insulin is an essential hormone that allows glucose to enter insulin-dependent tissue such as skeletal muscle, liver, fat cells. Lack of available insulin results in catabolism and development of diabetic ketoacidosis.

B. Etiology.
   1. Beta cell mass in islets of Langerhans of pancreas are gradually destroyed in genetically susceptible child.
   2. Triggers, such as environmental, dietary, viral, bacterial, or chemical, that induce T-cell–mediated beta cell injury and production of humoral auto-antibodies.
   3. Pancreatic islet cell antibodies are found in 70–85% of newly diagnosed diabetes mellitus. Degree of beta cell destruction determined by first-phase insulin response during testing for glucose tolerance.

C. Occurrence.
   1. Annual incidence in United States is about 11.7–17.8/100,000 per year for child population.
   2. Peak ages for presentation of diabetes mellitus: 5–7 years of age, at time of puberty; however, present in growing number of children between 1 and 2 years of age.

D. Clinical manifestations.
   1. Polydipsia, polyphagia, enuresis in toilet-trained child.
   2. Polyuria, nocturia.
   3. Blurred vision.
   4. Weight loss, vomiting.
   5. Fatigue, decrease in activity.
   6. Cerebral edema in diabetic ketoacidosis warning signs:
      a. Headache.
      b. Lethargy.
      c. Incontinence.
      d. Seizures.
      e. Pupillary changes.
      f. Decreasing heart rate.
      g. Increasing blood pressure.

      7. Cerebral edema occurs in 1–5% of those with diabetic ketoacidosis.

E. Physical findings.
1. Ketonuria, ketonemia, glucosuria.
2. Vomiting.
3. Dehydration.
4. Slow, labored breathing, flushed face and cheeks.
5. Mental confusion, lethargy.
6. Fruity odor to breath.
7. High blood glucose levels.
8. Monilial vaginitis in adolescent females.

F. Diagnostic tests.
1. Fasting plasma glucose, casual plasma glucose.
2. Urine for ketones and glucose.
3. Electrolytes and pH.
4. Blood urea nitrogen.
5. CBC.

G. Differential diagnosis.

Hypoglycemia, 251.2	Salicylate intoxication, 535.4
Intracranial lesions, 784.2	Sepsis, 038.9

1. Hypoglycemia.
2. Salicylate intoxication.
3. Sepsis.
4. Intracranial lesions.

H. Treatment.
1. Multidisciplinary approach involving family with pediatric endocrinologist, PNP, diabetic nurse educator, social worker, nutritionist.
2. Educate child and family in stabilizing blood sugars, diabetes management. Due to complexity of illness, management requires incorporation into daily life.
3. Treatment replaces insulin that child is unable to produce—the cornerstone of management.
4. Insulin dosage is tailored to child's blood glucose and HbA1c levels (**Table 29-1**). Diabetic control: based on HbA1c levels, clinical symptoms. HbA1c levels provide information on glycemic control during past 60 days.
5. Insulin is categorized by peak of onset.
6. Various insulin injection devices available.

Table 29-1 HbA1c and Glycemic Targets

	Premeal (mg/dL [mmol/L])	Postmeal (mg/dL [mmol/L])	HbA1c
Infants, toddlers	< 7.5 to 8.5	100 to 180 (5.6 to 10)	< 200 (11.1)
School-aged children	< 8.0	70 or 80 to 150 (3.9 or 4.4 to 8.3)	< 200 (11.1)
Teens	< 7.5	70 to 140 or 150 (3.9 to 7.7 or 8.3)	< 180 (10)

Source: Kaufman, F. (2003). Type 1 diabetes mellitus. *Pediatrics in Review, 24,* 9.

I. Follow up.
  1. Review medical, nutritional, insulin therapy, daily blood glucose monitoring (**Table 29-2**).
  2. Follow up every 3 months to review management plans, physical/psychosocial needs (**Table 29-3**).
J. Complications.

Eating disorders, 307.5	Neuropathy, 357.2
Ketoacidosis, 250.1	Retinopathy, 362.1
Nephropathy, 583.9	Vaginal yeast infections, 112.9

  1. Ketoacidosis.
  2. Vaginal yeast infections.
  3. Retinopathy.
  4. Nephropathy.
  5. Neuropathy.
  6. Lipid profile.
  7. Eating disorders.
K. Education.
  1. Prevention of diabetic ketoacidosis.
  2. Knowledge of onsets of action, peak action, duration of action of five types of insulin (**Table 29-4**).
  3. Recognition of hypoglycemia and hyperglycemia.
  4. Management of hypoglycemia: evening protein or fat snack to prevent hypoglycemia.

Table 29-2 Principal Adjustments in Basic or Set Insulin Dose

Rapid-, short-, intermediate-, or long-acting insulin is adjusted after a pattern has been identified over 3–7 days.

Increase or decrease by 0.5, 1.0, 1.5, or 2.0 units (10% of dose).

Time of test	Change this insulin
2 or 3 insulin injections	
Before breakfast	Evening intermediate- or long-acting
Before lunch	Morning rapid- or short-acting
Before dinner	Morning intermediate- or long-acting
Before bedtime	Evening rapid- or short-acting
In the night	Evening intermediate- or long-acting
Multiple insulin injections	
Same as above except:	
Before dinner	Lunch rapid- or short-acting
Insulin pump	
Change bolus dose if blood glucose abnormal	< 2–3 hours after the meal
Change basal dose if blood glucose abnormal	> 3 hours after the meal

Recheck to be sure the changes made return blood glucose levels to the target range.

Source: Kaufman, F. (2003). Type 1 diabetes mellitus. *Pediatrics in Review, 24,* 9.

5. Prevention of long-term complications.
6. Role of exercise in management: Exercise improves glucose utilization.
7. Insulin therapy and monitoring of glucose levels.
8. Meal planning, nutrition: Eat meals and snacks within 1 hour of usual time.
9. School issues and coping skills.
10. Monitoring weight: Maintain ideal body weight.

Table 29-3 The Outpatient Visit for Patients with Diabetes

Physical examination	Frequency recommendations
Weight, height, body mass index (BMI)	Every 3 months/assess changes in percentile
Sexual maturity rating stage	Every 3 months/note pubertal progression
Blood pressure	Every 3 months/target < 90th percentile for age
Eye	Dilated funduscopic examination every 12 months after 5 years of diabetes
Thyroid	Every 3 months/presence of goiter, signs of thyroid dysfunction
Abdomen	Every 3 months/presence of hepatomegaly, fullness, signs of malabsorption, inflammation
Foot, peripheral pulses	Every 3 months inspection/after 12 years of age, thorough
Skin, joints, injection sites	Every 3 months/injection sites, joint mobility, lesions associated with diabetes
Neurologic	Every 12 months/signs of autonomic changes, pain, neuropathy
Laboratory test	Frequency
HbA1c	Every 3 months
Microalbuminuria	Every 12 months after puberty or after 5 years of diabetes
Urinalysis, creatinine	At presentation and with signs of renal problems
Fasting lipid profile	After stabilization at diagnosis and every few years
Thyroid function tests, including antithyroid antibodies	Every 12 months
Celiac screen	At time of diagnosis; if symptoms, at puberty
Islet antibodies	At diagnosis

Source: Kaufman, F. (2003). Type 1 diabetes mellitus. *Pediatrics in Review, 24,* 9.

Table 29-4 Onset of Action, Peak Action, and Duration of Action in Five Types of Insulin

Insulin preparation	Duration of action (hours)	Maximal duration (hours)	Onset of action (hours)	Peak action (hours)
Rapid-acting				
Lispro	¼–½	1–2	3–5	4–6
Aspart	¼–½	1–2	3–6	5–8
Short-acting				
Regular	½–1	2–4	3–6	6–8
Intermediate-acting				
NPH (isophane)	2–4	8–10	10–18	14–20
Lente (zinc suspension)	2–4	8–12	12–20	14–22
Long-acting				
Ultralente (extended zinc suspension)	6–10	10–16	18–20	20–24
Basal Glargine	1–2	None	19–24	24

Source: Kaufman, F. (2003). Type 1 diabetes mellitus. *Pediatrics in Review, 24,* 9.

V. TYPE 2 DIABETES

Acanthosis nigricans, 701.2	Polydipsia, 783.5
Dyslipidemia, 272.5	Polyuria, 788.42
Dysuria, 788.1	Sleep apnea, 780.57
Family history of type 2 diabetes, V18	Type 2 diabetes, 250
Hypertension, 401.9	Vaginal infection, 616.1
Obesity, 278	Weight loss, 783.2

A. Chronic metabolic disorder characterized by insulin resistance.

B. Etiology.
   1. Most common clinical factor for type 2 diabetes is obesity/body mass index (BMI) > 85% for age and sex.
C. Occurrence.
   1. Female-to-male ratio is 1.7:1 regardless of race. Youths between 8–19 years of age.
D. Clinical findings.
   1. Obesity.
   2. Polyuria.
   3. Polydipsia and weight loss.
   4. Vaginal infection as chief complaint.
   5. Dysuria.
   6. Family history.
   7. Sedentary lifestyle, sleep apnea.
E. Physical findings.
   1. Obesity.
   2. Acanthosis nigricans: darkened thick, velvety pigmentation in skin folds.
   3. Hypertension.
   4. Dyslipidemia.
   5. Vaginal infection.
F. Diagnostic tests.
   1. Clinical impression with urinalysis.
   2. Plasma insulin.
   3. C-peptide concentrations.
   4. Autoantibodies to islet cell.
   5. Glutamic acid decarboxylase and tyrosine phosphatase helpful in distinguishing between type 1 and type 2 diabetes.
   6. Androgen levels.
   7. Serum testosterone levels.
G. Differential diagnosis.

Type 1 diabetes, 250.01

   1. Type 1 diabetes.
   2. Polycystic ovarian syndrome.
H. Treatment.
   1. Whenever possible, manage child with multidisciplinary team.
   2. Treat underlying cause of disorder: obesity.
   3. Increase physical activity/moderate exercise is of primary importance.

4. Diet should aim for gradual, sustained weight loss (eat smaller portions, lower caloric foods).
5. Treat hypertension if it exists.
I. Follow up.
 1. Routine health visits including dilated eye exam, foot exams, blood pressure, lipids, albuminuria.
 2. Assistance with lifestyle changes.
J. Complications.

Type 1 diabetes, ketoacidosis, 250.11
---

1. Type 1 diabetes, ketoacidosis.
K. Education.
 1. Lifestyle changes: most important, challenging issues.
 2. Near normalization of blood glucose and glycohemoglobin.
 3. Control lipids.
 4. Set outcome goals of mutual agreement.
 5. Review medication usage and insulin or oral medication if prescribed.

VI. STEROID USE WITH ATHLETES

Acne, 706.1	Mood swings, 296.99
Aggressiveness, 301.3	Ovulation, inhibition of, 628
Alopecia, 704	Prostate hypertrophy, 600.9
Breast atrophy in females, 611.4	Seborrhea, 706.3
Depressed libido, 799.81	Skin sensation, disturbance of, 782
Depression, 311	Sustained penile erection/priapism, 607.3
Early male baldness, 704	Testicular atrophy, 608.3
Headaches, 784	Torn or ruptured tendons, 845.09
Hirsutism, 704.1	Voice change, 784.49
Hypercholesterolemia, 272	Weight gain, 783.1
Hypertension, 401.9	Weight loss, 783.21
Jaundice, 782.4	Water retention, 782.3
Menses abnormalities, 626.4	

A. Anabolic, androgenic steroids: synthetic hormones used to develop bulk, muscle strength.

B. Etiology.
   1. Administration of or use by competing athletes for sole intention of increasing performance in artificial, unfair manner.
   2. Anabolic and androgenic steroids mimic action of hormones normally present.
   3. Anabolic compounds stimulate building of muscle.
   4. Androgenic compounds stimulate development of masculine characteristics.
   5. Steroids refer to class of drugs; known as performance-enhancing drugs.
   6. In males, testosterone is produced by testes and adrenal gland.
   7. In females, testosterone is produced only by adrenal gland; much less testosterone than males.
C. Occurrence.
   1. The prevalence of self-reported use of anabolic steroids in adolescence has ranged from 5–11% of males and up to 2.5% in females.
   2. Athletes in nonschool sports as well as nonathletes have been shown to represent a significant portion of the user population.
D. Clinical manifestations.
   1. Improbable gains in lean body mass, muscle bulk, definition.
   2. Behavioral changes/mood swings.
   3. Advanced stages of acne on chest and back.
   4. Headaches.
   5. Depressed libido.
   6. Early male baldness.
   7. Sustained penile erection/priapism.
   8. Deepening voice with laryngeal changes.
   9. Abnormal menses.
   10. Inhibition of ovulation.
   11. Depression, aggressiveness/combativeness.
E. Physical findings.
   1. Yellowing of eyes/jaundice.
   2. Oily skin.
   3. Water retention in tissue.
   4. Unexplained weight gain or loss.
   5. Breast development in males.
   6. Testicular atrophy.
   7. Seborrhea.
   8. Hypertension.
   9. Increased total cholesterol.
   10. Prostate hypertrophy.

11. Weakened tendons resulting in tearing or rupture.
12. Damage to growth plate at end of bones, permanently stunting growth.
13. Baldness/alopecia.
14. Clitoral enlargement.
15. Hirsutism.
16. Breast atrophy in females.
17. Acne.
F. Diagnostic tests.
  1. Urine for steroids.
  2. Electrolytes.
  3. Alkaline phosphatase.
  4. Serum glutamic oxaloacetic transaminase (SGOT), serum glutamic pyruvic transaminase (SGPT).
  5. Liver enzymes.
  6. Cholesterol profile.
  7. CBC.
G. Differential diagnosis.

Bipolar disease, 297.7
Brain tumor, 784.2
Pituitary gland dysfunction, 253.9

  1. Bipolar disease.
  2. Brain tumor.
  3. Pituitary gland dysfunction.
H. Treatment.
  1. Discontinuance of steroids, psychologic counseling.
I. Follow up.
  1. Emphasize benefits of proper training and nutrition.
  2. Provide effective role models for athlete.
  3. Evaluate hypertension, lipids.
J. Complications.

Coronary heart disease, 414
Liver tumors, 573.8

  1. Anabolic steroid psychologic addiction (addiction syndrome).
  2. Epiphyseal plate closure if adolescent continues to grow while taking steroids.

3. Liver tumors.
4. Risk of coronary heart disease directly related to low-density lipoprotein.
K. Education.
   1. Risks of steroid use; long-term health effects of continued use.

VII. POLYCYSTIC OVARIAN SYNDROME/DISEASE

A. Etiology.
   1. Endocrine disorder characterized by symptoms of obesity, amenorrhea, hirsutism, polycystic ovaries, and excessive androgen production.
B. Occurrence.
   1. High during adolescence and prevalence ranges from 8–26% of females age 12–45 years.
C. Clinical manifestation.
   1. Obesity.
   2. Hirsutism.
   3. Acne.
   4. Menstrual irregularities.
   5. Acanthosis nigricans suggesting insulin resistance.
D. Physical findings.
   1. Obesity/weight above 95% for age and sex.
   2. Hyperpigmentation of skin/neck, axillae, skin folds, and vulva.
   3. Acne.
   4. Dysfunctional bleeding/delayed menarche or amenorrhea.
E. Diagnostic tests.
   1. Serum testosterone levels free and total.
   2. Fasting insulin levels.
   3. Ultrasound of ovaries "pearl necklace appearance."
   4. LH and FSH levels.
   5. DHEA-S.
   6. 17 hydroxy-progesterone level.
   7. T3, T4.
   8. Triglycerides and cholesterol levels.
   9. Glucose tolerance.
F. Differential diagnosis.
   1. Type 2 diabetes.
   2. Pituitary thalamus disorder.
   3. Thyroid disease.

4. Adrenal cortex disease.
5. Ovarian dysfunction.
G. Treatment.
   1. Referral to endocrinologist.
   2. Regulate menses with oral contraceptive. Oral contraceptives such as norgestimate/ethinyl estradiol (Ortho-Cyclen) and norgestimate ethinyl estradio (Ortho Tri-Cyclen) help regulate menses, help with hirsutism, reduce acne, increase bone density, reduce follicular activity, and reduce ovarian and endometrial cancer risk. Oral contraceptives act by suppressing plasma androgens and inhibit ovarian function. If the patient cannot tolerate oral contraceptives, the next therapy would be medroxyprogesterone acetate (Depo Provera) for irregular menses.
   3. Stabilize or reduce body weight/manage lifestyle changes.
   4. Spironolactone (Aldactone) in daily doses of 50–2000 mg orally. Acts by binding at sites of androgen receptors and inhibiting testosterone biosynthesis.
   5. Cosmetic treatment for unwanted hair: either laser or electrolysis.
   6. Acne treated with clindamycin (Cleocin) or other antibacterial medications as indicated.
   7. Insulin resistance may be treated with glucophage (Metformin).
   8. Cholesterol- and triglyceride-lowering drugs as indicated.
H. Follow up.
   1. Monitor for prevention of long-term health problems such as cardiovascular disease.
   2. Lifestyle modification such as diet and exercise for obesity.
I. Complications.
   1. Hypertension.
   2. Hyperlipidemia.
   3. Hyperinsulinemia.
   4. Endometrial hyperplasia.
   5. Type 2 diabetes mellitus.

BIBLIOGRAPHY

Alemzadeh R, Wyatt D. Diabetes mellitus in children. In Kleigman R, Behrman, R, et al., eds. *Nelson textbook of pediatrics*. 18th ed. Philadelphia, PA: W.B. Saunders; 2007:2404–2431.

Barron A, & Falsette D. Polycystic ovary syndrome. *Advance for Nurse Practitioners*. 2008;16(3):49–54.

Binns H, & Ariza J. Guidelines help clinicians identify risk factors for overweight in children. *Pediatric Annals*. 2004;33:1.

Cohen P, Rogol AD, Deal CL, Rogol A, Dean C, Saenger E, et al. Consensus statement on diagnosis and treatment of children with idiopathic short stature: Summary of the Growth Hormone Research Society. *Journal of Clinical Endocrinology Metabolism.* 2008;93(11):4210–4217.

Congeni J, & Miller S. (2002). Supplement and drugs used to enhance athletic performance. *Pediatric Clinics of North America.* 2002;49(2):435–461.

Cox D, & Polvado K. Type 2 diabetes in children and adolescents. *Advance for Nurse Practitioner.* 2008; 16(11):43–45.

Greydanus DE, & Patel DR. (2010). Sports doping in adolescent: The Faustian conundrum of hors de combat. *Pediatric Clinics of North America.* 2010;57(30):729–750.

Gunder L, & Haddow S. Laboratory evaluation of thyroid function. *The Clinical Advisor.* 2009;12(12):26–32.

Ho J, Loh C, Pacoud D, & Liung A. Type 1 diabetes mellitus in children and adolescents: Part 1, overview and diagnosis. *Consultant for Pediatricians.* 2010;9(2):55–57.

Jenkins R, Adger H. Anabolic steroids. In: Kliegman R, Behman R, et al., ed. *Nelson textbook of pediatrics,* 18th ed. Philadelphia, PA: W.B. Saunders; 2007:833–834.

Kaufman F. Type 1 diabetes mellitus. *Pediatric Review.* 2003;24:9.

LaFranchi S. Disorders of the thyroid gland. In Saunders. 833–834.

Pinhas-Hamiel O. Type 2 diabetes: Not just for grownups anymore. *Contemporary Pediatrics.* 2001;18:1.

Sanfilippo J. Hirsuitism and polycystic ovarian syndrome in Kliegman R, Behman R, et al., eds. *Nelson textbook of pediatrics,* 18th ed. Philadelphia, PA: W.B. Saunders; 2007:2282–2283.

Sanfilippo J. Hirsuitism and polycystic ovarian syndrome. In Kliegman R, Behman R, et al., eds. *Nelson textbook of pediatrics,* 18th ed. Philadelphia, PA: W.B. Saunders; 2007:2316–2337.

Samuels C, & Cohen L. Understanding growth patterns in short stature. *Contemporary Pediatrics.* 2001;18:6.

Witchel S, & Finegold D. Endocrinology. In B. Zitelli & H. Davis, eds. *Atlas of pediatric physical diagnosis:* St. Louis: Mosby; 2002.

Wong K, Potter A. Mulbaney S, Russell W, Schlundt D, & Rothman R. Pediatric Endocrinologist's Management of Children with Type 2 Diabetes. *Diabetes Care.* 2010;33(3):512–514.

CHAPTER 30

Musculoskeletal Disorders

Miki M. Patterson

I. INJURIES: SPRAIN, STRAIN, OVERUSE

Ankle sprain, 845	Ligament tear, 848.9
Dislocation, 839.8	Sprain, 848.9
Finger sprain, 842.1	Wrist sprain, 842
Fracture, 829	

A. Etiology.
1. Damage or disruption to tendon (attaches muscle to bone), ligament (attaches bone to bone), from overstretching, exertion, repetitive application of excessive forces.
B. Occurrence.
1. Wrist, finger, ankle sprains are common among children.
C. Clinical manifestations.
1. Limp or pain with extremity or joint use.
2. Felt tearing or heard a "pop" during activity or with trauma.
D. Physical findings.
1. Pain, tenderness to palpation, swelling, discoloration (ecchymosis or erythema).
E. Diagnostic tests.
1. Radiograph in two planes to ensure no fracture and to assess bony relationships. May need views of unaffected side to compare ossification centers and normal alignment.
2. Physical exam: stress joints to varus, valgus, anterior, posterior. If a "give" is felt (e.g., at a knee or ankle joint "opening up"), refer patient to orthopedist. Palpation over physis should be pain free.
F. Differential diagnosis.

Dislocation, 839.8	Ligament tear, 848.9
Fracture, 829	Neurologic deficit, 781.99

1. Fracture, dislocation, ligament tears, neurologic deficit, vascular condition.
G. Treatment.
 1. Protect, rest, ice, compression, elevation (PRICE) and medication for pain as needed:
  a. *Protect:* with splint/brace or relief of weight bearing with crutches.
  b. *Rest:* do not use extremity.
  c. *Ice:* apply ice immediately for 10–20 minutes then every 3–4 hours for the first 24–48 hours.
  d. *Compression:* with ACE wrap; do not pull tightly when wrapping; compression will decrease amount of blood allowed to seep from injured tissues and decrease range of motion at joint.
  e. *Elevation:* above level of heart will decrease swelling accumulating from gravity.
  f. Identify and alter factors that contributed to overuse.
  g. May continue to do activities that do not cause pain.
  h. Pain relievers such as ibuprofen or narcotic, if needed.
H. Follow up.
 1. Return in 1 week to ensure resolution of majority of pain, swelling, and return of function.
 2. Pain and swelling after 2 weeks requires further workup.
I. Complications.

Compartment syndrome, 958.8
Skin abrasion, 919

 1. Missed fracture.
 2. *Caution:* Salter fractures (through the growth plate) may not be visible on X-ray; if physis is tender, treat as fracture (**Figure 30-1**).
 3. Compartment syndrome.
 4. Skin breakdown (presents as burning sensation under brace or splint; results from ischemia of tissue; pressure should be relieved immediately).
J. Education.
 1. Teach family to call immediately for any burning or worsening of pain, neurovascular changes such as paresthesias (numbness or tingling), pallor, paralysis, pulselessness, cyanosis—these 4 Ps are signs of compartment syndrome.
  a. Considered a surgical *emergency*.
  b. Most important: worsening pain and tightness.
  c. Compartment syndrome is accumulation of pressure in tissues, not relieved with elevation.
  d. Most common areas: calves, forearms, hands, feet.

Figure 30-1 Salter I fracture. Note the increased width compared to the distal tibial physis.

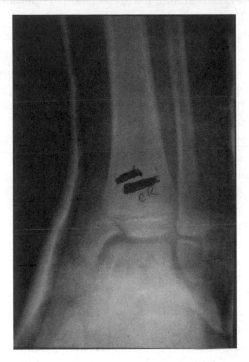

Source: Courtesy of Miki Patterson.

2. Range of motion, stretching should be pain free before beginning strengthening rehabilitation exercises then gradual return to regular activity.

II. INJURIES: FRACTURE, DISLOCATION

Dislocation, 839.8	Fracture, 829
Ecchymosis, 459.89	Point skin tenderness, 782
Erythema, 695.9	

A. Etiology.
1. Damage/disruption to bone or joint, respectively, from trauma, exertion, overuse.
2. Most common causes: child abuse and neglect, sports, falls, motor vehicle or pedestrian/bicycle events.

B. Occurrence.
1. All age groups can be affected.
2. Fractures are most common presentation of child abuse; 70% of fractures in children younger than 6 months are inflicted.
3. Fractures suggestive of nonaccidental trauma in children: metaphyseal, rib (seen in 5–20% of abused children), scapular/distal clavicle/night stick (midshaft ulna), vertebral fracture or subluxation, fingers in nonambulating child, humerus (except supracondylar) in those younger than 3 years of age, bilateral/multiple fractures in different stages of healing as well as complex skull.
C. Clinical manifestations.
1. Felt tearing or heard "pop" or "crack."
2. Most affect function.
3. Findings suspect for abuse:
   a. Fracture in child younger than 1 year of age.
   b. Unknown or unwitnessed injury.
   c. Delay in seeking medical attention.
   d. Changing story of how injury occurred.
   e. Fracture does not fit mechanism described (e.g., twisting an extremity will result in spiral fracture, whereas direct blow produces transverse fracture).
D. Physical findings.
1. Pain, point tenderness, swelling, ecchymosis or erythema, loss of function, obvious deformity.
E. Diagnostic tests.
1. Radiographs in two planes: AP and lateral or both obliques.
2. May require computed tomography (CT) scan or MRI for complex injuries (i.e., pelvis or spine).
F. Differential diagnosis.

Sprain, 848.9

1. Sprain.
G. Treatment.
1. Protect with immobilization/splinting, compression, ice, elevation.
2. Do not use extremity.
3. Pain medication (typically narcotic) such as acetaminophen (Tylenol) with codeine at 1 mg/kg of body weight every 4–6 hours for small children

or hydrocodone (Vicodin), oxycodone (Percocet), or morphine by weight for those > 100 pounds.

4. Dislocation and displaced fractures refer stat to orthopedist. Oral medication should not be used if surgical intervention is an imminent possibility.

H. Follow up.
1. Should be per orthopedist.
2. Many will not allow use of extremity for a period of time while healing.
3. Muscles will spasm around fracture to try to pull bone ends together for healing.
4. Fractures without fixation move for 10–14 days after injury while granulation occurs (even in casts).
5. Frequent X-rays may be needed to ensure alignment of fractures.
6. In 2–6 weeks: callus develops, bone ends become "sticky," pain is reduced.
7. Consolidation begins at 3 weeks in infants, may take 3–6 months in older children, adults.
8. Weight bearing, casting, splinting, bracing, or full use are all related to fracture configuration, healing, patient specifics.
9. Remodeling of bone that occurs in children younger than 8 years of age allows acceptance of angulated fractures.
10. Increased circulation to fractured bone causes some overgrowth (basis for 1-cm overlap of fractured femurs in young children).

I. Complications.

Compartment syndrome, 958.8

Loss of alignment, 781.2

Skin abrasion, 919

---

1. Compartment syndrome.
2. Loss of alignment.
3. Shortening, angulation, delayed or nonunion of fracture.
4. Skin breakdown.
5. Neurovascular problems.
6. Infection.
7. Missed abuse.

J. Education.
1. Same as for sprains.
2. Family should seek medical attention for neurovascular changes or pain inside cast/splint/brace.

III. BACK PAIN

Scoliosis, 737.3

Back pain, 724.5

A. Etiology.
   1. See Differential Diagnosis (below).
B. Occurrence.
   1. Most common in preadolescent and adolescent.
C. Clinical manifestations.
   1. Complaint of back pain, sometimes night pain (red flag), with/without numbness or tingling.
D. Physical findings.
   1. May or may not have:
      a. Deformity of spine.
      b. Pain with motion.
      c. Positive straight leg raise sign.
      d. Tight hamstrings (unable to sit upright with legs extended straight out in front).
      e. Neurologic changes or skin lesions.
E. Diagnostic tests.
   1. Radiographs: AP and lateral thoracolumbar and/or lumbosacral spine.
   2. Other testing as exam or history indicates (e.g., bone scan, MRI, labs: complete blood count (CBC) with differential, erythrocyte sedimentation rate [ESR], antinuclear antibodies [ANA], rheumatoid factor, or human leukocyte antigen B27 [HLA-B27]).
F. Differential diagnosis.

Ankylosis spondylitis, 720	Psoriatic arthritis, 696
Degenerative disk disease, 722.6	Reiter syndrome, 099.3
Discitis, 722.9	Scheuermann's kyphosis, 737.1
Inflammatory bowel disease, 569.9	Scoliosis, 737.3
Fracture, back, 805.8	Sickle cell crisis, 282.6
Kidney infection, 590.9	Spondylolisthesis, 756.12
Menstrual cramping, 625.3	Spondylolysis, 756.11
Osteoma, 213.9	

   1. Overuse (heavy backpacks).

Figure 30-2 (a) Spondylolisthesis (slipped forward) L-5 on S-1 with (b) spondylolysis (fractured).

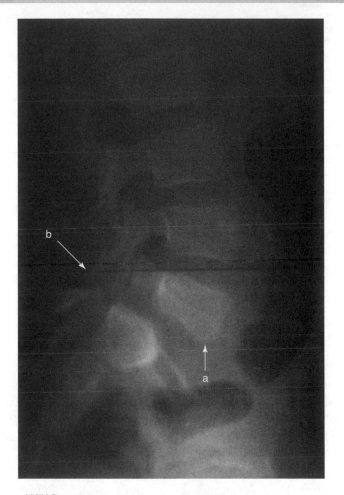

Source: Courtesy of Miki Patterson.

2. Fracture, spondylolysis (defect or separation of pars interarticularis), and spondylolisthesis (anterior slippage of vertebral body) typically occur at L-5 (**Figure 30-2**).
3. Scheuermann's kyphosis (anterior wedging > 5° of 3 or more adjacent vertebrae).
4. Scoliosis (see later discussion).
5. Degenerative disk disease, infection, discitis.

6. Inflammatory conditions, such as ankylosis spondylitis, psoriatic arthritis, inflammatory bowel disease, Reiter's syndrome (morning stiffness is hallmark sign).
7. Neoplastic such as osteoid osteoma (hallmark sign: night pain or constant pain independent of motion).
8. Other: sickle cell crisis, functional illness, referred pain such as kidney infection or menstrual cramping.

G. Treatment.
1. Depends on diagnosis: rest, nonsteroidal anti-inflammatory drugs (NSAIDs), stretching, abdominal strengthening, proper posture and backpack use, or referral to orthopedist.

H. Follow up.
1. Symptoms should improve in 2 weeks for overuse or strains.

I. Complications.
1. Missed diagnosis (see Differential Diagnosis).

J. Education.
1. Demonstrate exercises to help ensure that they are done correctly.
2. Work with family on medication schedule.
3. If symptoms persist or new symptoms occur, call healthcare provider.

IV. SCOLIOSIS

Embryonic malformation, 759.9

A. Abnormal lateral curvature of spine, typically with vertebral rotation.
B. Etiology.
1. Idiopathic: 90% (most common), unknown etiology, familiar pattern has been noted.
C. Occurrence.
1. Idiopathic: 3–5% in adolescents screened; males = females.
2. 0.6% require treatment; however, females are treated more often (1%) than males (0.1%).
D. Clinical manifestations.
1. Does not typically cause back pain (< 14%).
E. Physical findings.
1. Difficulty with fitting clothes.
2. S- or C-shape curve of spine.

3. Prominent: scapular, ribcage, paraspinal musculature (especially on forward bend test) or breast.
4. Asymmetric waistline or shoulder level.
5. Plumb line dropped from C-7 does not correlate with gluteal crease.

F. Diagnostic tests.
1. Inspection with minimal clothing.
2. Radiographs: scoliosis series, which is standing postero-anterior (PA) and lateral views of entire spine on one cassette.

G. Differential diagnosis.

Cerebral palsy, 343.9	Neurofibromatosis, 237.7
Emotional disturbance, 313.9	Polio, 045.1
Muscular dystrophy, 359.1	Spina bifida, 741.9
Myopathies, 359.9	Vertebra fracture, 805.8

1. Congenital: embryonic malformation.
2. Paralytic: polio, muscular dystrophy, cerebral palsy, spina bifida, myopathies, neurofibromatosis.
3. Traumatic: fracture of vertebrae.
4. Hysterical: rare, nonstructural, result of emotional disturbance.

H. Treatment.
1. Orthopedic referral all curves > 10°.
2. Orthopedic treatment for curves 10–20° observation.
3. Curves 20–40°: bracing (controversial) to prevent further curvature.
4. Curves > 40°: surgical intervention, posterior spinal fusion with segmental instrumentation occasionally requires anterior release.

I. Follow up.
1. Per orthopedics: until skeletal maturity (about 1 year after menstruation for girls).

J. Complications.

Lumbar back pain, 724.2

1. Progressive untreated scoliosis may result in significant deformity, cardiopulmonary compromise, debilitating lumbar back pain.

K. Education.
1. If braces and/or exercises ordered, ensure compliance.
2. Bracing helps delay progression of curve.

3. Frequent skin inspection necessary with brace use.
4. Continue usual activities if pain free in brace.

V. HIP PAIN

Hip pain, 719.45

A. Differential diagnosis.
  1. Infection: septic arthritis, osteomyelitis, Lyme disease, psoas abscess, appendicitis.
  2. Inflammatory: transient synovitis, systemic arthritis, juvenile rheumatoid arthritis (JRA), Kawasaki disease, idiopathic chondrolysis.
  3. Orthopedic conditions: Legg-Calvé-Perthes disease, avascular necrosis (AVN), slipped capital femoral epiphysis (SCFE), stress fracture, apophyseal injuries, trochanteric bursitis, muscular strain.
  4. Neoplastic: osteoid osteoma, leukemia, solid tumor primary, pigmented villonodular synovitis (PVNS), or sickle cell crisis pain.

VI. SEPTIC HIP/SEPTIC ARTHRITIS

Appendicitis, 541	Psoas abscess, 015
Avascular necrosis, 733.4	Septic arthritis, 711
Chondrolysis, 733.99	Sickle cell crisis, 282.6
Juvenile rheumatoid arthritis, 714.3	Slipped capitol femoral
Kawasaki disease, 446.1	epiphysis, 732.2
Legg-Calvé-Perthes disease, 732.1	Systemic arthritis, 716.9
Leukemia, 208.9	Transient synovitis, 727
Lyme disease, 088.81	Trochanteric bursitis, 726.5
Muscular strain, 848.9	Fever, 780.6
Osteoma, 213.9	Hip pain, 719.45
Osteomyelitis, 730.2	Septic arthritis hip, 711.08
Pigmented villonodular synovitis (PVNS), 719.2	

A. Infection in joint; hip joint is infected often, second only to knee in children.

B. Etiology.
   1. Bacterial infection spread hematogenously or from osteomyelitis of the femoral head.
   2. Most common organisms are *Staphylococcus* and *Streptococcus*.
C. Occurrence.
   1. Males = females; infancy to 6 years.
D. Clinical manifestations.
   1. Hip pain.
   2. Refusal to bear weight.
   3. Fever.
   4. Ill-appearing child with extreme pain and resistance to hip motion. Infection builds up pressure in hip capsule and can impede blood flow.
E. Physical findings.
   1. Fever > 37°C, typically lie with hip flexed and externally rotated.
   2. Infants may be irritable with pseudoparalysis of lower extremity.
F. Diagnostic tests.
   1. Elevate white blood cells (WBC) and ESR.
   2. Ultrasound or radiographs demonstrate widening of joint space.
   3. Diagnosis confirmed with CT or ultrasound-guided aspiration.
G. Differential diagnosis.

Septic sacroiliac joint, 711.08

---

   1. Septic sacroiliac joint.
H. Treatment.
   1. Emergent referral to hospital for surgical drainage of hip joint.
   2. Intravenous antibiotics tailored to culture results.
   3. Make sure child receives nothing by mouth (NPO).
I. Follow up.
   1. Per orthopedics, usually 1–2 weeks postop and 3–6 months to follow hip maturity.
J. Complications.

Joint destruction, 718.9

Osteomyelitis, 730.2

Septicemia, 038.9

---

   1. Septicemia, osteomyelitis, joint destruction.

K. Education.
   1. Prepare family for child's hospitalization and treatment with IV antibiotics.

VII. DEVELOPMENTALLY DISLOCATED HIP

> Breech birth, 763
>
> Dislocated hip, 835
>
> Hip dysplasia, 755.63

A. Broad spectrum of hip dysplasia regarding dislocated or dislocatable or sub-luxing femoral head in relation to acetabulum at birth or early development.
B. Etiology.
   1. Genetic, intrauterine position, postnatal positioning.
C. Occurrence.
   1. Most common hip disorder in children.
   2. 1 in 100 infants have hip instability at birth and true dislocation is seen in 1 of 1000 births.

Figure 30-3 Barlow maneuver: knees flexed and brought to midline with gentle downward pressure to see if hip "clunks" out posteriorly.

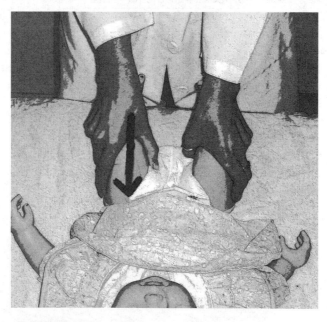

Source: Courtesy of Miki Patterson.

     3.   Ratio: 6 female: 1 male.

     4.   Left hip > right.

     5.   Higher frequency in firstborn children.

  D. Clinical manifestations.

     1.   Breech birth commonly associated with this condition.

     2.   Difficulty diapering (abducting leg).

     3.   Older children may have awkward Trendelenburg gait, leg length discrepancy, pain with ambulation.

  E. Physical findings.

     1.   Difficult in infants due to variety of levels of hip dysplasia.

     2.   Unequal thigh skin creases/gluteal folds.

     3.   Limited abduction.

     4.   Positive Barlow maneuver (to see if dislocatable with femur flexed and midline: adduct 10° gentle pressure posterior feel click with telescoping; **Figure 30-3**).

     5.   Positive Ortolani maneuver (abducting hip, feel it clunk back into place; **Figure 30-4**).

     6.   Galeazzi test (prone with knees flexed and heels at buttock): positive when knee heights are different (**Figure 30-5**).

Figure 30-4 Ortolani maneuver: Abduct hip while pushing up posteriorly with fingers trying to pop hip into the socket. A click is a positive finding.

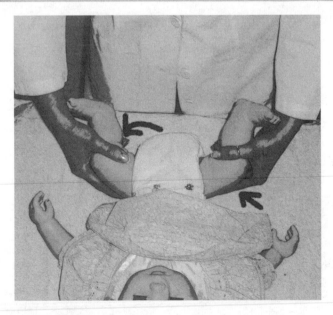

Source: Courtesy of Miki Patterson.

Figure 30-5 Positive Galeazzi test. Note knee height difference.

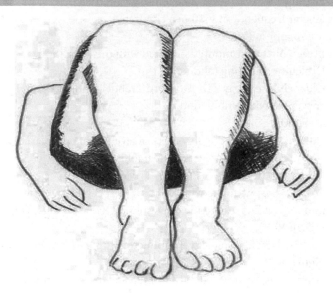

Source: Courtesy of Miki Patterson.

F. Diagnostic tests.

> Arthrogryposis, 728.3
>
> Congenital anomalies, 759.9
>
> Leg length discrepancy, 736.81
>
> Septic hip, 711.08

    1. Ultrasound of hips. Radiographs less helpful because femoral heads have not ossified.

G. Differential diagnosis.

    1. Congenital anomalies, arthrogryposis, septic hip, leg length discrepancy.

H. Treatment.

    1. Refer to orthopedist.

    2. Treatment goal: Reduce femoral head to anatomic position.

    3. May need Pavlik harness, hip spica cast, or surgical intervention.

I. Follow up.

    1. Reexamine hips each visit.

J. Complications.

Degenerated changes, 721.9	Scoliosis, 737.3
Dysplasia, 755.63	Unstable gait, 781.2
Low back pain, 724.2	

1. Delayed treatment affects normal growth of hip joint.
2. If untreated: residual dysplasia, limited range of motion, unstable gait, pain, functional scoliosis, low back pain, early degenerated changes.

K. Education.
1. Report any range-of-motion or neurovascular changes.
2. Important to hold and cuddle baby even in braces and casts.

VIII. TRANSIENT SYNOVITIS

Fever, low-grade, 780.6
Transient synovitis, 727
Urinary tract infection, 599

A. Etiology.
1. Unknown theory of post-traumatic or allergic cause.
2. Infection frequently assumed because 32–50% follow upper respiratory tract infection.

B. Occurrence.
1. 0.2–3% of children 3–8 years of age; 6:1 male-to-female ratio.

C. Clinical manifestations.
1. Pain and limp.

D. Physical findings.
1. Symptoms present < 1 week to 1 month.
2. Fever absent or low grade. Do not appear severely ill.

E. Diagnostic tests.
1. Negative CBC and ESR.
2. Ultrasound positive: effusion.

F. Differential diagnosis.

Legg-Calvé-Perthes disease, 732.1
Osteomyelitis, 730.2
Septic arthritis, 711

1. Septic arthritis *must* be ruled out. Osteomyelitis, Legg-Calvé-Perthes disease.
G. Treatment.
    1. Conservative.
    2. NSAIDs, rest, return to activity as tolerated.
H. Follow up.
    1. If concerned, follow up in 1–2 days to be sure symptoms are resolving.
I. Complications.

Legg-Calvé-Perthes disease, 732.1

Septic arthritis, 711

---

1. Missed septic arthritis (rare).
2. 1–2% may develop Legg-Calvé-Perthes disease.
J. Education.
    1. Any fever > 38.4°C or ill appearance of child should prompt reexamination.

IX. HIP PAIN: LEGG-CALVÉ-PERTHES DISEASE

Hip pain, 719.45

Legg-Calvé-Perthes disease, 732.1

Transient synovitis, 727

A. Idiopathic AVN of femoral head in children.
B. Etiology.
    1. Unknown cause of avascularity; however, multiple theories include trauma, transient synovitis, systemic abnormalities, vascular disturbances from intraosseous venous hypertension and venous obstruction.
C. Occurrence.
    1. 1 in 1200 in general population.
    2. 4:1 male-to-female ratio.
    3. Typically 4–8 years of age.
    4. Bilateral in only 15%; reported to be associated with attention-deficit/hyperactivity disorder (ADHD).

D. Clinical manifestations.
   1. Pain of groin, medial thigh, or knee.
E. Physical findings.
   1. Pain with weight bearing.
   2. Limited internal rotation or abduction of hip.
   3. Muscle spasm may have atrophy of thigh, calf, or buttock from disuse.
   4. Leg length inequality.
F. Diagnostic tests.
   1. Radiographs: AP pelvis and frog lateral hips.
   2. Initial X-rays may be normal; may need CT to see early changes.
   3. Four stages:
      a. Initial: interruption of blood supply, "crescent sign" areas of hyper- and hypodense appearance of femoral head.
      b. Fragmentation: epiphysis appears fragmented.
      c. Reossification: normal bone density returns, deformity becomes apparent.
      d. Healed: healing complete, residual deformity common.
G. Differential diagnosis.

Knee fracture, 822	Slipped capital femoral epiphysis (SCFE), 732.2
Septic hip, 711.08	Transient synovitis, 727

   1. Knee problem, fracture.
   2. Transient synovitis.
   3. Septic hip, SCFE.
   4. Neuromuscular condition.
H. Treatment.
   1. Refer to orthopedist.
   2. Goal: prevent femoral head deformity, alter growth disturbances.
   3. Generally try to unload femoral head while allowing motion.
   4. Abduction brace and bed rest, home traction with progressive abduction of legs.
   5. Surgical adductor release or derotational femoral or pelvic osteotomies and spica body cast occasionally needed.
I. Follow up.
   1. Per orthopedics.
   2. Patients will be followed long term, bed rest with traction, bracing, and surgery performed as indicated.

J. Complications.

Degenerated changes, 721.9
Unstable gait, 781.2

1. May not show on initial films.
2. Delayed treatment affects normal growth of hip joint.
3. Residual deformities (coax magna), limited range of motion, unstable gait, pain, early degenerated changes seen with treated and untreated.

K. Education.
1. Progressive until body replaces "dead" femoral head with new bone; younger it occurs, longer body has to replace collapsing bone and remodel femoral head.
2. No pressure should be put on rebuilding bone, but should be able to move in joint for shaping.

X. HIP PAIN: SLIPPED CAPITAL FEMORAL EPIPHYSIS

Slipped capital femoral epiphysis, 732.2

A. Femoral neck "slips" (displaces anteriorly) at physis (growth plate), leaving femoral head behind in acetabulum (**Figure 30-6**).

B. Etiology.
1. Unknown; however, suspect multifactorial cause, biomechanical, obesity, endocrine, metabolic, trauma, genetics, and other causes (e.g., kidney disorders or radiation).

C. Occurrence.
1. Most common hip disorder of adolescents, 3 of 100,000 are 8–17 years of age.
2. Males (10–17 years of age) affected 2–3 times more often than females (8–15 years of age).
3. Left hip most often affected; bilateral 25–70%.

D. Clinical manifestations.
1. Hip, groin, medial thigh, knee pain; sometimes for months.
2. May be brought on by very minor trauma (chronic/acute or acute on chronic).
3. Antalgic gait (limp to keep weight off painful extremity) or inability to bear weight.

Figure 30-6 Slipped capital femoral epiphysis. Note the appearance of ice cream falling off the cone.

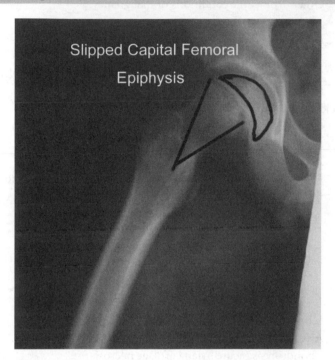

Slipped Capital Femoral

Epiphysis

Source: Courtesy of Miki Patterson.

   E. Physical findings.
      1. Range of motion may be limited depending on severity of slip, may have limited internal rotation and abduction of the hip.
   F. Diagnostic tests.
      1. Radiographs AP pelvis and true lateral (not frog lateral because may cause more femoral head displacement).
   G. Differential diagnosis.

Appendicitis, 541

Hip pain, 719.45

Testicular torsion, 608.2

      1. Knee problem.
      2. Infection.

3. Inflammation.
4. Referred pain such as appendicitis, testicular torsion.
5. Other orthopedic conditions or malignancy.
H. Treatment.
   1. Immediate referral to orthopedist.
   2. *Do not* allow further weight bearing because femoral head can "slip" further.
   3. Surgical intervention with "pinning" by screw(s) to fuse physis between femoral head and neck.
I. Follow up.
   1. Orthopedics typically allow partial weight bearing with crutches for 6–8 weeks.
   2. Return in 2 weeks for wound check, staple removal.
   3. Follow healing clinically and radiographically for several months/years.
J. Complications.

Avascular necrosis, 733.4

Chondrolysis, 733.99

Degenerative changes, 721.9

Malunion, 733.81

---

   1. Missed on X-ray 25% of time.
   2. Avascular necrosis.
   3. Chondrolysis (acute hylan cartilage necrosis).
   4. Loss of range of motion.
   5. Limb shortening.
   6. Early degenerative changes.
   7. Malunion.
K. Education.
   1. High incidence of recurrence of other hip.
   2. Parents or child should report any similar findings and be seen immediately.

XI. KNEE PAIN: OSGOOD-SCHLATTER DISEASE

Knee pain, 719.46

Osgood-Schlatter disease, 732.4

A. Painful swelling of tibial tubercle, caused by traction and resulting in apophysitis.

B. Etiology.
  1. Overuse by chronic repetitive knee flexion.
C. Occurrence.
  1. 11–14 years of age during rapid growth.
  2. Males > females, but ratio changing with increased female participation in sports.
  3. Frequently bilateral.
D. Clinical manifestations.
  1. Pain with running, jumping, kneeling. Resolves/fades with rest.
E. Physical findings.
  1. Pain in anterior knee; warmth, swelling, and tenderness over tibial tubercle, especially with resistive knee extension (kicking motion) or squatting.
F. Diagnostic tests.
  1. Radiographs of knee: AP and lateral and 10° obliques to rule out tumor or fracture.
  2. Classic prominent tibial tubercle above physis (**Figure 30-7**).

Figure 30-7 Osgood-Schlatter disease: apophysitis of the tibial tubercle.

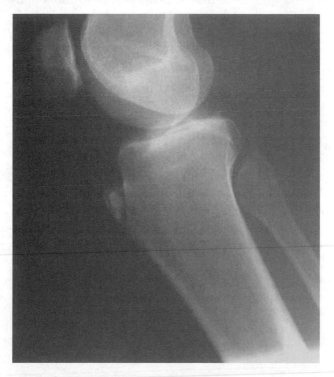

Source: Courtesy of Miki Patterson.

G. Differential diagnosis.

Knee fracture, 822

Sinding-Larsen-Johansson syndrome, 732.4

---

1. Tumor.
2. Fracture.
3. Sinding-Larsen-Johansson syndrome (apophysitis of distal pole of patella).

H. Treatment.
   1. Limit activities, especially sports; ice after activity.
   2. Hamstring and quadriceps stretching and strengthening.
   3. Knee immobilizer or cylinder casting for brief periods to manage severe pain.
   4. Ibuprofen.

I. Follow up.
   1. Teach patients, families to decrease activity; wear knee immobilizer when painful.
   2. Follow up until skeletal maturity seen in closure of physis or growth plate.

J. Complications.

Apophysis deformity, 738.9

Enlargement of tibial tubercle, 718.86

Tibia fracture, 823.8

---

1. Enlargement of tibial tubercle (bony prominence).
2. Pain may continue into adulthood.
3. Fracture of tibial tubercle.
4. Premature closure of apophysis causing recurvatum deformity.

K. Education.
   1. "Bump" made because body thinks there is injury to bone which is being pulled apart at growth plate by patella; tendon bump will *not* go away.
   2. Continued use while painful typically increases size of "bump"; this is cosmetically unappealing for most and may interfere with kneeling. Condition ceases to exacerbate on skeletal maturity.

XII. PHYSIOLOGIC GENU VARUM (BOW LEGS)

Genu varum, 736.42

A. Etiology.
1. Physiologic genu varum or bowing is part of normal development.
B. Occurrence.
1. Most common cause of bow legs in toddlers.
2. Varum is greatest at 6 months of age, may progress to neutral by 18–24 months of age.
3. Adult physiologic valgus (knock knee): about 8°, typically reached by 5–6 years of age.
C. Clinical manifestations.
1. Pain-free bowing appearance to legs of toddler.
D. Physical findings.
1. Gentle curve to entire leg.
2. Normal knee flexion, extension without pain.
3. Normal progression: 15° genu varum at birth (Figure 30-8); 0° (straight) 18–24 months; 10–12° genu valgum (knock knees) at 30 months to 4 years; 0° (straight) to 4–6° genu valgum normal at 4–6 years.
E. Diagnostic tests.
1. Radiographic bowing of entire limb, no acute angulation seen (**Figure 30-8**).
2. Medial proximal tibial physeal changes suggestive of pathology (Blount's disease), refer to orthopedist.
F. Differential diagnosis.

Achondroplasia, 756.4	Osteogenesis imperfecta, 756.51
Blount's, 732.4	Osteomyelitis, 730.2
Chondrodysplasia, 756.4	Renal failure, 593.9
Leg fracture, 827	Rickets, 268

1. Blount's, vitamin D–resistant rickets, renal failure, chondrodysplasia, achondroplasia, osteogenesis imperfecta, osteomyelitis, neoplasm, fracture.
G. Treatment.
1. Generally resolve spontaneously.

Figure 30-8 Physiologic genu varum. Normal "beaking" of distal femur and proximal tibial metaphysis.

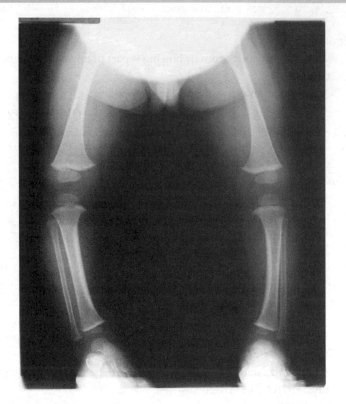

Source: Courtesy of Miki Patterson.

2. Refer to orthopedics for obvious asymmetry, clear progressive deformity, or if associated with pain.
3. Osteotomy and correction of angulation may be performed using internal or external fixation devices.

H. Follow up.
1. Return visits every 3–6 months.

I. Complications.

Blount's, 732.4

Tibia vara, 732.4

1. Tibial vara or Blount's disease (abrupt deformity medial proximal tibia).

    2. May be seen in younger than 5 years of age but more common in adolescents.

    3. Females > males.

    4. Bilateral 80% of time.

    5. Higher incidence in obese and African American children.

    6. Will not correct with age.

J. Education.

    1. Reassurance of normal finding.

    2. Encourage child not to sleep or sit with legs tucked underneath; position might delay spontaneous correction.

XIII. IN-TOEING: METATARSUS ADDUCTUS

> Metatarsus abductus varus, 754.53

A. Etiology.

    1. Unknown, theory of intrauterine position.

B. Occurrence.

    1. Most common childhood foot problem.

    2. 1 in 5000 births.

    3. 1:20 in sibling.

    4. Males, twins, preterm infants have higher incidence.

    5. Seen first year of life; left > right, often bilateral.

C. Clinical manifestations.

    1. Medial deviation of forefoot on hindfoot, in-toeing gait.

D. Physical findings.

    1. C-shaped foot.

E. Diagnostic tests.

    1. No radiographs needed for infants.

    2. Children older than 4 years of age should have standing foot films, 3 views.

F. Differential diagnosis.

> Spastic anterior tibialis, 781
>
> Talipes equinovarus, 754.51

    1. Spastic anterior tibialis.

    2. Talipes equinovarus (clubbed foot).

G. Treatment.
   1. Most will correct with normal use.
   2. Severe deformity: Refer to orthopedist for stretching, serial casting of flexible conditions; surgical intervention is rare.
H. Follow up.
   1. Per orthopedics until deformity is corrected.
   2. Serial casting may be done weekly. Have parents remove semirigid cast night before appointment. Teach to stretch, then apply new cast with orthopedist holding position.
I. Complications.
   1. Cast/skin complications.
   2. Neurovascular problems.
   3. Incorrect position, especially if cast slips and toes are no longer visible (common with infants).
J. Education.
   1. Most resolve spontaneously.
   2. Return to orthopedist if circulation problems, irritability (e.g., suspect cast is bothering child), or if child kicks cast off.

XIV. IN-TOEING: TIBIAL TORSION

Tibial torsion, 736.89

A. Etiology.
   1. Normal development in utero, genetic influence.
B. Occurrence.
   1. Birth 0–20° internal tibial rotation normal: 90% correct with growth, adults achieve 0–20° of external rotation.
C. Clinical manifestations.
   1. Curved appearance to tibia or in-toeing or out-toeing gait.
   2. If knees are pointing forward, feet may either point in (internal tibial torsion) or out (external tibial torsion); becomes less noticeable with running.
D. Physical findings.
   1. Thigh-foot angle (**Figure 30-9**). Child prone with knee bent at 90° angle of imaginary line drawn down thigh and middle of foot. Normal 0–30° external.
   2. Foot progression angle is angle of foot compared to line extended in front of ambulating child. Best observed from directly behind patient (**Figure 30-10**).

Figure 30-9 Thigh-foot angle. A line drawn along the axis of the femur bisects the foot.

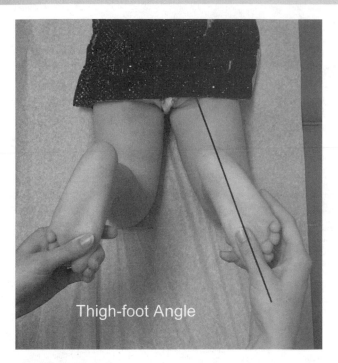

Thigh-foot Angle

Source: Courtesy of Miki Patterson.

E. Diagnostic tests.
   1. None if younger than 8 years of age and symmetrical pain-free appearance.
   2. If needed, standing leg length X-ray (scanogram) done on long cassette.
F. Differential diagnosis.

Hip dysplasia, 755.3

   1. Developmental dysplasia of hip, neuromuscular conditions.
G. Treatment.
   1. Observation.
   2. None unless unilateral or severe or remains after age 8 years.
   3. Tibial osteotomy rare but may be performed for severe cases.
H. Follow up.
   1. If persists at 8 years of age, refer to orthopedist.

Figure 30-10 Foot progression angle: normal variations.

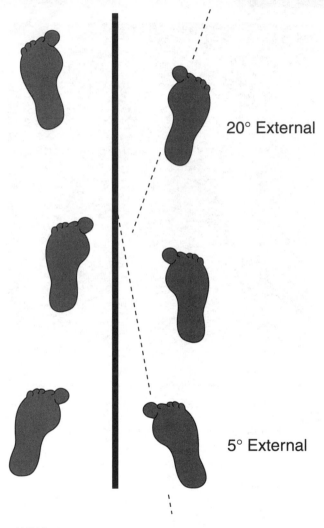

20° External

5° External

Source: Courtesy of Miki Patterson.

    I. Complications.
        1. Rare and related to surgical intervention.
    J. Education.
        1. Reassurance and handouts.
        2. Despite grandparents' (or older relatives'/caregivers') insistence, braces are not effective. Studies show same improvement or correction through normal growth without braces.

3. Many athletic children, adults have tibial torsion; does not result in any increased incidence of arthritis or interfere with activity.

XV. IN-TOEING: FEMORAL ANTEVERSION

Femoral anteversion, 755.63

A. Etiology.
   1. Normal and appears when child begins walking, causing ligaments to get looser; thus hips are allowed more internal rotation, especially in children 2–6 years of age.
B. Occurrence.
   1. Normal in 2- to 4-year olds, usually corrects spontaneously by 8 years of age.
C. Clinical manifestations.
   1. In-toeing gait.
   2. Children tend to "W" sit pain free.
D. Physical findings.
   1. Knees and toes point inward when standing.
   2. Able to internally rotate hips up to 90°.
E. Diagnostic tests.
   1. None.
F. Differential diagnosis.

Hip dysplasia, 755.63

Tibial torsion, 736.89

   1. Tibial torsion, hip dysplasia.
G. Treatment.
   1. Discourage "W" sitting.
   2. Observation unless functional deformity after 8 years old.
   3. Refer to orthopedist for unilateral, severe, or painful deformity.
   4. Surgical intervention with femoral derotational osteotomy.
H. Follow up.
   1. Yearly if not progressive.
I. Complications.
   1. None unless surgical intervention.
J. Education.
   1. Normal, child will grow out of it. Braces or shoe modification are ineffective.

XVI. FOOT PROBLEMS: TALIPES EQUINOVARUS (CLUBBED FOOT)

Clubbed foot, 754.51

Talipes equinovarus, 754.51

A. Rigid fixed foot deformity with inverted heel, forefoot adduction, and down-facing toes.
B. Etiology.
   1. Unknown; possibly genetic, mechanical, chemical embryologic insults.
C. Occurrence.
   1. Age: newborn.
   2. 2:1 males to females.
   3. 1.24 in 1000 live births.
   4. Increased incidence in families where parents/siblings have same disorder.
D. Clinical manifestations.
   1. Tight Achilles tendon, joint capsule, medial ligaments.
   2. Short angulated talus, thin atrophic muscles.
E. Physical findings.
   1. Small foot and calf, with rigid equinus deformed foot with heel in varus.
   2. Prominent crease in arch of foot.
   3. Adducted forefoot.
F. Diagnostic tests.
   1. Clinical exam of newborn; radiographs are of little use.
G. Differential diagnosis.

Arthrogryposis, 728.3

Calcaneovalgus, 755.67

Spastic hemiplegia, 342.1

   1. "Positional clubbed foot," arthrogryposis, spastic hemiplegia, calcaneo-valgus.
H. Treatment.
   1. Refer to orthopedist. Serial casting and surgical intervention may be necessary.
I. Follow up.
   1. Per orthopedist.
   2. Treatment soon after birth: weekly visits for manipulation and casting by orthopedist experienced in this form of treatment.

3. If rigid deformity, surgical intervention may be necessary; may entail heel cord and joint capsule releases and casting typically at 6 months of age.
4. Casting or braces may be used for a period of time; follow up is ongoing because deformity may recur until about age 7 years.
J. Complications.

Leg length discrepancy, 736.81
---

1. Progressive deformity, leg length discrepancy, surgical complications.
K. Education.
1. Affected foot will always be smaller but may function near normal after correction.

XVII. PES PLANUS: FLAT FOOT

Pes planus flat foot, 734

A. Etiology.
1. Flexible normal (asymptomatic) genetic etiology or rigid (symptomatic) tarsal coalition (fusion of calcaneus with talus or navicular) common cause.
B. Occurrence.
1. Normal occurrence younger than 2 years of age due to medial fat pad. Rigid is rare.
C. Clinical manifestations.
1. Flat foot while standing; normal arch that returns while sitting and hanging over exam table is flexible pes planus.
2. Bilateral.
3. Hereditary expression.
4. May cause some discomfort for older children.
D. Physical findings.
1. Loss of normal plantar arch while standing.
2. Limited subtalar joint motion for rigid pes planus.
3. Look at parents' feet!
E. Diagnostic tests.
1. If rigid: radiographs, three standing views of both feet, CT or MRI looking for coalition.

F. Differential diagnosis.

Arthritis, 716.97

Arthrogryposis, 728.3

Foot fracture, 825.2

---

1. Overuse.
2. Arthrogryposis.
3. Neuromuscular condition.
4. Arthritis.
5. Infection.
6. Trauma/fracture.

G. Treatment.
1. Refer rigid pes planus to orthopedist, orthotics may decrease symptoms of older child with flexible pes planus.
2. Apply before sling.

H. Follow up.
1. May require further workup or referral if not pain free after 1 month.

I. Complications.
1. None known.

J. Education.
1. Proper shoe wear. Sneakers with built-in arch preferred.

XVIII. NURSEMAID'S ELBOW: RADIAL HEAD SUBLUXATION

Nursemaid's elbow, 832

A. Etiology.
1. Traction along axis of extended pronated arm resulting in radial head subluxation with annular ligament displacement.
2. Typically "pulling" child's hand/arm to prevent from falling or pulling away or swinging child by arms.

B. Occurrence.
1. Most common elbow injury of children age 1–4 years.
2. Female > males.
3. Left > right.

C. Clinical manifestations.
1. Will not use arm.

   2. Holds arm close to body with elbow slightly flexed and pronated (palm down).
D. Physical findings.
   1. Restricted supination of elbow.
   2. Typically nontender or swollen; however, exhibits distress if tries moving elbow.
E. Diagnostic tests.
   1. Radiographs AP and lateral of elbow if questionable success of reduction (*note:* many times these are reduced when arm is rotated to get lateral X-ray).
F. Differential diagnosis.

Elbow fracture, 813.01
---

   1. Fracture.
G. Treatment.
   1. Reduction maneuver.
      a. Child in parent's lap.
      b. Flex child's elbow to 90° with gentle pressure of thumb over radial head.
      c. Fully or "hyper" pronate wrist then fully supinate wrist; typically click will be felt and child will stop resisting (**Figure 30-11**).
   2. Sling and refer to orthopedist if child fails to use arm.
H. Follow up.
   1. Call or visit to ensure child is using arm normally within 1 week.
I. Complications.
   1. Unreduced radius.
J. Education.
   1. Teach parents mechanism of injury to prevent reoccurrence (30–40%).

XIX. GROWING PAINS

Growing pains, 781.99

A. Etiology.
   1. Unknown theory of periosteal irritation.
B. Occurrence.
   1. Peak in 3–5 and 8–12-year olds.

Figure 30-11 Reduction maneuver for "nursemaid's elbow." Flex elbow to 90°, fully pronate wrist (palm down), then with gentle pressure over radial head supinate the wrist (palm up).

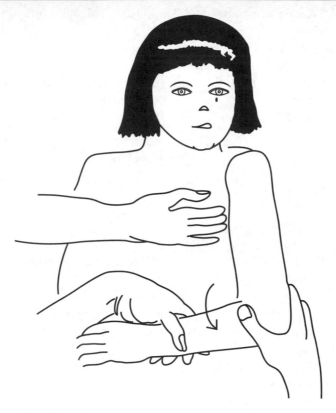

Source: Courtesy of Miki Patterson.

    C. Clinical manifestations.
        1. Muscular pain (not joint): thighs, calves, behind knee.
        2. Typically late afternoon, early evening after physically active day.
        3. Can wake child from sleep.
    D. Physical findings.
        1. None.
    E. Diagnostic tests.
        1. Only if suspicious, X-ray to exclude fracture/lesion.
    F. Differential diagnosis.
        1. Diagnosis of exclusion:

       a. No fever.

       b. Not in joint.

       c. No swelling, erythema, warmth.

       d. No trauma.

       e. No weight loss, rashes, unusual fatigue or behavior.

G. Treatment.

    1. Massage, heat, acetaminophen/ibuprofen.

H. Follow up.

    1. Follow up if lasts > 24 hours at time.

    2. Follow up if child does not respond to medications and massage.

I. Complications.

    1. None.

J. Education.

    1. Normal, may come and go, child is not "faking."

XX. COSTROCHONDRITIS

Costochondritis, 733.6

A. Etiology.

    1. Diagnosis of exclusion.

B. Occurrence.

    1. Unknown.

C. Clinical manifestations.

    1. Insidious and persistent lasting hours to days.

    2. Worse with position change and deep breathing. May be diffuse or localized. Common after repetitive new activity of upper trunk and arms.

D. Physical findings.

    1. Skin lesions, chest wall syndrome tests, "crowing rooster," "horizontal arm flexion," "hooking maneuver" diagnostic: if pain is reproduced, test is positive (**Figure 30-12**).

    2. Chest expansion test (tape measure around chest at fourth intercostal level max)—exhale then inhale = 5 cm excursion; < 2.5 cm abnormal.

E. Treatment.

    1. NSAIDs, rest.

F. Diagnostic tests.

    1. Radiographs of chest to rule out fracture or tumor.

    2. CT, bone scan (most sensitive to rule out arthropathies, tumors, infection).

Figure 30-12 "Crowing rooster." Elbows are pulled back and up to expand chest. A positive test is when pain is reproduced with this maneuver.

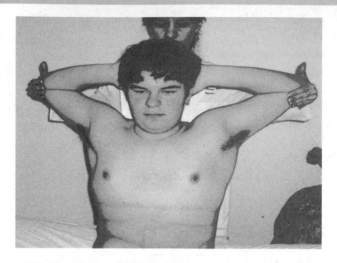

Source: Courtesy of Miki Patterson.

3. ESR, ANA, rheumatoid factor purpose to rule out: cardiopulmonary, abdominal sources associated with rheumatologic condition or assess structure of chest wall.

G. Differential diagnosis.

Ankylosing spondylitis, 720
Fibromyalgia, 729.1
Sternoclavicular hyperostosis, 733.3

1. Cardiopulmonary.
2. Esophagus, head, neck, and interior chest wall.
3. Ankylosing spondylitis.
4. Sternoclavicular hyperostosis.
5. Infection.
6. Fibromyalgia.

H. Follow up.
1. Within 2 weeks to document resolution of symptoms.

I. Complications.
1. Missed diagnosis.

J. Education.
1. Call for changes in symptoms.

XXI. OSTEOPOROSIS

Osteoporosis, 733

A. Etiology.
1. Bony calcium deficit from various causes including lack of intake while prepubertal, absorption or metabolic origin.
B. Occurrence.
1. Disease of childhood with severe adulthood complications.
C. Clinical manifestations.
1. Majority (50–66%) of total body calcium is deposited to bone by end of puberty.
2. Earlier in females than males.
3. Highest velocity of increased bone mineral content within 9–12 months of menarche.
D. Physical findings.
1. Stress fractures, fractures with minimal trauma or no findings in childhood.
E. Diagnostic tests.
1. Lack of calcium in past 3-day diet history.
2. Poor dietary habits.
3. High suspicion in lactose-intolerant or anorectic children.
F. Differential diagnosis.
1. None.
G. Treatment.
1. Increase dietary calcium intake or supplementation.
H. Follow up.
1. Continue to assess calcium intake, stress importance to prepubertal/pubescent children.
I. Complications.

Dowager's hump (kyphosis), 737.1
Degenerative joint changes, 721.9
Fractures, 829
---

    1. Fractures.

    2. Dowager's hump (kyphosis).

    3. Early adulthood degenerative joint changes.

J. Education.

    1. Three servings of milk, cheese, yogurt daily: 1200 mg of calcium.

BIBLIOGRAPHY

American Academy of Pediatrics. Clinical practice guideline: Early detection of developmental dysplasia of the hip. *Pediatrics.* 2000;105(4):896–905.

Clark MC. Approaches to child with a limp; 2003. Retrieved June 11, 2011, from: http://www.uptodate.com/contents/approach-to-the-child-with-a-limp.

Flynn JM, & Mehta S. An evidence-based approach to the evaluation and management of hip pain in children. *Pediatric Case Review.* 2002;2(1):26–32.

Gregory PL, Biswas AC, & Batt ME. Musculoskeletal problems of the chest wall in athletes. *Sports Medicine.* 2002;32(4):235–250.

Gunner KB, & Scott AC. Evaluation of a child with a limp. *Journal of Pediatric Health Care.* 2001;15(1):38–40.

Hawk D & Bailie S. Pediatric/congenital disorders. In: *Core curriculum for orthopaedic nursing* Boston: Pearson Custom Publishing; 2009:259–326.

Kleposki RW, & Sehgal K. Common pediatric hip diseases in primary care. *Clinical Advisory.* 2010;13(6): 21–26.

Lincoln TL, & Suen PW. Common rotational variations in children, *J Am Acad Orthopaedic Surgeons.* 2003;11(5):312–320.

Proulx AM, & Zryd TW. Costochondritis: diagnosis and treatment. *Am Fam Physician.* 2009;80(6):617–620.

Shelton YA, & Mortimer E. Orthopaedic problems in the pediatric patient. In G Steinberg, C Akins, & D Baran, eds. *Orthopaedics in primary care.* 3rd ed. Philadelphia, PA: Lippincott Williams & Wilkins; 1999.

Staheli LT. *Fundamentals of pedicatric orthopaedics.* 4th ed. India: Lippincott Williams & Wilkins; 2008.

CHAPTER 31

Neurologic Disorders: Altered States of Consciousness

Kristin Miller

I. MENINGITIS

A. Inflammation of the protective membranes covering the brain and spinal cord, collectively called the meninges, usually due to the spread of infection.

Altered consciousness, 780.09	Meningitis, 322.9
Brain dysfunction, 314.9	Papilledema, 377
Bulging fontanel, 756	Seizure, 780.39
Fever, 780.6	Stiff neck, 723.5
Headache, 784	Vomiting, 787.03
Intracranial pressure, 781.99	Irritability, 799.2

B. Etiology.
  1. Infectious.
      a. Viral infections—most common cause, usually termed *aseptic meningitis* when no bacterial cause can be found
        • Enteroviruses (90%).
        • Herpes simplex virus type 2.
        • Varicella zoster virus.
      b. Bacterial.
        • Newborns to 3 months of age.
            i. Group B streptococci.
            ii. *Escherichia coli.*
            iii. Listeria monocytogenes.
        • Older children.
            i. *Neisseria meningitidis.*
            ii. Streptococcus pneumonia.

        iii. *Haemophilus influenzae* type B especially in countries that do not offer vaccinations.

  c. Parasitic.
  - *Angiostrongylus cantonensis.*
  - Gnathostoma spinigerum.

2. Noninfectious.
   a. Cancer.
   b. Drugs.
      - Nonsteroidal anti-inflammatory drugs (NSAIDs).
      - Antibiotics.
      - Intravenous immunoglobulin.
   c. Inflammatory conditions.
      - Sarcoidosis.
      - Systemic lupus erythematous.
      - Vasculitis.

C. Occurrence.
   1. Viruses more likely in late summer and fall.
   2. Bacterial: 3 per 100,000.
   3. Viral: 10.9 per 100,000.
   4. Increased risk with crowding and prolonged exposure such as daycare, military, college dorms, and those with compromised immune systems.
   5. Age—most cases occur in children younger than 5 years, but decreased incidence with increased vaccination rates.
   6. Race—higher incidence in African Americans than Caucasians.
   7. Sex—viral 3 times more likely in males than females.

D. Clinical manifestations.
   1. General population.
      a. Classic triad of severe headache, nuchal rigidity, high fever.
      b. Altered mental status.
         - Confusion.
         - Extreme irritability.
         - Sleepiness.
         - Abnormal cry.
         - Seizures.
      c. Sensitivity to light.

E. Physical findings.
   1. Signs in newborns.
      a. Constant cry.
      b. Excessive sleepiness or irritability.
      c. Poor feeding.

      d. Bulging fontanel (increased ICP).

      e. Stiffness of body and/or neck.

      f. Difficult to comfort, cries harder when picked up.

  2. Positive Kernig's sign or Brudzinski's sign.

F. Diagnostic tests.

  1. Lumbar puncture (LP)—definitive test for diagnosis, will see low glucose, increased white blood cells (WBC), increased protein, culture and Gram stain should be done.

  2. Complete blood count (CBC), blood culture, C-reactive protein, polymerase chain reaction (PCR), erythrocyte sedimentation rate (ESR).

  3. CT or MRI before LP since LP contraindicated with tumor, abscess, or increased intracranial pressure (ICP); MRI often done later to assess complications/sequelae.

G. Differential diagnosis.

Brain abscess, 324	Head injury, 959.01
Brain lesion/tumor, 348.8	Subdural empyema, 324.9
Encephalitis, 323.9	

H. Treatment.

  1. Viral.

      a. Supportive care—bed rest, fluids, analgesics.

      b. Antiviral drugs—acyclovir for herpes simplex and varicella zoster.

      c. May need to be admitted to monitor ICP or complications.

  2. Bacterial.

      a. Early intervention with antibiotics critical.

      b. Always treat with antibiotic for most commonly known pathogens until diagnosis confirmed.

      c. May need to be admitted to manage ICP, complications, administration of IV fluids and antibiotics.

      d. Birth to 6 weeks—ampicillin and third-generation cephalosporin (Cefotaxime or Ceftriaxone).

      e. Older than 6 weeks—vancomycin and third-generation cephalosporin.

      f. Prophylactic treatment of contacts with patients with *Neisseria meningitidis*—sulfadiazine or rifampin.

I. Complications.

  1. Increased ICP.

  2. Deafness—may be prevented with prophylactic steroids.

  3. Hydrocephalus.

4. Seizures.
5. Venous or cerebral infarction.
6. Cranial nerve palsies.
7. Up to 70% sustain sequelae from bacterial meningitis.
8. Most children with nonherpetic viral meningitis recover completely.
J. Follow up.
1. Frequent visits when cared for at home.
2. Immediately for any decline in neurological condition or respiratory distress.
3. Shortly after hospitalization to follow neurological status and assess pan for treatment of any sequelae.
K. Education.
1. Importance of prevention via immunizations.
2. Handwashing and infection-control measures, especially in crowded locations.
3. Prophylaxis for certain exposures.
4. Support and coordination of comprehensive services may be needed.

II. ENCEPHALITIS

A. Inflammation of the brain due to a viral infection.

Altered consciousness, 780.9	Lethargy, 780.79
Confusion, 298.9	Meningitis, 322.9
Encephalitis, 323.9	Seizure, 780.39
Headache, 784	Stiff neck, 723.5
Irritability, 799.22	Vomiting, 787.03

B. Etiology.
1. Primary form: direct viral infection of the brain and spinal cord.
2. Secondary form: viral infection that first occurs elsewhere in the body and travels to the brain.
3. Exposure to viruses through:
   a. Breathing in respiratory droplets from infected person.
   b. Contaminated food or drink.
   c. Insect bites or animal bites (rabies).
   d. Specific viruses:
      • Arboviruses—most common cause, carried by mosquitoes or ticks.
      • Enteroviruses—coxsackievirus, echovirus, poliovirus.

- Others: herpes simplex encephalitis (most common and worst prognosis—10–40% mortality).
- Eastern equine: 70–90% mortality.
- Western equine.
- St. Louis encephalitis: 30% mortality.
- West Nile.
- California and Venezuela equine.
4. Allergic reaction to vaccinations (extremely rare).
5. Effects of cancer and treatments.
6. Autoimmune or immune response problems (immunocompromised, HIV).
C. Occurrence.
1. Seasonal: more common summer and fall.
2. Age: more prevalent or severe in young children and elderly.
3. Higher in those with weakened immune system.
4. Geographic: higher in areas where mosquito-borne viruses are common.
5. Outdoor activities increase risk.
D. Clinical manifestations.
1. Headache.
2. Nausea.
3. Lethargy.
4. Behavioral changes—confusion, disorientation, irritability, personality changes.
5. Joint pain, stiff neck.
E. Physical findings.
1. Fever.
2. Positive Brudzinski's sign or Kernig's sign.
3. Abnormal reflexes.
4. Rash.
5. Emergency symptoms:
   a. Low level of consciousness (LOC), poor responsiveness.
   b. Muscle weakness or paralysis.
   c. Seizure.
   d. Sudden change in mental functions.
   e. Bulging fontanel.
F. Diagnostic tests.
1. LP with CSF exam may show hemorrhagic component and increase WBC.
2. Electroencephalogram (EEG)—periodic sharp waves at 2- to 3-second intervals on a background of diffuse or lateralized slowing if characteristic but nonspecific.

    3. MRI—often abnormal, showing limited or massive areas of inflammation and necrosis.

    4. PCR and blood antibodies—can show positive DNA for viruses.

    5. CBC, toxicology screen.

G. Differential diagnosis.

Autoimmune disorder, 279.4	Intracranial hemorrhage, 432.9
Brain mass/lesion/tumor, 191.9	Metabolic disorder, 279.49
Demyelination, 341.9	Seizure, 780.39
Ingested or inhaled toxins, 977.9	

H. Treatment.
    1. Antiviral medications.
        a. Acyclovir—herpes encephalitis or varicella zoster virus.
        b. Ganciclovir—cytomegalovirus (CMV).
    2. Antibiotics if bacterial cause.
    3. Seizure medications as needed.
    4. Steroids to reduce swelling.
    5. Acetaminophen for fever and headache.
    6. Rest and fluids.

I. Complications.
    1. Acute phase lasts 1–2 weeks, may take several months to fully recover.
    2. Permanent brain damage can occur in severe cases—can affect hearing, memory, muscle control, sensation, speech, vision.
    3. Outcomes vary—high recovery (Rocky Mountain spotted fever), high morbidity (herpes encephalitis) definite mortality, especially if untreated (rabies).

J. Follow up.
    1. Emergency for sudden fever or other symptoms of encephalitis.
    2. Call for decline in neurological condition.
    3. 2–4 weeks to assess for sequelae.

K. Education.
    1. Importance of vaccinations: measles-mumps-rubella (MMR), varicella, meningococcal.
    2. Immunizations specific for foreign travel.
    3. Take steps to prevent genital herpes.
    4. Avoidance of mosquitoes.
        a. Apply DEET products, not on face, hands, or infants younger than 2 months.

      b. Remove sources of standing water.

      c. Wear long-sleeve shirts and pants when outside, especially at dusk.

   5. Avoidance of ticks.

      a. Avoid woods, clear brush in yard, and keep grass mowed.

      b. Inspect body after return inside.

      c. Avoid contact with vector/host animals.

   6. Thoroughly cook meat and wash fruits/vegetables, especially in endemic areas.

III. HEAD INJURY

A. Any trauma that leads to injury to scalp, skull, or brain.

Alterations in consciousness, 780.09	Nausea, 787.02
Confusion, 298.9	Skull fracture, 803
Head trauma, 959.01	Vomiting, 787.03
Intracranial pressure, 781.99	

B. Etiology.
1. Trauma from motor vehicle accident (MVA), physical assaults, falls, accidents at home, work, outdoors, or while playing sports.
2. Common causes include biking, skating, skateboarding, and contact sports.
3. Types.
    a. Closed head—did not break the skull, more common.
    b. Penetrating or open—break in skull where objects enter brain (50% mortality rate).
    c. Focal brain injury—acute epidural, subdural, or subarachnoid hemorrhage.
C. Occurrence.
1. 1.7 million people sustain traumatic brain injury (TBI) annually. Majority are concussions or other forms of mild traumatic brain injury.
2. Contributes to substantial number of deaths and causes of permanent disability.
3. Range from mild with brief change in mental status or consciousness to severe with extended period of unconsciousness.
4. Falls cause 50% of TBI in children age 0 to 14 years.

   5. Strike by moving or stationary object causes 25% of TBI in children ages 0 to 14 years.
   6. Males more often sustain TBI (59%).
   7. High-risk age groups—0 to 4 years and 15 to 19 years.
D. Clinical manifestations.
   1. Occur immediately or over several hours to days.
   2. Minor head injury symptoms:
      a. Headache.
      b. Dizziness.
      c. Impaired concentration, thinking, and memory.
      d. Blurred vision.
      e. Distractibility.
      f. Noise sensitive.
      g. Depression.
      h. Anxiety.
   3. Severe head injury symptoms:
      a. Impaired hearing, smell, taste, or vision.
      b. Irritability, personality changes, unusual behavior.
      c. Severe headache.
E. Physical findings.
   1. Minor head injuries.
      a. Unsteadiness.
      b. Fatigue.
      c. Irritability.
   2. Severe head injuries.
      a. Changes in or unequal pupils.
      b. Convulsions.
      c. Fracture in skull or face, bruising of face, swelling at site of injury.
      d. Inability to move one or more limbs.
      e. Loss of consciousness, confusion, drowsiness.
      f. Restlessness, clumsiness, lack of coordination.
      g. Stiff neck or vomiting.
F. Diagnostic tests.
   1. Important to obtain history of exact details of injury.
   2. Glasgow Coma Scale.
   3. Head CT to identify significant contusion, hemorrhage, and swelling.
   4. Skull and cervical plain films to evaluate skull or neck trauma.
   5. Angiogram to evaluate blood vessels in cases of bleeding.
   6. Certain cases may require CBC, comprehensive metabolic panel (CMP), blood alcohol level, drug screen, prothrombin time (PT), partial thromboplastin time (PTT), fibrinogen.

G. Differential diagnosis.

Brain tumor, 191.9	Meningitis, 320.9
Encephalitis, 323.9	Migraine, 346.9
Ingested or inhaled toxins, 977.9	Seizures, 780.39

H. Treatment.
   1. Mild head injury—treated at home as long as someone available to monitor.
   2. Acetaminophen for pain. No aspirin or ibuprofen due to increased risk of bleeding.
   3. *Do not:*
       a. Wash head wound that is deep or profusely bleeding.
       b. Remove any object sticking out of wound.
       c. Move the person unless absolutely necessary.
       d. Shake the person to arouse.
       e. Remove helmet if you suspect a serious head injury.
       f. Pick up a fallen child with any sign of head injury.
   4. Apply ice to reduce swelling.
   5. Roll on side if vomiting.
   6. Cover bleeding area with clean cloth, only press firmly if no concern for skull fracture.
   7. Always treat as if spinal injury if patient unconscious, keep head midline and immobile.
   8. Maintain airway and vital signs, CPR if needed.
   9. Admit to hospital for severe injury, monitor for progression of symptoms or concern for increased ICP.
I. Complications.
   1. Increased ICP.
   2. Surgery to remove objects, control hemorrhage, or decompress brain.
   3. Seizures.
   4. Resulting focal deficits.
       a. Weakness, aphasia, personality and intellectual changes, depression, anxiety, aggression, loss or change in: sensations, hearing, vision, taste, smell, speech, or language.
   5. Paralysis.
   6. Chronic headaches.
J. Follow up.
   1. Seek care immediately for:
       a. Vomiting more than once.
       b. Confusion.
       c. Drowsiness, unable to awaken.

        d. Weakness or inability to walk.

        e. Severe headache.

        f. Severe head trauma or fall from more than height of the person.

        g. LOC for > 1 minute.

        h. Stops breathing.

        i. Severe head or facial bleeding.

    2. Follow up in 1 week after injury and every few weeks to monitor for and manage any sequelae.

K. Education.

    1. Wear helmets for biking, skating, and other similar sports.

    2. Wear proper sports equipment, and make sure in good condition.

    3. Wear seat belts, use age-appropriate car seats.

    4. Prevent falls by childproofing home—stairs, bathtubs, rugs, furniture.

    5. Be visible and obey traffic laws when biking.

    6. Safe areas to play.

    7. Know signs and symptoms of head injury/concussion and know when to seek medical care.

IV. CONCUSSION

A. Alteration in mental status after a blow to the head, consciousness may or may not occur.

Altered consciousness, 780.09	Confusion, 298.9
Concussion, 850.9	Dizziness, 780.4
Concussion, syndrome, 310.2	Head trauma, 959.01

B. Etiology.

    1. Type of traumatic brain injury caused from: bump, blow, or jolt to the head.

    2. Blow to body can cause head and brain to move rapidly back and forth, resulting in head injury.

    3. Results from falls, MVA, and players that collide with each other, ground, or obstacles.

C. Occurrence.

    1. 135,000 sports- and recreation-related TBIs come to emergency departments (EDs) each year (includes concussions in children age 5–18 years).

    2. Athletes who have had a concussion are at increased risk for another.

3. Children and teens are more likely to get a concussion and take longer to recover than adults.
4. More than 2 million concussions happen per year, 85% never diagnosed.
5. 50% of football players may experience one concussion per year.

D. Clinical manifestations.
1. Hallmark signs—confusion and amnesia that may occur immediately or several minutes after injury occurs.
2. Early (minutes and hours) symptoms experienced:
   a. Headache.
   b. Dizziness or vertigo.
   c. Lack of awareness of surroundings.
   d. Nausea or vomiting.
3. Late (days to weeks) symptoms experienced:
   a. Persistent low-grade headache.
   b. Light-headedness.
   c. Poor attention and concentration.
   d. Memory dysfunction.
   e. Easy fatigability.
   f. Irritability and low frustration tolerance.
   g. Intolerance to bright light or loud noises.
   h. Anxiety or depressed mood.

E. Physical findings.
1. Vacant stare.
2. Delayed verbal and motor responses.
3. Confusion and inability to maintain focus.
4. Disorientation.
5. Slurred or incoherent speech.
6. Incoordination.
7. Memory deficits.
8. Emotional.
9. Any period of unconsciousness.
10. Grade 1 concussion.
    a. Transient confusion.
    b. No loss of consciousness.
    c. Concussion symptoms or mental status abnormalities resolve in less than 15 minutes.
11. Grade 2 concussion.
    a. Transient confusion.
    b. No loss of consciousness.

        c. Concussion symptoms or mental status abnormalities last more than 15 minutes.

    12. Grade 3 concussion.

        a. Any loss of consciousness, either brief (seconds) or prolonged (minutes).

F. Diagnostic tests.

    1. Sideline/immediate evaluation.

        a. Orientation—to time, place, person, and situation.

        b. Concentration—digits backward, months of year in reverse.

        c. Memory—recall 3 words or objects, details of contest, names.

        d. Physical tests—40-yard sprint, pushups, knee bends.

          • Any associated symptoms with these tests are abnormal findings.

        e. Neurological tests.

          • Pupils, coordination, sensation.

    2. Head CT—for Grade 2 concussion with symptoms that worsen or last longer than 1 week and for Grade 3 concussions.

    3. Immediate post-concussion assessment and cognitive testing (ImPACT) testing to assess cognitive functioning, done soon after concussion and before return to activities, mostly for Grade 3 concussions.

G. Differential diagnosis.

Migraine, 346.9

Seizure, 780.39

Transient alteration in awareness, 780.02

Transient ischemic attack, 435.9

H. Treatment.

    1. Remove from contest.

    2. Monitor for progressive neurological changes.

    3. ED for Grade 3 concussions.

    4. When to return to play: need to be asymptomatic with normal neurological assessment at rest and with exertion.

        a. Grade 1—after 15 minutes same day.

        b. Multiple Grade 1—1 week.

        c. Grade 2—1 week.

        d. Multiple Grade 2—2 weeks

        e. Grade 3 with brief LOC—1 week.

        f. Multiple Grade 3—1 month or longer.

I. Complications.

    1. Seizures.

    2. Second impact syndrome—repeat concussion that occurs before the brain recovers from the first, can slow recovery or increase likelihood of long-term problems including brain damage, brain swelling, and even death.

    3. Depression—not being able to participate in their sport.

    4. Rare case for development of blood clot on brain.

J. Follow up.

    1. See return to sports guidelines above, need to be cleared first.

    2. Call or go to ED for:

      a. Unequal pupils.

      b. Drowsy and cannot awaken.

      c. Worsening headache.

      d. Weakness, numbness.

      e. Repeated vomiting.

      f. Seizure.

      g. Slurred speech.

      h. Increased confusion.

      i. Unable to recognize people or places.

      j. LOC.

K. Education.

    1. Use protective equipment that fits properly and is well maintained.

    2. Practice safe playing techniques/good sportsmanship.

    3. Know signs and symptoms of concussion, when to sit out and when to return.

V. STATUS EPILEPTICUS

A. 30 minutes or more of continuous seizure activity or a series of seizures without return to full consciousness between seizures.

Alteration in consciousness, 780.09   Status epilepticus, 345.3

B. Etiology.

    1. Idiopathic.

    2. Central nervous system (CNS) neoplasms, stroke, infections, electrolyte abnormalities, trauma, metabolic disorders, toxic ingestion, hypoxic insult.

    3. History of epilepsy.

    4. Noncompliance with antiepileptic medications.

    5. History of injury—MVA, fall.

C. Occurrence.
  1. 50,000—200,000 cases per year.
  2. Mortality rate 20%, mostly from underlying case of brain injury.
  3. Can occur in all age groups, more in elderly.
  4. Males and females affected equally.
D. Physical findings.
  1. Absence status.
     a. Confusion, lethargy.
     b. EEG with continuous or intermittent but frequent spikes and slow wave discharges.
  2. Focal motor status.
     a. Continuous jerking of restricted muscle groups.
  3. Complex partial status.
     a. Confused, dazed, automatisms often present.
     b. Most often series of seizures, remaining confused between seizures.
  4. Generalized tonic-clonic status.
     a. Continuous convulsions or repetitive convulsions without resolution of postictal depression between episodes.
E. Diagnostic tests.
  1. EEG.
  2. Head CT initially, may do MRI later if warranted.
  3. CMP (focus on glucose, Na+, Ca++), toxicology screen, WBC.
  4. LP if CNS infection in differential.
F. Differential diagnosis.

Encephalitis, 323.9	Stroke/ischemia, 434.91
Hypoglycemia, 251.2	Subarachnoid hemorrhage, 430
Hyponatremia, 276.1	Toxicity, 292.89
Meningitis, 320.9	

G. Treatment.
  1. Maintain vital signs and ABCs.
  2. Administer DIASTAT AcuDIAL after 5 minutes of seizure activity. Call 911 if seizure continues.
  3. Ativan IV: 0.1 mg/kg at 2 mg/min.
  4. Diazepam IV: 0.3–0.5mg/kg at 2 mg/min.
  5. Fosphenytoin, phenobarbital, phenytoin (Dilantin), divalproex sodium (Depakote IV). Monitor for respiratory depression.
  6. Correct any abnormal laboratory findings.
  7. Treat any underlying infection.

H. Complications.
    1. Respiratory failure.
    2. Aspiration.
    3. Hypotension.
    4. Acidosis.
    5. Hyperthermia.
I. Follow up.
    1. Coordinate with specialists for any associated injuries or complications.
    2. See neurologist in 2 weeks.
    3. Start maintenance antiepileptic medication, call for any side effects or further seizures.
J. Education.
    1. Know signs and symptoms and when and how to give DIASTAT AcuDIAL.
    2. Medication information and compliance.
    3. Avoidance of any seizure triggers: sleep deprivation, alcohol.
    4. Seizure safety: no tub baths unsupervised, monitor closely with swimming, helmets appropriate for sports, no driving until seizure free for 6 months, what to do during a seizure—lay on side on ground, do not put anything in mouth, time event, and keep safe.

VI. CONFUSIONAL MIGRAINE

A. Characterized by a typical migraine aura, headache, and confusion.

Confusion, 298.9	Irritability, 799.22
Headache, 784	Migraine variant, 346.2

B. Etiology.
    1. Idiopathic.
    2. Triggered by head trauma.
C. Occurrence.
    1. Rare, only 5% of migraine patients.
    2. Single attacks are most common, multiple attacks are rare.
    3. May evolve into typical migraine episodes.
D. Clinical manifestations.
    1. Inattention
    2. Distractibility.
E. Physical findings.
    1. Impaired speech and motor activities.

    2. Can last 10 minutes to 20 hours. A more profound, disturbed level of consciousness may lead to migraine stupor, which can last hours up to 5 days.

    3. Confusional state is usually followed by sleep.

F. Diagnostic tests.

    1. Complete neurological exam.

    2. MRI and MRA to evaluate arteries within the brain.

    3. History may include family history, history of trauma, and classic symptoms.

G. Differential diagnosis.

Acute psychosis, 298.9	Metabolic encephalopathies (Reye's syndrome, hypoglycemia), 348.31
Complex partial seizures, 345.4	
Drug ingestion, 977.9	Viral encephalitis, 049.9

H. Treatment.

    1. Sleep.

    2. Typical migraine-abortive medications.

I. Follow up.

    1. Reoccurrence of episodes.

    2. Change in neurological status (resulting from any head trauma).

J. Education.

    1. Avoidance of migraine triggers.

    2. Keep a headache/episode diary.

    3. Limit use of over-the-counter analgesics.

    4. Keep a regular schedule: meals, sleep, hydration, exercise, and minimize stress.

VII. HEADACHES: MIGRAINES

A. Episodic headache disorder characterized by various combinations of neurological, gastrointestinal, psychophysiological, and autonomic changes.

Benign paroxysmal vertigo, 386.11	Migraine, 346.9
Blurred vision, 368.8	Motion sickness, 994.6
Cyclic vomiting, 536.2	Nausea with vomiting, 787.01
Dizziness, 780.4	Photophobia, 368.13

Headache, 784	Presence of aura, 346
Irritability, 799.2	Vertigo, 780.4
Mental confusion, 298.9	

B. Etiology.
1. Generally inherited disorder, 70–80% familial.
2. Leading hypothesis for origin—neurovascular disturbance triggered by multiple stimuli and affecting serotonin transmission in the CNS.
3. Episodic brain malfunction—a central nervous system disorder of primarily the brain and nerves, and secondarily of the blood vessels. Malfunction is caused in part by changes in the level of circulating neurotransmitters and involving serotonin in particular.
4. Head trauma.
5. Illness and infection.
6. Environmental and emotional factors.
7. Certain foods and beverages.

C. Occurrence.
1. Mean age of onset is 7.2 years for boys and 10.9 years for girls.
2. 3% of children age 3–7 years.
3. 4–11% for children age 7–11 years.
4. 8–23% for children age 11–15+ years.
5. Risk factors:
   a. Children who have a family history of headaches or migraines.
   b. Boys before they reach puberty.
   c. Girls after they reach puberty.
   d. Children over age 10 years.

D. Clinical manifestations.
1. Pounding or throbbing head pain. In children, pain usually affects the front or both sides of the head. In adolescents, pain usually affects one side of head.
2. Pallor or paleness of skin.
3. Irritability.
4. Phonophobia or sensitivity to sound.
5. Photophobia or sensitivity to light.
6. Loss of appetite.
7. Nausea and/or vomiting, abdominal pain.
8. Dizziness.

E. Physical findings.
1. May have none if not experiencing migraine at time of exam.

2. Due to pain, may see increase in heart rate or blood pressure.
3. Look of discomfort in facial expressions and demeanor.
4. Wanting to lie down in quiet, dark room.
F. Diagnostic tests.
   1. Most important aspect of diagnosing migraine is the headache history.
      a. Description of current and previous headaches, when started.
      b. Headache frequency, duration, and associated symptoms.
      c. What medications have been taken and are currently being taken.
      d. Family and medical history.
      e. Pain location, quality, and severity—how disabling?
      f. Social history—psychological symptoms.
      g. Precipitating factors.
   2. Complete neurological exam—including fundoscopic exam to rule out papilledema.
   3. Head CT.
      a. Recent/new onset.
      b. Evolution or change in headaches.
   4. Head MRI.
      a. Papilledema present.
      b. Focal neurological signs—abnormal exam, hemiparesis.
      c. Complicated migraine—examine blood vessels that supply the brain.
   5. Evaluation as needed if concern for infectious cause.
      a. LP if concern for increased intracranial pressure/papilledema present; generally need to do head MRI prior to LP.
G. Differential diagnosis.

Brain tumor, 239.6	Papilledema, 377
Head trauma, 959.01	Pseudotumor cerebri, 348.2
Intracranial bleed, 432.9	Psychological, 300.9
Intracranial pressure, 781.99	Sinusitis, 473.9
Meningitis, aseptic, 047.9	Stroke, 436

H. Treatment.
   1. Treat underlying pathology if present.
      a. Diamox for pseudotumor cerebri.
   2. Goals of treatment.
      a. Reduce attack frequency, severity, and duration.
      b. Improve responsiveness to treatment of acute attacks.
      c. Improve function, reduce disability, and improve quality of life.

3. Nonpharmacologic treatments.
    a. Relaxation techniques, biofeedback, stress management.
    b. Rest, quiet dark room, applying ice packs to forehead or neck.
    c. Lifestyle/behavioral interventions.
        * Maintain routine sleep pattern with adequate sleep hours.
        * Regular routines, meal, exercise, school attendance.
        * Staying hydrated.
        * Avoidance/discontinuation of caffeine.
        * Avoidance/discontinuation of overuse of abortive medications.
        * Stress reduction.
4. Acute medication treatment.
    a. Medication should not be used more than 2, or at most, 3 days a week to prevent development of rebound headaches.
    b. Prevents or stops progression of headache.
    c. Use medication as early as possible to prevent escalation and to increase the drug's effectiveness.
    d. Mild to moderate pain: ibuprofen (NSAIDs with or without caffeine) or acetaminophen (Tylenol).
    e. Moderate to severe pain: triptans (contraindicated for migraine variant such as hemiplegic or basilar migraine), ergotamine, dihydroergotamine (DHE).
    f. Antiemetics to help relieve pain, nausea, vomiting.
    g. Steroid dose pack to break migraine status, prolonged migraine.
5. Preventative medication treatment.
    a. Use when:
        * Recurring migraine that interferes with daily routine despite acute treatment (two or more attacks/month that produce disability and can last up to 3 days or more).
        * Failure, contraindication, or side effects from acute medications.
        * Overuse of acute medications.
        * Frequent headaches (more than 2/week) with risk for rebound headache syndrome.
    b. Medication options:
        * Antidepressants: amitriptyline (Elavil), fluoxetine (Prozac), duloxetine (Cymbalta).
        * Beta blockers: propranolol (Inderal).
        * Antihistamines: cyproheptadine (Periactin) (most effective in toddlers).
        * Calcium channel blockers: verapamil.
        * Anticonvulsants: valproic acid (Depakote), topiramate (Topamax).

I. Follow up.
1. Assess medication effectiveness, monitor for any possible side effects.
2. When abortive medications do not elevate migraine, may need IM or IV abortive medications and fluids such as ketorolac (Toradol) or promethazine (Phenergan).
3. Any neurological changes or progression in headaches.
J. Complications.
1. Comorbid anxiety and/or depression.
2. Medication side effects.
3. Acute vascular disorder.
4. High incidence of motion sickness.
5. Sleep disturbance.
6. Drop in school performance due to missed days, and inability to concentrate with a headache.
K. Education.
1. Migraine diagnosis and treatment (medications/possible side effects).
2. Keep a headache diary, look for headache triggers.
3. Know symptoms and when to treat headache.
4. Limit use of abortive medications.
5. Behavioral modifications, follow routine schedule.
6. Daily school attendance.
7. Reduce stress and avoid triggers.
8. Empower patient and family to be involved and take control of their headaches and treatment.

VIII. TENSION-TYPE HEADACHES

A. Headache that presents with pressure/tightening quality and lacks migraine criteria.

Headache, 784	Pain, neck, 723.1
Irritability, 799.2	

B. Etiology.
1. Behavioral.
2. Muscular.
3. Vascular.
4. May coexist with otherwise typical migraine headaches.

C. Occurrence.
1. Most common benign headache disorder.
2. 10–25% prevalence in childhood and adolescence.
3. Boys and girls tend to suffer equally until age 11 or 12 when female preponderance occurs.
D. Clinical manifestations.
1. Episodic headaches occur less than 15 days/month.
2. Chronic headaches occur more than 15 days/month.
3. Can last 30 minutes to 7 days.
4. Pain is mild to moderate (not severe).
5. Pain is bilateral and described as pressing or tightening, may occur in a hat band distribution.
6. Pain not aggravated by physical activity (unlike migraine).
7. No nausea or vomiting.
8. May have photophobia or phonophobia, but not both.
E. Physical findings.
1. Normal neurological exam, worrisome if abnormal.
2. May see signs of pain: facial expressions, demeanor, increased heart rate and blood pressure.
3. May be misdiagnosed as sinus headache.
F. Diagnostic tests.
1. Same as migraine.
2. History/complaints consistent with tension-type headache criteria.
G. Differential diagnosis.

Allergies, 995.3	Sinusitis, 473.9
Glaucoma, 365.9	Subarachnoid hemorrhage, 430
Hypertension, 401	Temporomandibular joint dysfunction
Migraine, 346.90	(TMJ), 524.6

H. Complications.
1. Depression.
2. Poor academic performance, difficulty concentrating, missed school days and other activities.
I. Treatment.
1. Nonpharmacologic treatments.
   a. Healthy habits.
   • Adequate routine sleep schedule.
   • Balanced meals.

- Regular exercise.
- No caffeine.
  b. Psychophysiological therapy.
  - Reassurance.
  - Counseling.
  - Stress management.
  - Relaxation therapy.
  - Biofeedback.
  - Treatment of anxiety and/or depression.
2. Pharmacotherapy.
   a. Acute treatment—not to be used more than 2 days/week.
   - NSAIDs.
   - Acetaminophen.
   b. Preventative treatment.
   - Amitriptyline (Elavil).
   - Selective serotonin reuptake inhibitors (SSRIs).
   - Muscle relaxers (tizanidine [Zanaflex]).
J. Follow up.
1. Assess medication effectiveness and any possible side effects.
2. Any neurological change or headache progression.
K. Education.
1. As with migraines.

IX. COMMON MEDICATIONS TO TREAT HEADACHES IN CHILDREN

A. Preventative:
1. Cyproheptadine (Periactin): 0.25–0.4 mg/kg or 2–4 mg daily bid.
2. Amitriptyline: start 10 mg at bedtime. Up to 1–2 mg/kg at bedtime.
3. Propranolol (Inderal): 1–2 mg/kg/day up to 4 mg/kg/day bid. Unless using LA form.
4. Tizanidine (Zanaflex): 2–4 mg at bedtime up to 12 mg. Monitor hepatic panel at 1, 3, and 6 months.
5. Valproic acid (Depakote): 10–20 mg/kg bid up to 60 mg/kg.
6. Topiramate (Topamax): titrate to 50 mg bid.
7. Verapamil: 40 mg tid or SR 120 mg, 180 mg, 240 mg daily.
B. Abortive:
1. Sumatriptan (Imitrex NS): 5–10 mg (1–2 sprays). Oral 25 mg up to 100 mg.

2. Rizatriptan (Maxalt): 5–10 mg tab.
3. Dihydroergotamine mesylate (Migranal): 1 spray each nostril, may repeat in 15 minutes.
4. Zolmitriptan (Zomig): 2.5–5 mg tab; 5 mg NS.
5. Eletriptan (Relpax): 20–40 mg tab.
6. Metoclopramide (Reglan): 0.1–0.2 mg/kg/dose up to 4 times a day.
7. Promethazine (Phenergan): 0.25 mg/kg/dose (max 25mg) up to 4 times a day.
8. Ibuprofen: 15 mg/kg/dose every 6 hours.
9. Acetaminophen (Tylenol): 10 mg/kg/dose every 4 hours.

X. FEBRILE SEIZURES

A. Seizure in association with a febrile illness in the absence of central nervous system infection or acute electrolyte imbalance in children older than 3 months of age without a prior afebrile seizure.

Altered level of consciousness, 780.09	Fever, 780.6
Febrile seizure, 780.31	Seizure, 780.39

B. Etiology.
   1. Benign age-dependent epilepsy syndrome, seizure in early life in presence of fever without intracranial infection.
   2. Genetic disposition—two to three times more common among family members of affected children than general population.
C. Occurrence.
   1. 2–5% of children will have a febrile seizure.
   2. Most common between ages of 6 months to 3 years, with peak incidence at 18 to 24 months of age.
   3. Risk factors.
      a. High peak temperature during illness.
      b. Family history of febrile seizures in a first- or second-degree relative.
      c. Developmental delay.
      d. Neonatal nursery stays longer than 30 days.
      e. Attendance at daycare.
D. Physical findings.
   1. Temperature of at least 39°F.
   2. Simple febrile seizure.
      a. Generalized tonic-clonic movements.

      b. Eyes roll back.

      c. Loss of consciousness.

      d. Last few seconds to minutes (less than 15 minutes).

      e. Postictal depression is brief.

   3. Complex febrile seizures.

      a. Last longer than 15 minutes.

      b. May reoccur within the same day.

      c. Prolonged period of postictal drowsiness or neurological abnormalities.

      d. Focal seizure manifestations.

E. Diagnostic tests.

   1. Simple febrile seizure.

      a. Extensive history taking.

      b. Evaluation for cause of fever, CBC.

      c. LP for infants younger than 6 months of age.

   2. Complex febrile seizure.

      a. CSF evaluation.

      b. Head CT if warranted.

      c. EEG if concerned.

F. Differential diagnosis.

Encephalitis, 323.9	Metabolic disorder, 277.9
Generalized seizure, 345.1	Sepsis, 995.91
Meningitis, 322.9	

G. Treatment.

   1. Control fever with antipyretic medication.

   2. Antibiotics appropriate for any bacterial infections.

   3. Treat cause of fever, fluids.

   4. Diazepam rectally or lorazepam (Ativan) IV for seizures lasting longer than 5 minutes.

   5. No need for anticonvulsant medication.

H. Complications.

   1. Rare, no neurological sequelae.

   2. Fewer than 10% of patients experience severe or recurrent attacks.

   3. Likelihood of developing epilepsy less than 5%.

   4. Possible complications if septic nature is cause for fever and seizure.

   5. Risk for reoccurrence.

      a. Neurological or developmental abnormality.

      b. Positive family history.

      c. Onset of febrile seizures before age 1 year.

      d. Low peak temperature at onset of seizure.

      e. Duration of fever.

I. Follow up.
1. Any seizure without fever.
2. As needed for treatment of cause of fever.

J. Education.
1. Reassurance of the benign nature.
2. First aid during a seizure.
3. When to call the doctor or go to the emergency room: Need to find and treat cause of fever, to stop seizure that continues past 5 minutes and does not stop with diazapam rectal (Diastat).

XI. GENERALIZED SEIZURES

A. Seizure in which the first clinical changes indicate initial involvement of both hemispheres.

Absence seizure, 345	Seizure, 780.39
Epilepsy, 345.9	
Primary generalized seizure, 345.1	

B. Etiology.
1. Up to 80% have unclear etiology.
2. Hereditary.
3. Perinatal: infectious, hypoxia, trauma.
4. Metabolic, toxic, nutritional.
5. Infectious.
6. Vascular.
7. Neoplastic.

C. Occurrence.
1. Children account for about 15% of all epilepsy cases.
2. Generalized seizures account for one-third of all epilepsies.
3. Most often start in childhood or adolescence.

D. Clinical manifestations.
1. Generalized tonic-clonic (grand mal).
    a. Starts suddenly with stiff muscles (tonic phase) and then rhythmic contractions (clonic phase).
    b. Impaired consciousness.

      c. Loss of bladder control common.
      d. Can last a few minutes.
      e. Postictal phase that can include drowsiness, confusion, and headache.
   2. Atonic seizure (drop attack).
      a. Sudden drop to the floor, head may nod/drop.
      b. Brief episode, loss of consciousness brief.
      c. Injuries are common.
   3. Absence seizures.
      a. Abrupt sudden loss of consciousness with cessation of all motor activity.
      b. Brief periods of staring blankly into space.
      c. Ends abruptly, no postictal state.
      d. Can be induced by hyperventilation.
      e. May see lip smacking, chewing, eye fluttering.
   4. Myoclonic.
      a. Brief contraction of a muscle group.
      b. Can drop objects.
      c. Recovery is immediate and often maintains consciousness.
   5. Infantile spasms.
      a. Clusters of seizures involving flexion jerk of the neck, trunk, and extremities.
      b. Range from subtle head drop or shoulder shrug to more violent action.
      c. Decreased responsiveness may follow spasms.
      d. Spasms are brief, lasting just a few seconds.
E. Physical findings.
   1. Seizure rare to happen in office to observe, can have family video episodes.
   2. May be "normal" between seizures.
   3. Low-grade fever, up to 101°F may occur after seizure.
   4. Injuries possible, especially with atonic seizures.
F. Diagnostic tests.
   1. EEG in awake and sleep states.
   2. MRI if focal spike on EEG or abnormal neuro exam.
   3. May do CMP, CBC if concerned abnormalities might be a cause.
   4. EKG for concern for cardiac disorder (syncope).
   5. Prolonged EEG to catch episodes if warranted.

G. Differential diagnosis.

Apnea, 786.03	Hyperventilation, 786.01
Arrhythmia, 427.9	Migraine, 346.9
Behavior disorder, 312.9	Pseudoseizures, 780.39
Breath holding, 786.9	Sleep disorder, 780.5
Daydreaming, 300.13	Syncope, 780.2

H. Treatment.
   1. Anticonvulsant medication.
      a. Absence seizures—ethosuximide (Zarontin), lamotrrgine (Lamictal), divalproex (Depakote).
      b. Generalized—divalproex (Depakote), lamotrigine (Lamictal), topiramate (Topamax), levetiracetam (Keppra), felbamate (Felbatol), zonisamide (Zonegran).
      c. Infantile spasms—ACTH, topiramate (Topamax), Vigabitrin (Sabril).
   2. 70% of patients with epilepsy will gain seizure freedom with medications.
   3. Vagal nerve stimulator or ketogenic diet for intractable seizures.
I. Follow up.
   1. Medication management, anticonvulsant therapeutic levels, and possible need for CMP, liver functions, CBC for some medications.
   2. Medication side effects.
   3. Continued seizures.
J. Complications.
   1. High risk for depression in epilepsy patients.
   2. Medication side effects.
   3. Developmental delay.
   4. Anxiety, intellectual underachievement.
K. Education.
   1. Seizure/epilepsy etiology and prognosis.
   2. Seizure safety.
   3. Psychosocial comorbidities.
   4. Medication management and possible side effects.
   5. Reevaluation parameters.

XII. PARTIAL SEIZURES

A. Seizure, electrical disturbance, arising from one area of the brain; consciousness may or may not be preserved. Can spread to become generalized.

Autonomic phenomena, 337.9	Partial simple seizure, 345.5
Partial complex seizure, 345.4	Seizure, 780.39

B. Etiology.
   1. Idiopathic (most common in children).
   2. Brain injury/trauma.
   3. Developmental brain abnormality.
   4. Tumors (rare).
   5. Infectious or hypoxic injuries.
C. Occurrence.
   1. Most common type of seizure experienced by people with epilepsy.
   2. Risk factors—developmental and brain abnormalities.
D. Clinical manifestations.
   1. Depends on which part and how much of the brain is affected.
   2. Virtually any movement, sensory, or emotional symptom can occur.
   3. Simple partial.
      a. No loss of consciousness.
      b. Motor signs.
         • Focal nature.
         • Postural.
         • Phonatory (vocalizations or arrest of speech).
         • Eye or truncal deviations.
      c. Somatosensory symptoms.
         • Visual.
         • Auditory.
         • Olfactory.
         • Gustatory.
         • Vertiginous.
      d. Autonomic symptoms.
         • Epigastric sensations.
         • Pallor.
         • Sweating.
         • Flushing.
         • Papillary dilation.

4. Complex partial.
   a. Impairment of consciousness.
   b. Can start as simple and evolve to loss of consciousness.
   c. May also progress to generalized seizure (partial seizure that secondarily generalizes).
E. Physical findings.
   1. Generally none on office exam, unless cause of seizure leaves or is cause of a neurological deficit.
F. Diagnostic tests.
   1. As with generalized seizures, but head MRI warranted.
G. Differential diagnosis.

Abnormal involuntary movements, 781	Myoclonus, 345.1
Dystonias, 333.89	Pseudoseizures, 780.39

H. Treatment.
   1. Anticonvulsant medications.
      a. Oxcarbazepine (Trileptal), or broad-spectrum anticonvulsant medication.
   2. Surgical intervention if intractable to medications.
   3. Vagal nerve stimulator or ketogenic diet.
I. Follow up.
   1. As with generalized seizures.
J. Complications.
   1. As with generalized seizures.
K. Education.
   1. As with generalized seizures.

XIII. COMMON ANTICONVULSANT MEDICATIONS FOR CHILDREN

A. Divalproex (Depakote): Start 10–20 mg/kg/day given bid, liquid tid; maintenance dose 30–60 mg/kg/day. Monitor CBC with platelets and liver enzymes every 6 months for liver failure, thrombocytopenia.
B. Levetiracetam (Keppra): Start 10–20 mg/kg/day bid; maintenance dose 30–60 mg/kg/day.
C. Lamotrigine (Lamictal): Titrate slowly over 8–12 weeks to starting dose. Risk for Stevens-Johnson syndrome. Maintenance dose 5–15 mg/kg/day bid; lower dose when on enzyme inducer anticonvulsant.

    D. Topiramate (Topamax): Start 1 mg/kg/day bid; maintenance 3–9 mg/kg/day. Monitor bicarb for metabolic acidosis.

    E. Oxcarbazepine (Trileptal): Start 10 mg/kg/day bid; maintenance 30–60 mg/kg/day.

    F. Ethosuximide (Zarontin): Start 10–15 mg/kg/day bid; maintenance dose 15–40 mg/kg/day. Monitor CBC for leucopenia, aplastic anemia.

    G. Zonisamide (Zonegran): Start 1–2 mg/kg/day daily or bid; maintenance dose 5–8 mg/kg/day.

XIV. GLOBAL DEVELOPMENTAL DELAY

    A. Subset of developmental disabilities defined as significant delay in two or more of the following developmental domains: gross/fine motor, speech/language, cognition, social/personal, and activities of daily living.

Abnormal brain development, 742.2	Language disorder, 315.31
Developmental delay, 783.42	Mitochondrial disorder, 758.89
Hypotonia/lack of coordination, 781.3	

    B. Etiology.
        1. Genetic abnormalities.
        2. Early environmental deprivation.
        3. Metabolic abnormalities.
        4. Abnormal CNS/brain development.
        5. Idiopathic/unknown.
    C. Occurrence.
        1. Developmental disabilities of early onset affect 5–10% of children.
        2. Refers to younger children younger than 5 years of age.
        3. 1–3% of children younger than 5 years of age are affected.
    D. Clinical manifestations.
        1. Two standard deviations or more below the mean on age-appropriate standardized norm-referenced testing.
    E. Physical findings.
        1. Not walking independently by 18 months of age.
        2. Poor/clumsy fine motor skills.
        3. No two-word sentences by 2 years of age.
        4. Does not follow two-step commands at age 2 years.
        5. Does not know 6 body parts by 2 years of age.

6. Unable to feed, dress, or do activities of daily living.
7. May see poor feeding, poor weight gain, dysmorphic features, cardiac or liver, kidney, bowel abnormalities.

F. Diagnostic testing.
   1. Obtain detailed history and examination.
   2. Refer for auditory and ophthalmologic screening.
   3. Consider metabolic studies/T4 if newborn screening not done.
   4. EEG if history suspects seizures.
   5. If close family member with global developmental delay due to a known cause, test for that disorder and obtain cytogenetic screen.
   6. Head MRI.
   7. Lead screen.
   8. Complete metabolic panel.
   9. Lactic acid.
   10. High resolution chromosomes, fragile X, Rett syndrome.
   11. Urine genetic screen.
   12. Microarray if other tests negative .
   13. Mitochondrial testing, muscle biopsy, if suspected and other testing inconclusive or negative.

G. Differential diagnosis.

Autism, 299	Genetic syndrome, 759.89
Cerebral palsy, 343.9	Progressive neurological disease, 330.9
Chromosomal abnormality, 758.9	
Encephalopathy, 348.3	

H. Treatment.
   1. Therapy—speech, physical, occupational, developmental, and/or nutritional.
   2. Medications as needed for any underlying cause.
   3. Genetic counseling.

I. Follow up.
   1. Discussion of test results.
   2. For any regression or loss of developmental milestones.
   3. Every 3 months to assess progression/development.
   4. To obtain further recommendations for testing in step-wise approach.
   5. For need for additional resources: referral to genetics, metabolism, developmental pediatrics, therapies, psychiatry, neurology, and other services as needed.

J. Complications.
1. Progressive loss of skills or lack of progression if untreated.
2. Seizures.
3. Behavioral disturbances.
4. Some disorders may affect systemic organs/systems.
K. Education.
1. Explaining test results, possible outcomes, prognosis.
2. Possible complications.
3. Medications if needed/treatment plan.
4. Resources.
5. Genetic and other counseling.

XV. TOURETTE SYNDROME

A. Neurobiological disorder characterized by tics—involuntary, rapid, sudden movements and/or vocal outburst that occur repeatedly.

> Involuntary movements, 781
> Tourette syndrome, 307.22

B. Etiology.
1. No known cause has yet been established.
2. Evidence points to abnormal metabolism of dopamine.
3. Genetic studies indicate that Tourette syndrome is inherited as a dominant gene.
C. Occurrence.
1. Estimated that 200,000 people in United States are affected—up to 18% of children.
2. Often undiagnosed or misdiagnosed.
3. 50% chance of affected parent passing to child.
4. Sons are 3 to 4 times more likely to be affected than daughters.
5. Peak severity of symptoms between 8–12 years and adolescents.
6. Can occur as early as 2 years of age, mean age of onset 6–7 years.
7. More common in males.
8. Exacerbated by anxiety, excitement, anger, fatigue, tension, stress.
9. Can decrease with relaxation or concentrating on an absorbing task.
D. Clinical manifestations.
1. Motor tics—involuntary rapid repetitive stereotyped movements of muscle groups.

a. Simple—involves one muscle group: eye blinking, facial grimacing, head jerking, shoulder shrugging.
b. Complex—involves either a cluster of simple movements or more coordinated sequence of movements: hopping, clapping, tensing arm or neck muscles, touching people or objects.
2. Vocal tics—transient vocalizations, meaningless sounds or noises or even words or phrases.
a. Simple vocal tics: sniffing, humming, clearing throat, coughing, squeaking.
b. Rare, complex vocal tics:
• Echolalia—repeating others' words.
• Palilalia—repeating one's own words.
• Coprolalia—obscene words.
3. Symptoms vary in children by type of specific tic and degree of severity.
E. Physical findings.
1. May or may not see tics exhibited on exam while in office because some children can temporarily suppress them, but still have urge.
2. May complain of muscle pain due to frequent motor tics.
F. Diagnostic testing.
1. Based on observing symptoms and evaluating history.
2. Must meet *Diagnostic and Statistical Manual of Mental Disorders* (DSM–IV) criteria:
a. Both motor and vocal tics must be present at same time.
b. Tics occur many times a day (usually in bouts) nearly daily or intermittently for more than 1 year without a tic-free period of 3 months or more.
c. Tics cause marked distress or significant impairment in social or daily functioning.
d. Onset is before age 18.
e. Tics are not due to physiological effects of medication or underlying medical condition.
G. Differential diagnosis.

Akathisia, 781	Meige syndrome, 333.82
Autism, 299	Neuroacanthocytosis, 363.2
Dystonia, 333.6	Paroxysmal kinesigenic
Huntington's disease, 333.4	Seizure, 780.39
Hyperekplexia, 759.89	Stereotypies, 307.3
Medication side effect or overdose, 977.9	Tardive dyskinesia, 781.3

H. Treatment.
   1. None if tics are not disruptive to patient/child.
   2. Teach coping skills and relaxation techniques.
   3. Maintain adequate sleep hours and routine.
   4. Treat with medication if disruptive, causes pain, decreases self-esteem, child is teased, child is frustrated, interferes socially or academically.
      a. Guanfacine (Tenex)—low side effects, but effective only 50% of time.
      b. Clonidine—sedating.
      c. Haloperidol (Haldol).
      d. Risperidone (Risperdal)—can cause weight gain.
      e. Pimozide (Orap)—monitor EKG for prolonged QT interval.
      f. Topiramate (Topamax)—limited studies, but can be effective.
I. Follow up.
   1. To monitor progression of symptoms to see if they become disruptive.
   2. For education and assessment of comorbidities.
   3. Medication management.
J. Complications.
   1. ADHD: seen in up to 70% of patients who have tics/Tourette syndrome.
   2. Obsessive compulsive disorder: seen in up to 50% of patients who have tics/Tourette syndrome.
   3. Depression.
   4. Anxiety.
   5. Muscle pain.
K. Education.
   1. Explanation of tics and Tourette syndrome, no known specific cause and no harm to brain, most often "normal" child and IQ.
   2. Do not criticize child or draw attention to tics.
   3. Be sensitive to child's feelings, child unable to fully stop tics.
   4. Teach coping skills and relaxation techniques.
   5. Most children have tics for only a few months or less.
   6. One-third of children will outgrow Tourette syndrome.
   7. Discuss possible complications and when to treat.

BIBLIOGRAPHY

Arizona Sports Concussion Center. Heads up: Concussion in youth sports. Retrieved July 5, 2011, from: www.azsportsconcussion.com/concussion.php.

Bruun R, Cohen D, & Leckman J. *A physician's guide to the diagnosis and treatment of Tourette syndrome.* 3rd ed. Bayside, NY: Tourette Syndrome Association; 1997.

Center for Disease Control and Prevention. Concussion and TBI; 2010. Retrieved July 5, 2011, from: www.cdc.gov/Concussion.

Centers for Disease Control and Prevention. Traumatic brain injury; 2010. Retrieved July 5, 2011, from: www.cdc.gov/TraumaticBrainInjury/index.html.

Cleveland Clinic Staff. Migraines in children and adolescents; 2009. Retrieved July 5, 2011, from: http://my .clevelandclinic.org/disorders/headaches/hic_migraines_in_children_and_adolescents.aspx.

Devinsky O, Feldmann E, Weinreb H, & Wilterdink J. *The resident's neurology book*. New York: F. A. Davis; 1997.

Epilepsy Foundation. Types of seizures. Retrieved July 5, 2011, from: http://www.epilepsyfoundation.org/ about/types/types/index.cfm.

Fusco E. Head injury causes, symptoms, diagnosis, and treatment; 2010. Retrieved July 5, 2011, from: http:// www.emedicinehealth.com/head_injury/article_em.htm.

Goldenberg L. Beyond a single seizure, identification and treatment of epilepsy. *Advance for Nurse Practitioners*. 2004;12(6):61–65.

Goldstein J. (2004). Evaluating new onset of seizures in children. *Pediatric Annals*. 2004;33(6):368–374.

Heller J. Head injury. *Medline Plus;* 2011. Retrieved July 5, 2011, from: www.nlm.gov/medlineplus/ency/ article/000028.htm.

Hershey A, Kabbouche M. & Powers S. Treatment of pediatric and adolescent migraine. *Pediatric Annals*. 2010;39(7):416–423.

Huff J. Status epilepticus; 2010. www.emedicine.medscape.com

Leung A, & Robson W. Febrile seizures. *Journal of Pediatric Health Care*. 2006;21(4):250–255.

Lewis D, Ashwal S, Hershey A, Hirtz D, Yonker M, & Silberstein S. Practice Parameter: Pharmacological treatment of migraine headache in children and adolescents: Report of the American Academy of Neurology Quality Standards Subcommittee and the Practice Committee of the Child Neurology Society. *American Academy of Neurology*. 2004;63:2215–2224. Retrieved July 5, 2011, from: www.neurology.org/cgi/ content/full/63/12/2215.

Mayo Clinic staff. Meningitis; 2008. Retrieved July 5, 2011, from: www.mayoclinic.com/health/meningitis/ ds00118.

Mayo Clinic Staff. Encephalitis; 2009. Retrieved July 5, 2011, from: www.mayoclinic.com/health/ encephalitis/DS00226/DSECTION=symptoms.

Mayo Clinic Staff. Headaches in children; 2009. Retrieved July 5, 2011, from: www.mayoclinic.com/health/ headaches-in-children/DS01132/DSECTION=symptoms.

Pakalnis A, & Yonker M. 'Other' headache syndromes in children. *Pediatric Annals*. 2010;39(7):440–446.

Panayiotopoulos C. Idiopathic generalized epilepsies; 2008. Retrieved July 1, 2011, from: http://professionals. epilepsy.com/page/ideopathic_generalized_epilepsies.html.

Saper J, Silberstein S, Gordon C, & Hamel R. *Handbook of headache management: A practical guide to diagnosis and treatment of head, neck, and facial pain*. Philadelphia, PA: Lippincott Williams & Wilkins; 1993.

Shevell M, Ashwal S, Donley D, Flint J, Gingold M, Hirtz D, et al. Practice parameter: Evaluation of the child with global developmental delay: Report of the quality standards subcommittee of the Child Neurology Society. *Neurology*. 2010;60:367–380.

Shinnar S, & O'Dell C. Febrile seizures. *Pediatric Annals*. 2004;33(6):394–401.

Silberstein S, & Lipton R. Variants confused with epilepsy; 2004. Retrieved July 5, 2011, from: www.professional .epilepsy.com/page/migraine_variants.html.

Silberstein S, Lipton R, & Goadsby P. Headache in clinical practice. London, UK: Thomson; 2002.

Tourette Syndrome Association website: www.tsa-usa.org

Vyas J. Encephalitis. *Medline Plus;* 2008. Retrieved July 5, 2011, from: www.nlm.nih.gov/medlineplus/ency/ article/001415.htm.

Wikipedia. Meningitis; 2010. Retrieved July 5, 2011, from: www.en.wikipedia.org/wiki/Meningitis.

Wyllie E, Gupta A, & Lachhwani D. *The treatment of epilepsy principles and practice*, 4th ed. Philadelphia, PA: Lippincott Williams & Wilkins; 2006.

Hematologic Disorders

Betsy Atkinson Joyce

I. IRON-DEFICIENCY ANEMIA (IDA)

Anemia, 280.9	Palmar pallor, 782.61
Anemia, mild, 285.9	Poor weight gain, 263.9
Fatigue, 780.79	Splenomegaly, 789.2
GI bleeding, 578.9	Systolic flow murmurs, 785.2
Headaches, 784	Tachycardia, 785
Irritability, 799.2	

A. Most common anemia of childhood. Anemia is defined as reduction in red blood cell (RBC) mass or in hemoglobin concentration to a level that is > 2 standard deviations below mean in healthy children. Can be determined in primary care setting by physical examination, important aspects of history, and hemoglobin concentration. Screening should occur routinely around 9 months to 1 year. High-risk infants: screen earlier, more often.

B. Etiology.
   1. Microcytic anemia reflecting defect in production of hemoglobin during erythrocyte maturation, resulting from defect in heme synthesis due to inadequate quantities of iron:
      a. Inadequate supply of iron at birth, inadequate dietary iron.
      b. High demand for iron associated with growth.
      c. Blood loss without replacement.
      d. Inflammatory bowel disease.
      e. Menstruation.

C. Occurrence.
   1. Common between 1 and 3 years of age because of inadequate dietary iron due to cow's milk being major staple in most children's diets.
   2. Lack of adequate iron stores to meet needs for growth.
      a. Affects 9% of children younger than 2 years of age.
      b. Affects 9–11% of adolescent females.

3. Lack of adequate iron to meet needs for RBC production.
    a. Affects 3% of children younger than 2 years of age.
    b. Affects up to 3% of adolescent females and < 1% of adolescent males.
D. Clinical manifestations.
    1. Mild anemia (hemoglobin of 9.5–11): may be asymptomatic; sometimes only minimal symptoms when severe anemia (hemoglobin of 8–9.5 or lower) is present. May only be detected on routine screening or discovered when blood count ordered for another reason.
    2. History of fatigue, irritability, excessive milk intake, headaches.
E. Physical findings.
    1. Mild anemia (normal physical exam).
    2. More severe anemia.
        a. Poor weight gain.
        b. Sclera or palmar pallor.
        c. Splenomegaly: 15% of affected children.
        d. Tachycardia.
        e. Systolic flow murmurs: with progression of the iron deficit.
F. Diagnostic tests.
    1. Hemoglobin concentration (**Table 32-1**).
    2. Complete blood count (CBC).
        a. RBC hypochromic, microcytic.
        b. Mean cell volume (MCV) decreased.
        c. Ratio of MCV/RBC > 13 (Mentzer index).
            • > 13 = iron-deficiency anemia.
            • < 13 = thalassemia trait.
    3. Iron studies if need further information.
        a. Serum iron: decreased.
        b. Total iron-binding capacity: increased.
        c. Ferritin: decreased.
        d. Percentage of iron saturation: decreased.
G. Differential diagnosis.

Lead poisoning, 984.9
Sideroblastic anemia, 285
Thalassemia, 282.49

1. Thalassemia trait.
2. Lead poisoning.

Table 32-1 Maximum Hemoglobin Concentration and Hematocrit Values for Iron-Deficiency Anemia

Sex/age, years	Hemoglobin (g/dL)	Hematocrit (%)
Both genders		
1 to < 2 years	11.0	32.9
2 to < 5 years	11.1	33.0
5 to < 8 years	11.5	34.5
8 to < 12 years	11.9	35.4
Females		
12 to < 15 years	11.8	35.7
15 to 18 years	12.0	35.9
≥ 18 years	12.0	35.7
Males		
12 to < 15 years	12.5	37.3
15 to 18 years	13.3	39.7
≥ 18 years	13.5	39.9

Source: Adapted from Centers for Disease Control and Prevention. (1998, April 3). Recommendations to prevent and control iron deficiency in the United States. *Morbidity and Mortality Weekly Report, 47*(RR-3), 1–36.

   3. Chronic infection.
   4. Sideroblastic anemia.
  H. Treatment.
   1. Nutritional strategies.
   2. Reduce milk to no more than 16–24 oz/day.
      a. Increase intake of high-iron foods (e.g., beans, whole cereals, dried fruit, pork, beef).
      b. Iron therapy for infants and children:
         • Ferrous sulfate.
            i. Mild to moderate iron deficiency: elemental iron 3 mg/kg/day in 1–2 divided doses.

            ii. Severe iron deficiency: elemental iron 4–6 mg/kg/day in 3 divided doses.

I. Follow up.
1. Recheck hemoglobin in 1 month.
2. Treat until hemoglobin and hematocrit reach normal ranges. Then give at least 1 month additional treatment to replenish iron stores.
3. If response not adequate within 1–2 months, consider further diagnostic testing for GI bleeding or other microcytic hypochromic anemias.

J. Complications.

Anemia, 280.9	Developmental delays, 783.4
Behavioral delays, 312.9	Poor growth, 253.2

1. Result from long-standing iron-deficiency anemia.
   a. Increased susceptibility to infection.
   b. Poor growth.
   c. Developmental delays (lower mental and motor test scores).
   d. Behavioral delays.

K. Education.
1. Need for balanced diets and foods containing iron.
   a. Cereal, egg yolks, green/yellow vegetables, yellow fruits, red meat, potatoes, tomatoes, raisins.
2. Amount of milk necessary/day (age dependent).
3. Information about iron medications:
   a. Give after meals with orange juice to enhance absorption.
   b. Do not give with milk (inhibits absorption of iron).
   c. Give with straw or brush teeth after giving (may stain teeth).
   d. May cause abdominal discomfort, constipation, black stools.
   e. Extremely poisonous if taken in excessive amounts.
   f. Keep out of reach of small children.

II. THALASSEMIA

A. An inherited anemia that can affect both males and females and can be mild or severe. Hemoglobin has two types of protein chains, alpha globin and beta globin, which are needed to properly form the red blood cell and allow it to then carry enough oxygen. Therefore one can have either an alpha thalassemia or a beta thalassemia. It occurs most often in people of Italian, Greek, Middle Eastern, Asian, and African descent. Severe form is usually diagnosed in early childhood and is a lifelong condition.

B. Etiology.
  1. Alpha thalassemia: need 4 genes (2 from each parent) to make enough alpha protein chains, located on chromosome 16.
     a. Mild anemia.
        • One missing gene, silent carrier, no symptoms.
        • Two missing genes—carrier and mild anemia.
     b. Moderate to severe anemia.
        • Three missing genes—hemoglobin H disease.
        • Four missing genes—alpha thalassemia major or hydrops fetalis.
  2. Beta thalassemia—need 2 genes (one from each parent) to make enough beta globin protein—located on chromosome 11.
     a. Mild anemia.
        • One missing or altered gene—carrier status.
     b. Moderate or severe anemia.
        • Two missing or altered genes.
          i. Beta thalassemia intermedia—moderate anemia.
          ii. Beta thalassemia major—Cooley's anemia, severe.
C. Occurrence.
  1. Family history and ancestry are the two risk factors.
     a. Alpha thalassemias most often affect ancestry origin of Indian, Chinese, Filipino, or Southeast Asian.
     b. Beta thalassemias most often affect ancestry origin of Mediterranean (Greek, Italian, Middle Eastern), Asian, or African.
D. Clinical manifestations.
  1. No symptoms if a silent carrier as in alpha thalassemia.
  2. May or may not have symptoms with mild anemia—usually fatigue—most often mistaken for IDA.
  3. More severe symptoms with moderate anemia that may include slowed growth and development and physical problems with bones and the spleen.
  4. Symptoms of severe anemia due to thalassemias occur during the first 2 years of life and include other serious health problems besides the severe anemia.
E. Physical findings.
  1. Mild anemia—normal physical exam.
  2. More severe anemia.
     a. Pale and listless appearance.
     b. Poor appetite.
     c. Dark urine.
     d. Jaundice.
     e. Enlarged spleen, liver, and heart.

      f. Bone problems, especially the bones of the face.

      g. Delayed puberty.

      h. Slowed growth.

F. Diagnostic tests.

    1. CBC with differential.

    2. Iron tests—to rule out IDA.

    3. Hemoglobin tests.

    4. Genetic studies.

G. Differential diagnosis.

    1. IDA.

    2. Other anemias.

H. Treatment.

    1. Mild forms need no treatment.

    2. Moderate to severe forms.

      a. Regular blood transfusions—RBCs live 120 days so may need transfusions for severe anemia every 2 to 4 weeks.

      b. Iron chelation therapy—transfusions can lead to a build up of iron in the blood.

        • Deferoxamine—liquid given slowly under the skin with a pump; takes time and is often painful and side effects include loss of vision and hearing.

        • Deferasirox—pill taken once a day; side effects include headache, nausea, vomiting, diarrhea, joint pain, and fatigue.

      c. Folic acid supplements—a B vitamin that helps build healthy RBCs.

      d. Bone marrow/stem cell transplant—only cure for thalassemia.

I. Follow up.

    1. Well-child physical as indicated.

    2. Vaccines as scheduled.

    3. Follow with hematology physicians on routine basis.

J. Complications.

    1. Heart disease—caused by iron overload from the transfusions.

    2. Heart attack.

    3. Arrhythmias.

    4. Heart failure.

    5. Liver disease—also caused by iron overload and damage to the organ.

    6. Infection—risk of infection higher in persons whose spleen has been removed.

    7. Osteoporosis.

K. Education.

    1. Follow the treatment plan as outlined by the doctor/clinic.

        a. Blood transfusions as needed.
        b. Chelation medications to be taken as prescribed.
        c. Take your folic acid supplements.
    2. Routine maintenance.
        a. Yearly well child checks (WCC).
            • Height and weight.
            • Test for iron build up in the liver.
            • Vision and hearing tests.
        b. Monthly CBCs.
        c. Quarterly tests for iron build up in the blood.
    3. Measures to stay healthy.
        a. Healthy eating.
        b. Vaccinations as scheduled.
        c. Watch for signs of infection.
        d. Wash hands.
        e. Avoid crowds during cold and flu season.
        f. Call clinic/doctor if develop fever.
    4. Support groups—parents and children.

III. LEAD POISONING

Headache, 784	Poor attention span, 314
Irritability, 799	Seizures, 780.39
Lead poisoning, 984.9	Sleep disorders, 780.5
Loss of visual motor coordination, 781.3	Stomachache, 789
Muscular weakness, 728.87	Tiredness, 780.79
Poor appetite, 783	Weight loss, 783.2

A. Most common, widespread environmental health concern, especially for children younger than 6 years of age. Can cause decrease in gestational weight and age; may increase possibility of stillbirths and miscarriages.
B. Etiology.
    1. Increased lead levels in children occur by exposure to deteriorating paint, household dust, bare soil, air, drinking water, food, ceramics, home remedies, hair dyes, other cosmetics. Usually exposure is in child's own home.
    2. Manufacture, use, disposal of modern products containing lead results in fine lead particles that release into environment. Lead particles enter air, water, food; also contaminate soil, dust.

       3. Lead containing toys, crayons, soft vinyl lunch boxes.

C. Occurrence.

    1. Estimated at least 400,000 children younger than 6 years of age have too much lead in their bodies.

    2. Questions for assessing risk of lead poisoning:

       a. Live in, regularly visit, or have lived in a place with peeling or chipping paint built before 1960?

         • Includes daycare, preschools, homes of babysitters, relatives.

         • Houses with recent, ongoing, planned renovation or remodeling.

       b. Brother or sister, housemate, playmate being followed or treated for lead poisoning (blood level > 15 mcg/dL)?

       c. Live with adult whose job or hobby involves exposure to lead?

         • Ceramics, furniture refinishing; stained glass work; construction workers.

       d. Taking home remedies such as azarcon and greta?

       e. Live near active smelter, battery-recycling plant, other industry likely to release lead into air?

    3. Lead toxicity is decreasing in the United States but approximately 25% of children still live in housing with deteriorating lead-based paint.

D. Clinical manifestations.

    1. Many symptoms resemble common childhood complaints: headache, stomachache, irritability, tiredness, poor appetite.

    2. Other subtle symptoms: poor attention span and memory, sleep disorders.

    3. All of these can lead to coma and death because not noticed until brain damage has already occurred. Once organ systems are damaged, damage often irreversible.

E. Physical findings.

    1. Weight loss, decreased growth.

    2. Muscular weakness (diminished reflexes).

    3. Seizures (signs of anemia).

    4. Loss of visual motor coordination.

    5. Irritability.

    6. Constipation, abdominal pain.

    7. Learning difficulties/cognitive impairment.

F. Diagnostic tests.

    1. CBC.

    2. Lead blood levels: < 10 mcg/dL. Screening tests as recommended by Centers for Disease Control and Prevention (CDC) (**Table 32-2**).

    3. Free erythrocyte protoporphyrin (FEP): elevated.

Table 32-2 CDC Recommendations for Follow-Up Lead Blood Level Measurements

Class	Blood lead level	Comment
I	≤ 9 mcg/dL	Not lead poisoned
		Low risk: 6–35 months of age, retest at 24 months
		High risk: 6–35 months of age, retest every 6 months
		Older than 36 months of age: retest yearly until 6 years of age
IIA	10–14 mcg/dL	Rescreen frequently and consider prevention activities 6–35 months of age, retest every 3–4 months
		Older than 36 months of age, retest yearly
IIB	15–19 mcg/dL	Institute nutritional and educational interventions
		Retest every 3–4 months
III	20–44 mcg/dL	Evaluate environment and consider chelation therapy
		Retest every 3–4 months
IV	45–69 mcg/dL	Institute environmental intervention and chelation therapy within 48 hours
V	> 70 mcg/dL	Medical emergency; requires immediate treatment

Source: Data from Centers for Disease Control and Prevention. Recommendations for follow-up lead blood level measurements. Retrieved March 2004, from: www.cdc.gov; Cohen, S. (2001). Lead poisoning: A summary of treatment and prevention. *Pediatric Nursing, 27,* 125.

G. Differential diagnosis.

Abdominal pain, unspecified, 789	Iron-deficiency anemia, 280.9
Behavioral disorders, 312.9	Unexplained seizures, 780.39

  1. Neurologic problems (unexplained seizures, behavioral disorders).
  2. IDA.
  3. Unexplained abdominal pain.
H. Treatment.
  1. Lead blood level determines treatment (Table 32-2).
  2. Alteration in environment; stop unusual exposure to lead.

3. Good nutrition.
4. Chelation therapy.
   a. British anti-Lewisite (BAL).
   b. Edetate calcium disodium (CaNa2EDTA).
   c. Dimercaptosuccinic acid (DMSA) or Succimer.
   d. D-Penicillamine.

I. Follow up.
1. Follow recommendations in Table 32-2 for rescreening. Treatment time is lengthy: There will be rebound levels as stored lead releases from bones and teeth.
2. After chelation therapy: Obtain another blood lead level in 10–14 days.
3. Blood lead level determines subsequent treatment.

J. Complications.

Coma, 780.01	Learning disabilities, 315.2
Diminished fertility, 628.9	Lower sperm counts, 792.2
Elevated BUN, 790.6	Mental retardation, 319
Headache, 784	Persistent vomiting, 536.2
Hearing loss, 389.9	Seizures, 780.39
Hypertension, 401.9	Sterility, female, 628.9
Impaired growth, 253.2	Sterility, male, 606.9
Kidney diseases, 593.9	Toxicity, 323.7
Lead encephalopathy, 984.7	

1. Lead encephalopathy and toxicity:
   a. Headache, persistent vomiting.
   b. Seizures, coma, death.
   c. Mental retardation, learning disabilities.
   d. Impaired growth.
   e. Hearing loss.
2. Renal disorders: hypertension, kidney diseases (later in life), elevated blood urea nitrogen (BUN).
3. Reproductive system:
   a. Diminished fertility, abnormal sperm and lower counts, sterility—male and female.
   b. Increased chance of miscarriage.

K. Education.
1. Prevention.

2. Advice for families:
   a. If suspect exposure, test child.
   b. Use caution when purchasing older home.
   c. Maintenance to keep old lead-based paint intact.
   d. Watch for lead dust when doing home improvement projects: Protect furniture from lead dust, wet mop work area after projects using detergent.
   e. Wash work clothes separately from family's clothing.
   f. Encourage children to play in sand, grass rather than dirt.
   g. Wash hands, pacifiers before naps, bedtime.
   h. Avoid folk remedies or cosmetics containing lead.
   i. Test water supply for lead.
   j. Wash fruits, vegetables before eating.
   k. Eat healthy diet rich in iron: helps body to absorb less lead.
   l. Use only cold water from tap for drinking, cooking, making baby formula. Hot water more likely to contain higher levels of lead.

IV. SICKLE CELL DISEASE

Abdominal pain, unspecified, 789	Hepatitis C, 070.51
Angina, 413.9	Hepatitis D, 070.52
Aplastic crisis, 284.9	Hepatitis E, 070.53
Cardiomyopathy, 425.4	Increased lethargy, 780.79
Cerebral vascular accident, 436	Irritability, 799.2
Chest syndrome, acute, 517.3	Leg ulcerations, 707.1
Chronic hemolytic anemia, 282.9	Maxillary hyperplasia, 524.01
Cytomegalovirus, 078.5	Meningitis, 322.9
Dehydration, 276.5	Ocular retinopathy, 362.1
Delayed puberty, 259	Orthopnea, 786.02
Dental malocclusion, 534.9	Pallor, 782.61
Dyspnea, 786.09	Pallor/jaundiced skin, 782.61
Emesis, recurrent, 787.03	Persistent headaches, 784
Emotional stress, 308	Pneumonia, 486
Exercise intolerance, V47.2	Priapism, 607.3

Fatigue, 780.79	Pulmonary fibrosis, 515
Fever, 780.6	Sickle cell disease, 282.6
Gallbladder disease, 575.9	Splenomegaly, 789.2
Hemolytic anemia, 282.9	Tachycardia, 785
Hemolytic crisis, 283.9	Tightness in chest, 786.59
Hemoptysis, 786.3	Urinary tract infection, 599
Hepatitis A, 070.1	Visual/speech changes, 784.49
Hepatitis B, 070.3	Weakness/numbness in extremities, 780.79

A. Group of inherited heme disorders characterized by sickle hemoglobin (HbS); several variants within sickle cell disease. This section aimed at variant that results when one is homozygous for HbS, sometimes referred to as sickle cell anemia (HbSS).

B. Etiology.
  1. Due to single defective hemoglobin module inherited as gene from both parents (autosomal-recessive disorder).
  2. Abnormal HbS is produced instead of HbA, normal hemoglobin.
  3. The abnormal hemoglobin S, when deoxygenated, deforms red cells into sickle shapes that occlude small vessels, slowing blood flow, creating vaso-occlusive crises in blood vessels and in organs such as spleen.

C. Occurrence.
  1. Predominantly in African Americans with about 1 in 400 African Americans affected.
  2. Mediterranean or Arabic descendants also found to have sickle cell anemia, but in fewer numbers.

D. Clinical manifestations.
  1. Chronic hemolytic anemia (aplastic crisis, hemolytic crisis, sequestration crisis).
  2. Vaso-occlusion resulting in ischemia to tissues.
     a. Painful crisis: from infarcts of muscle, bone, bone marrow, lung, intestines.
     b. Cerebrovascular accident.
     c. Acute chest syndrome.
     d. Chronic lung disease such as pulmonary fibrosis.
     e. Priapism.
     f. Ocular retinopathy.
     g. Gallbladder disease.

   h. Renal.
   i. Cardiomyopathy.
   j. Leg ulcerations.
  3. Susceptibility to infection.
  4. Growth failure, delayed puberty.
  5. Psychologic problems (narcotic addiction, chronic illness, unusual dependence).
 E. Physical findings.
  1. Depends on which clinical manifestation is presenting.
  2. Chronic hemolytic anemia: pallor/jaundiced skin, tachycardia, fatigue.
  3. Susceptibility to infection: fever, other symptoms related to causative organism or system infected: e.g., meningitis; urinary tract infection (UTI); cytomegalovirus (CMV); hepatitis A, B, C, D, E; pneumonia.
  4. Vaso-occlusive crisis: again depends on location of occlusion.
  5. Splenomegaly.
  6. Maxillary hyperplasia and dental malocclusion result from compensatory bone marrow expansion.
 F. Diagnostic tests.
  1. Newborn screening for hemoglobinopathies. Electrophoresis on cellulose acetate indicates type of hemoglobin: fetal (F), normal adult (A), sickle (S), hemoglobin C (C).
  2. Repeat testing with abnormal hemoglobin (FS) pattern on newborn screen.
  3. CBC with hemoglobin MCV.
 G. Differential diagnosis.

Beta thalassemia anemia, 282.49
Sickle cell disease, 282.6

  1. Sickle cell trait (benign), beta-thalassemia anemia.
 H. Treatment.
  1. Preventive care.
   a. Education of the family.
    • Adequate fluid intake.
    • Immediate medical help for fevers.
    • Importance of prophylactic treatment.
   b. Immunizations per the schedule plus 23-valent pneumococcal vaccine at 2 and 5 years.

2. Pharmaceutical therapies.
   a. Penicillin prophylaxis:
      - 2 months to 3 years of age: Penicillin VK 125 mg PO bid.
      - 3 years to 5+ years of age: Penicillin VK 250 mg PO bid.
   b. Alternative to penicillin: erythromycin (EES) 20 mg/kg/day divided bid.
   c. Folic acid: 1 mg/day.
   d. Multivitamin once daily.
   e. Hydroxyurea drug therapy.
      - Anti-sickling effect of hydroxyurea can decrease frequency of vaso-occlusive crises.
      - Starting dose: 15 mg/kg/day, increase gradually by 5 mg/kg/day while monitoring for toxicity.
      - Toxicity manifested by falls in neutrophil count to < 2500/mm^3 or platelet count < 80,000/mm^3.
   f. Pain medications: acetaminophen or nonsteroidal anti-inflammatory drugs (NSAIDs) (mild pain), acetaminophen with codeine (moderate pain), morphine (severe pain).
I. Follow up.
   1. Routine well-child checks:
      a. Birth to 6 months: every 2 months, CBC every visit.
      b. 6 months to 2 years: every 3 months.
         - CBC every 3–6 months.
         - Urinalysis (UA) annually.
         - Ferritin or serum iron and total iron-binding capacity (TIBC) once at 1–2 years of age.
         - BUN, creatinine, liver function tests (LFTs) once at 1–2 years of age.
         - Influenza vaccine annually.
         - Start folic acid daily at 1 year of age.
      c. 2–5 years: visits every 6 months.
         - CBC and UA at least yearly.
         - BUN, creatinine, LFTs every 1–2 years.
         - 23-valent pneumococcal vaccine at 2 years of age, with booster at 5 years.
         - Hearing, vision, purified protein derivative (PPD) per standard practice.
      d. Older than 5 years: visits every 6–12 months.
         - CBC and UA at least annually.
         - BUN, creatinine, LFTs every 2–3 years.

- Influenza vaccine yearly.
- Continue folic acid.
- May opt to stop penicillin V.
  e. Adolescent: yearly visits.
- CBC and UA yearly.
- BUN, creatinine, LFTs every 2–3 years.
- Ferritin or serum iron and TIBC at least once.
- Hearing, vision, PPD as per standard practice.
- Influenza vaccine yearly.
2. Close monitoring by family for complications.
J. Complications.

Acute chest syndrome, 517.3	Priapism, 607.3
Anemia, 285.9	Renal dysfunction, 593.9
Aplastic crisis, 284.9	Renal failure, 586
Avascular necrosis of hips, 733.42	Retinal detachment, 361.9
Chronic lung disease, 518.89	Retinopathy, 362.1
Febrile events, 780.6	Splenic sequestration, 289.52
Gallstones, 574.2	Stroke, 436
Hemolysis, 283.9	Vaso-occlusive events, 459.9
Leg ulcers, 707.1	

1. Acute and chronic complications (hemolysis, anemia, gallstones) need early recognition, prompt treatment to reduce morbidity and mortality.
2. Acute events:
   a. Painful vaso-occlusive events.
   b. Febrile events.
   c. Acute chest syndrome.
   d. Splenic sequestration.
   e. Stroke.
   f. Aplastic crisis.
3. Chronic events:
   a. Avascular necrosis of hips/shoulders.
   b. Priapism.
   c. Chronic lung disease.
   d. Leg ulcers.
   e. Renal dysfunction or renal failure.
   f. Retinopathy and retinal detachment.

K. Education.
  1. When family/patient should seek immediate medical care:
      a. Fevers or persistent low-grade fever.
      b. Pain unrelieved by prescribed oral medications.
      c. Persistent abdominal pain, recurrent emesis.
      d. Dyspnea, pain with breathing, hemoptysis, or feelings of tightness in chest.
      e. Angina, exercise intolerance, or orthopnea.
      f. Visual/speech changes, weakness/numbness in extremities, persistent headaches.
      g. Sustained penile erections unrelieved by prescribed medications.
      h. Increased lethargy, irritability, or pallor.
  2. Factors that may precipitate painful vaso-occlusive crises:
      a. Inadequate rest, emotional stress, fatigue.
      b. Vasoconstrictive drugs, smoking, constrictive clothing.
      c. Dehydration, strenuous physical exercise.
      d. Extreme hot/cold temperatures, high altitudes, unpressurized aircraft.

V. BLEEDING DISORDERS

A. Usually bruising and bleeding are a part of active childhood. Bruises on the knees and shins and nose bleeds can simply be a fact of life. They become a health problem when the bleeding is hard to control or the bruising is in areas of the body that one does not normally hit, e.g., the back or stomach. Also, in adolescence, heavy menses could be the norm for many girls or it could signal a bleeding problem. The provider needs to decide when further studies would differentiate pathological or nonpathological causes of the bleeding and bruising. Normal clotting involves some 20 clotting factors that work together along with some other chemicals to form a substance called fibrin that leads to a clot.

B. Etiology.
  1. Platelets or clotting factors do not work in the right way.
  2. Supply of specified clotting factors are deficient.
  3. Physical abuse.
  4. Vitamin K deficiency.

C. Occurrence.
  1. Congenital.
      a. Hemophilia A or B—about 400 newborns a year are diagnosed in the U.S.

- X-linked recessive pattern of inheritance.
- Deficiencies in factor VIII (hemophilia A) and factor IX (hemophilia B).
- Males exclusively affected, some very rare cases of females with hemophilia.
  b. von Willebrand—affects 66–100 people/1 million of the population.
  - Autosomal inheritance with variable phenotypic expression.
  - Common in both men and women.
  - Deficiency in the von Willebrand clotting factor.
    i. Blood protein that affects platelet function.
    ii. Is a critical link between platelets and exposed vascular subendothelium.
    iii. Binds and stabilizes coagulation factor VIII.
2. Acquired.
  a. Acquired hemophilia.
  - Rare condition with no genetic inheritance.
  - Autoimmune etiology that results in development of autoantibodies to coagulation factors.
  b. Disseminated intravascular coagulation.
  - Acquired syndrome that activates the coagulation pathway.
  - Results in intravascular thrombi and depletion of platelets and coagulation factors.
  c. Idiopathic thrombocytopenic purpura.
  - Characterized by thrombocytopenia (platelet count less than 150,000/mcL) in the absence of other causes.
  - Thought to be secondary to an autoimmune phenomenon.
  d. Henoch-Schönlein purpura.
  - Results from autoimmune reaction where the body attacks its own tissues.
  - Small, bluish purple spots on feet, legs, arms, and buttocks.
  - Usually develops after respiratory infection but can occur after immunization, insect bite, or allergic reaction to drugs or food.
  - Rate at which disease develops and its duration vary.
D. Clinical manifestations.
  1. Excessive bruising or bleeding.
  2. Bleeding history.
    a. Location, duration, frequency, precipitating factors.
    b. What does it take to stop the bleeding?
    c. Reactions to injections, lacerations, toothbrushing, menstruation (as applicable).

    d. Medications taken that may increase tendency to bleed.

    e. Family history of unexpected or severe bleeding (surgery, childbirth, dental procedures).

    f. Consideration of abuse.

E. Physical findings—dependent upon site of bleeding and age of the child.

    1. Epistaxis—unilateral or bilateral—bleeding longer than 15 minutes.

    2. Menorrhagia—menses longer than 7 days, double pads, lightheadedness.

    3. Ecchymosis—where, clusters or not, especially in areas that are anatomically protected.

    4. Skin and mucous membrane bleeding—generalized petechial rash, subcutaneous hemorrhagic nodules, submucosal hemorrhages of the mouth.

    5. Spontaneous hemarthrosis—joints affected, amount of swelling/pain, limited range of motion.

    6. Intracranial bleeding in absence of elicited history of trauma—headache, nausea.

    7. Hepatosplenomegaly.

    8. Hematuria.

    9. Gastrointestional cramping/pain.

F. Diagnostic tests.

    1. Initial lab screening.

        a. CBC with differential and platelets.

        b. Prothrombin time (PT).

        c. Activated partial thromboplastin time (aPTT; see **Table 32-3**).

    2. Secondary lab screening.

        a. PT/aPTT mixing studies.

        b. von Willebrand panel.

        c. von Willebrand antigen.

        d. Factor VIII activity.

        e. Platelet function testing.

        f. Bleeding time.

        g. PFA-100.

        h. Platelet aggregation studies.

G. Differential diagnosis.

    1. Child abuse.

    2. Leukemia.

    3. Hemophilia.

    4. von Willebrand's disease.

    5 Idiopathic thrombocytopenia purpura.

    6. Thrombocytopenia.

    7. Henoch-Schönlein purpura.

Table 32-3 Common Causes of Prolonged PT/aPTT

Scenario	Common/Important Causes	Comments
Prolonged PT	Vitamin K deficiency Liver disease Warfarin Factor VII deficiency DIC	Isolated PT elevation is sensitive marker early in DIC development
Prolonged aPTT	vWD Hemophilia (FVIII, FIX or FXI deficiency) Heparin Antiphospholipid antibodies (associated with minor infections or, rarely, autoimmune thromboembolic disease)	Rare deficiencies of factor XII, HMWK, or PK may also elevate aPTT, but are not clinically significant Half of children with prolonged aPTT do not have a bleeding disorder
Prolonged PT and aPTT	Heparin Warfarin Liver disease DIC Hypofibrinogenemia Factor II, V, or X deficiency Underfilled specimen tube Severe vitamin K deficiency	Fibrinogen measurement can help distinguish among liver disease and DIC (decrease in fibrinogen) and vitamin K deficiency (no decrease in fibrinogen)

PT= prothrombin time

aPTT = activated partial thromboplastin time

DIC = disseminated intravascular coagulopathy

vWD = von Willebrand disease

HMWK = high-molecular-weight kininogen

PK = prekallikrein

Source: Savage, W., & Takemoto, C. (2009). Bleeding and bruising. *Contemporary Pediatrics, 26*(6), 66.

8. Acquired hemophilia—presence of inhibitory antibodies.
9. Scurvy.
10. Fabry disease.
11. Ehlers-Danlos syndrome.
12. Deficiency of other coagulation factors (V, VII, X, XI, or fibrinogen).

H. Treatment.
1. Dependent upon cause of bleeding or bruising and the site of the bleeding.
2. Referral to hematologist if deficient factors or platelet deficiency—chronic illness that needs to have specialist involved and be enrolled in a hemophilia treatment center.
   a. Treatment is prevention of bleeding by replacement therapy.
   b. Long-term management of joint and muscle damage.
   c. Management of complications from treatment.
3. Corticosteroids if Henoch-Schönlein purpura.
4. Child protective services if suspected child abuse.

I. Follow up.
1. Well child checks and immunizations as recommended.
2. Good communication between specialist and primary care.
3. Action plan for family—see Education section that follows.
4. Regular dental care.
5. Support groups.

J. Complications.
1. School absence.
2. Joint deformities.
3. Intracranial hemorrhage.
4. Complications from therapies like corticosteroids.

K. Education.
1. Importance of finding and knowing correct diagnosis.
   a. Untreated bleeding disorder leads to dangerous bleeding after childbirth, miscarriage, dental work, minor surgery, and injury.
2. Epistaxis.
   a. Know procedure to control nosebleeds.
   b. Know when to seek medical help.
   c. Vaseline around and in the nares at bedtime.
   d. Humidifier in bedroom to provide moisture.
3. Safety precautions with bleeding disorders to minimize long-term permanent damage to joints and muscles and the brain.
4. Importance of keeping regular checkups with primary care provider and the hematology provider if congenital/or acquired bleeding disorder.

5. Avoiding platelet-impairing medications such as aspirin and ibuprofen.
6. Limit alcohol as excessive intake, which can adversely affect blood clotting.
7. Exercise regularly.
8. Medic alert bracelet—if hemophilia, von Willebrand, platelet dysfunction.

BIBLIOGRAPHY

Abelsohn AR, Sanborn M. Lead and children: Clinical management for family physicians. *Canadian Family Physician.* 2010;56:531–535.

Berkowitz CD. *Berkowitz's pediatrics: A Primary care approach.* 3rd ed. Elk Grove Village, IL: American Academy of Pediatrics; 2008.

Burns CE, Brady MA, Dunn AM, et al., eds. *Pediatric primary care,* 4th ed. Philadelphia, PA: Elsevier Health Sciences; 2008.

Carter RC, et al. Iron deficiency anemia and cognitive function in infancy. *Pediatrics.* 126(2):e427–2434.

Center for Disease Control and Prevention. Prevention tips for lead; 2009. Retrieved July 1, 2011, from: www.cdc.gov/nceh/lead/tips.htm.

Committee on Environmental Health. Policy statement: Lead exposure in children: Prevention, detection, and management. Revision of June 1998 statement. *Pediatrics.* 2009;116(4):1036–1046.

Eden AN, et al. Contemporary pediatrics: Your voice: Hidden toddler iron deficiency; 2009. Retrieved July 1, 2011, from: http://www.modernmedicine.com/modernmedicine/Pediatrics/Your-Voice-Hidden-toddler-iron-deficiency-A-public/ArticleStandard/Article/detail/598172.

Environmental Protection Agency. Lead in paint, dust and soil; 2010. Retrieved July 1, 2011, from: http://epa.gov/lead/pubs/leadinfo.htm#facts.

Hay W, et al. Current diagnosis and treatment, pediatrics. 19th ed. New York: McGraw-Hill; 2009.

Janus J, & Moerschel SK. Evaluation of anemia in children. *American Family Physician.* 2010;81(12):1462–1471.

Kleinman RE, ed. *Pediatric nutrition handbook.* 6th ed. Elk Grove Village, IL: American Academy of Pediatrics; 2009.

Kulp JL, Mwangi CN, Loveless M. Screening for coagulation disorders in adolescents with abnormal uterine bleeding. *Journal of Pediatric Adolescent Gynecology.* 2008;21:27.

Lissauer T, Clayden G, eds. *Illustrated textbook of paediatrics.* 3rd ed. Philadelphia, PA: Elsevier Health Sciences; 2007.

Marcdante K, Kliegman RM, & Behrman RE, eds. *Nelson essentials of pediatrics.* Philadelphia, PA: W.B. Saunders; 2010.

Mayo Clinic Staff. Lead poisoning; 2011. Retrieved July 1, 2011, from: www.mayoclinic.com/health/leadpoisoning/FL00068/.

Merck Manual. Thrombocytopenia (ITP, TTP); 2008. Retrieved July 1, 2011, from: http://www.merck.com/mmhe/print/sec14/ch173/ch173d.html.

Merck Manual. Henock-Schonlein purpura. Retrieved May 3, 2010, from: www.merck.com/mmhe/print/sec14/ch173/ch173c.html.

National Institute of Health, National Heart, Lung, and Blood Institute. The management of sickle cell disease; 2004. Retrieved August 2, 2010, from: http://www.nhlbi.nih.gov/health/dci/Diseases/Sca/SCA_WhatIs.html.

National Institutes of Health, National Heart, Lung and Blood Institute. Thalassemias. Retrieved August 2, 2010, from: http://www.nhlbi.nih.gov/health/dci/Diseases/Thalassemia/Thalassemia_WhatIs.html

National Institutes of Health: National Heart Lung and Blood Institute. Iron deficiency anemia. Retrieved August 2, 2010, from: http://www.nhlbi.nih.gov/health/dci/Diseases/ida/ida_whatis.html.

Savage W, & Takemota C. Bleeding and bruising in children: Formulating your response. *Contemporary Pediatrics*, 2009;6:61–68.

CHAPTER 33

Pediatric Obesity

Julie LaMothe

I. INTRODUCTION

A. Obesity (BMI above the 95th percentile) is increasing among children and
    adolescents. Pediatric obesity has tripled since 1980. A majority of obese
    children remain obese as adults. The risk of pediatric obesity is related to
    childhood diet and sedentary time. Obesity is associated with higher blood
    pressure, elevated blood lipids, insulin resistance, impaired glucose tolerance,
    and increased risk of several chronic diseases of adulthood, including diabe-
    tes, hypertension, dyslipidemia, sleep apnea, cardiovascular disease (CVD),
    fatty liver, metabolic syndrome, hepatic stenosis, orthopedic complications,
    pseudotumor cerebri, and some cancers. In addition, obesity in childhood can
    have psychosocial implications including low self-esteem, impaired quality of
    life, and depression.

II. CODING FOR OBESITY

A. Many insurance carriers will deny claims submitted with obesity codes. The
    following is a guide to coding for obesity-related healthcare services: "Obesity
    and Related Comorbidites Coding Fact Sheet for Primary Care Pediatricians,"
    from the NICQUE Academy of Pediatrics.
B. Additional resources include:
    1. *Pediatric Coding Companion*, from the NICHQ Academy of Pediatrics.
    2. *Coding and reimbursement for children with abnormal weight gain in pri-
        mary care*, from the NICHQ Academy of Pediatrics.
    3. *Denials (Strategies and a Template letter for pediatric practices)*, from the
        AAP Member Center.
    4. *AAP Hassle Factor Form*, from the AAP Member Center.
C. Codes for procedures.
    1. Calorimetry, 94690.

   2. Glucose monitoring, 95250.
   3. Venipuncture, 36415.
D. Healthcare Common Procedure Coding System (HCPCS) education and counseling codes.
   1. S9445, patient education individual.
   2. S9446, patient education group.
   3. S9449, weight management class.
   4. S9451, exercise class.
   5. S9452, nutrition class.
   6. S9454, stress management class.
   7. S9470, nutrition counseling.
E. Common diagnosis codes, ICD-9-CM codes.
   1. Circulatory system.
       a. 401.9, hypertension.
       b. 429.3, cardiomegaly.
   2. Congenital anomalies.
       a. 758.0, Down syndrome.
       b. 759.81, Prader-Willi syndrome.
       c. 759.89, other specified anomalies.
   3. Digestive system.
       a. 530.81, esophageal reflux.
       b. 564.00, constipation.
       c. 783.3, feeding difficulties and mismanagement.
       d. 571.8, other chronic nonalcoholic liver disease.
       e. 789.1, hepatomegaly.
   4. Endocrine, nutritional, metabolic.
       a. 244.8, other specified acquired hypothyroidism.
       b. 244.9, unspecified hypothyroidism.
       c. 250, diabetes mellitus, type 2 or unspecified type, uncontrolled.
       d. 253.8, other disorders of the pituitary.
       e. 255.8, other disorders of the adrenal glands.
       f. 256.4, polycystic ovaries.
       g. 259.1, precocious sexual development and puberty.
       h. 259.9, unspecified endocrine disorder.
       i. 272, pure hypercholesterolemia.
       j. 272.1, pure hyperglyceridemia.
       k. 272.2, mixed hyperlipidemia.
       l. 272.4, other and unspecified hyperlipidemia.
       m. 272.9, unspecified disorder of lipoid metabolism.

n. 277.7, dysmetabolic syndrome X/metabolic syndrome.

o. 278, obesity, unspecified.

p. 278.01, morbid obesity.

q. 278.02, overweight.

r. 278.1, localized adiposity.

s. 783.1, abnormal weight gain.

t. 783.4, lack of normal physiological development.

u. 783.43, short stature.

v. 783.5, polydipsia.

w. 783.6, polyphagia.

5. Genitourinary system.

a. 611.1, hypertrophy of the breast.

6. Mental disorders.

a. 300, anxiety state, unspecified.

b. 300.02, generalized anxiety disorder.

c. 307.5, eating disorder, unspecified.

d. 307.51, bulimia nervosa.

e. 307.59, other and unspecified disorders of eating.

f. 311, depressive disorders.

g. 313.81, oppositional defiant disorder.

7. Nervous system.

a. 732.4, obstructive sleep apnea.

b. 327.26, sleep-related hypoventilation/hypoxemia in conditions classifiable elsewhere.

c. 780.51, insomnia with sleep apnea.

d. 780.52, insomnia, unspecified.

e. 780.54, hypersomnia.

f. 780.57, unspecified sleep apnea.

g. 780.71, chronic fatigue syndrome.

8. Skin and subcutaneous tissue.

a. 701.2, Acquired acanthosis nigricans.

9. Respiratory.

a. Asthma.

• 786.05, shortness of breath.

10. Orthopedic.

a. Hip pain.

b. Knee pain.

c. Blount's disease.

d. SCIFES.

III. OBESITY ASSESSMENT

A. Vital signs and BMI calculation.
1. Obesity is a chronic condition involving an excess of body fat. It is often defined by body mass index (BMI). BMI varies in children by age and sex. BMI for age is weight in kilograms divided by height in meters squared (kg/m^2).
   a. Measure height.
   b. Measure weight.
   c. Calculate BMI and plot on gender-specific growth chart (see 2000 CDC Growth Charts: www.cdc.gov/growthcharts/).
      • 85th–94th percentile for BMI is overweight and in need of consistent education on healthy eating and physical activity.
      • BMI at 95th percentile or above is obese and in need of intervention based on severity of obesity.
   d. BMI should be tracked at each well care visit.
   e. BMI calculators are available online (see: www.statcoder.com/growthcharts.htm; and for parents: www.nhlbisupport.com/bmi).
   f. Blood pressure, (correct cuff size) documented and compared to norms for age and sex, hypertension if systolic or diastolic blood pressure higher than 95th percentile for age, gender, and height on more than three occasions.
B. Patient history of current habits.
1. Nutrition.
   a. 24-hour recall.
   b. Fruits and vegetables.
   c. Sugar-sweetened beverages.
   d. Milk—type and quantity.
   e. Noncaloric beverages.
   f. Snacking—types and quantity.
   g. Portion size.
   h. Eat at home or eat out in sit-down restaurants or fast food—how often.
   i. Eat breakfast, lunch, and dinner or skip meals.
   j. Eat at table or in front of TV; eat alone or with other family members.
   k. Binge eating.
2. Physical activity.
   a. Assess family's physical activity habits.
   b. Type and quantity.
   c. Access to gym, playground, boys or girls club.

        d. Physical education.

        e. Organized sports.

        f. Walking to school or in daily activities.

        g. Any shortness of breath with activity.

        h. Joint pain, knee, hip, feet, type of footwear, any use of orthotics.

    3. Screen time.

        a. Type and quantity.

        b. TV/computer in room.

C. Review of systems.

    1. Constitutional; sleep habits, fatigue, and lethargy.

    2. Respiratory; snoring, wheezing, coughing, difficulty breathing.

    3. Cardiovascular; chest pain.

    4. Gastrointestinal; abdominal, pain, vomiting, constipation.

    5. Skin; striae.

    6. Neurologic; developmental delay, headache.

    7. Genitourinary; menarche, oligo/amenorrhea.

D. Family history.

    1. Obesity.

    2. Diabetes.

    3. Hypertension.

    4. Cardiovascular disease.

    5. Depression.

    6. Polycystic ovarian syndrome.

E. Social history.

    1. School/daycare.

    2. Who lives at home?

    3. Who helps parent?

    4. Are there multiple caregivers?

F. Past medical history.

    1. Birth weight—IUGR/LGA.

    2. Complications at birth.

    3. Mental health.

        a. Anxiety, school avoidance, social isolation.

        b. Sleepiness.

        c. Recent stressors.

G. Medications.

    1. Neuropsychiatric medications may affect weight gain.

H. Physical exam.

    1. Skin.

        a. Acanthosis nigricans indicates increased risk of insulin resistance.

        b. Hirsutism, acne may indicate polycystic ovary syndrome.

        c. Irritation and inflammation—a complication of severe obesity.

        d. Violaceous striae indicate possible Cushing's syndrome.

    2. Eyes.

        a. Papilledema, cranial nerve V1 paralysis—possible pseudotumor cerebri.

    3. Throat.

        a. Tonsillar hypertrophy—possible obstructive sleep apnea.

    4. Neck.

        a. Goiter may indicate hypothyroidism.

    5. Chest.

        a. Wheezing—possible asthma and exercise intolerance.

    6. Abdomen.

        a. Tenderness may indicate gastroesophageal reflux disorder, gall bladder disease, nonalcoholic fatty liver disease (NAFLD).

    7. Reproductive.

        a. Tanner stage—premature puberty age younger than 7 years in Caucasian girls, age younger than 6 years in African American girls, and age younger than 9.years in boys.

        b. Micropenis—may be normal penis buried in fat.

        c. Undescended testis/micropenis may be Prader-Willi syndrome.

    8. Extremities.

        a. Abnormal gait, limp, limited hip range of motion—possible slipped capital femoral epiphysis.

        b. Bowing of tibia—possible Blount's disease.

        c. Small hands and feet, polydactyl—possible Prader-Willi syndrome, Bardet-Biedl syndrome.

I. Laboratory tests.

    1. Complete blood count (CBC).

    2. Comprehensive metabolic panel (CMP).

    3. Fasting lipid profile.

    4. Fasting glucose.

    5. Fasting insulin.

    6. Hemoglobin A1C.

    7. Alanine aminotranferease (ALT), aspartate aminotransferase (AST).

    8. Sleep study if signs of snoring, napping, headaches, daytime sleepiness, restless sleep, and unrefreshed sleep.

J. Plan.

    1. Assess family's readiness to make changes.

        a. Motivational interviewing—patient-centered method for enhancing intrinsic motivation.

      b. Elicit patients' and families' motivation to change.

      c. Encourage patients to take responsibility for their behavior.

      d. Ambivalence needs to be resolved for change to occur.

2. Goal setting.

      a. Set measurable and achievable goals.

      b. Use small steps and gradual change.

      c. Aim for long-term healthy behaviors/lifestyle change with slow weight loss (1–2 pounds per week).

      d. Focus on success, what has worked in the past.

      e. Expect periods of relapse and be ready to help guide patient and family and troubleshoot situations and support return to plan in nonjudgmental way.

3. Logging of food intake.

      a. Provide a journal to log the diet, with beverages, meal time, food and portion size, snacks on a daily basis. This will increase awareness of intake and has proven to show weight loss if done consistently.

4. Nutritional goals.

      a. Promote three meals daily, not meal skipping, and emphasize that breakfast provides energy for the day.

      b. Increase fruit and vegetable intake; daily fruit recommendations from http://www.choosemyplate.gov/.

      c. Water and low-fat milk as main beverages; eliminate high-calorie, sugar-sweetened beverages; limit 100% fruit juice.

      d. Avoid distractions during meal time; eat as a family and not alone. This will promote good nutrition practices, increase awareness, and slow down mealtime.

      e. Provide age-appropriate information on portion size.

      f. Limit fast foods.

      g. Limit refined sugars, high-fat foods.

      h. Aim for reasonable daily target for calorie reduction and weight loss (1–2 pounds per week).

5. Physical activity goals.

      a. Assess present activity level, both individual and family.

      b. Promote increasing activity on a daily basis, such as increased outside activity—goal is 60 minutes or more daily.

      c. Gradually increase vigorous aerobic activity as tolerated.

      d. Limit total screen time to 2 hours or less per day (TV, computer, texting, video games).

      e. Remove TV from the bedroom; keep sleeping area free of distractions.

      f. Provide free pedometers with age-appropriate goals for steps; parents may also enjoy walking with children to encourage family activity.

    g. Provide information on community gyms, centers, after-school activity centers that promote increased physical activity. Look for scholarship opportunities or discounts based on family income in these centers. Promote activities provided by schools, sports, clubs, and year-round athletic activities.

6. Subspecialist referral for comorbidities.
    a. Provide referrals to orthopedics, physical therapy, or podiatrist for hip/knee pain or flat feet.
    b. Promote adequate sleep, early bedtime, and waking at the same time each morning; refer for a polysomnography if snoring, unrefreshed sleep, headaches, or daytime sleepiness.
    c. Refer to neurology for headaches, pseudotumor cerebri.
    d. Pediatric endocrinology for type 2 diabetes, metabolic syndrome, polycystic ovarian syndrome.
    e. Pediatric gastroenterology for progressive elevated ALT and AST levels and persistent stomach pain.
    f. Pediatric pulmonary for sleep study and asthma.
    g. Pediatric psychology for depression, anxiety, and low self-esteem, family dysfunction.
    h. Medical genetics for chromosome abnormalities, Prader-Willi syndrome, fragile X, developmental delay.

7. Follow up.
    a. Patients will set and reach healthy weight goals pertaining to physical fitness, activity level, and weight.
    b. Patients will develop individualized health plans to encourage increased activity and decreased caloric intake.
    c. Patients will participate in individual sessions, behavioral modification, and group activity sessions.
    d. Patients will be responsible for keeping a food log, wearing pedometer for 24 hours, and keeping activity log.
    e. BMI will be tracked at all clinical visits.
    f. Incentives will be offered to encourage program compliance.

BIBLIOGRAPHY

American Academy of Pediatrics *Pediatric Obesity Clinical Decision Support Chart* 5201; 2008.
Barlow SE, & Dietz WH. Obesity Evaluation and Treatment: Expert Committee Recommendations. *Pediatrics*, 2007;102:S164.

Daniels SR, Arnett DK, & Eckel RH. Overweight in children and adolescents: Pathophysiology, consequences, prevention, and treatment. *American Heart Association: Scientific Statement.* 2005;111:1999–2012.

Fennoy I. Metabolic and Respiratory Co morbidities of Childhood Obesity. *Pediatric Annuals.* 2010;39: 140–145.

Parks E. Practical application of the nutrition recommendations for the prevention and treatment of obesity in pediatric primary care. *Pediatric Annuals.* 2010;39:147–153.

Riley POWER Program Tool Kit: A comprehensive weight management program designed to improve health of obese children (ages 2-18) Riley Children's Hospital, A Clarian Health Partner. NICHQ National Initiative for Children's healthcare Quality.

Schwartz RP. Motivational Interviewing (Patient-Centered Counseling) to Address Childhood Obesity. *Annuals.* 39:154–158.

CHAPTER 34

Behavioral Disorders

Donna Hallas

I. BEHAVIORAL ASSESSMENT INSTRUMENTS

A. Various instruments are available for assessment of children with behavioral and emotional disorders in primary care settings. Based on the results of these assessments, referral to a psychiatrist, psychologist, or social worker for completion of additional assessment tools may be indicated. Data from these evaluations will assist in understanding dynamics of family functioning and behavioral management plan (**Boxes 34-1, 34-2, 34-3**).

Box 34-1 Behavioral Assessment Rating Scales

Achenbach Child Behavior Checklist System (CBCL)

- Parent Form (CBCL)
- Teacher Report Form (TRF)

Attention Deficit Disorders Evaluation Scales (ADDES)

- Home Version
- School Version

Behavior Assessment System for Children (BASC)

- Parent Rating Scale (PRS)
- Teacher Rating Scale (TRS)

Connor's Parent/Teacher Rating Scale
Personality Inventory for Children–Revised (PIC–R)
Social Skills Rating Scale (SSRS)
Walker Problem Behavior Identification Checklist (WPBIC)

Box 34-2 Behavioral Assessment: Self-Report Rating Scales

Achenbach Child Behavior Checklist System (CBCL)

Youth Self-Report
Behavior Assessment System for Children (BASC)

Self-Report of Personality
Child Anxiety Scale
Children's Personality Questionnaire (CPQ)
Early School Personality Questionnaire (ESPQ)
High School Personality Questionnaire (HSPQ)
Revised Children's Manifest Anxiety Scale (RCMAS)
Social Skills Rating System (SSRS)–Student Form

Box 34-3 Behavioral Assessment: Protective Measures

Draw a Person: Screening Procedure for Emotional Disturbance (DAP: SPED)
Minnesota Multiphasic Personality Inventory–A (MMPI-A)
Tell Me a Story (TEMAS)

II. ATTENTION DEFICIT HYPERACTIVITY DISORDER (ADHD)

Arithmetical disorder, 315.1	Emotional disorder, V40.9
Attention deficit/hyperactivity disorder, 314.01	Impulsivity, 314.01
Behavioral disorders, 312.9	Inattentive behavior, 314
Combined hyperactive/inattentive, 314.01	Language disorder, 315.31
Dyspraxia, 315.4	Learning disability, 315.2
ADHD–not otherwise specified, 314.9	Reading disorder, 315

A. ADHD is one of the most common chronic conditions of childhood and the most common neurobehavioral disorder in child health. ADHD is characterized by the children presenting with three core behavioral symptoms: hyperactivity, impulsive behaviors, and inattentive behaviors outside the normal parameters of the psychosocial development for child's age. Symptoms are displayed by the child before 7 years of age even though diagnosis may not be established until child enters the school setting. Three subtypes of ADHD are now recognized: (1) hyperactive/impulsive (ADHD-HI), (2) inattentive (ADHD-IA), and (3) combined (ADHD-CT).

B. ADHD–not otherwise specified: for children who present with symptoms predominantly of inattentive type but do not meet the full criteria.

C. The American Academy of Pediatrics (AAP) evidence-based guidelines for diagnosis and management of ADHD are limited to children 6 to 12 years of age with any coexisting conditions.

D. Etiology.
   1. Specific etiology unknown. Believed that abnormal dopamine transport and uptake at nerve synapse may account for symptoms displayed.

E. Occurrence.
   1. The prevalence of ADHD is 5%.
   2. Two-thirds of children with ADHD continue to have symptoms in adolescence.
   3. More prevalent in males than females—approximate ratio of 4:1.
   4. Prevalence of comorbid conditions ranges from 9–50% depending on specific comorbid condition. Refer to **Table 34-1.**

F. Clinical manifestations.
   1. Child displays and/or parents and teachers report inappropriate degrees of:
      a. Hyperactivity.
      b. Impulsivity.
      c. Inattentive behaviors.
   2. *Diagnostic and Statistical Manual of Mental Disorders* (DSM-IV) diagnostic criteria delineate clinical manifestations of ADHD and clarify criteria utilized to make definitive diagnosis (**Box 34-4**).

Table 34-1 Prevalence of Comorbid Conditions in Children with ADHD

Comorbid condition	Prevalence rate (%)
Conduct disorder, 312.81	25
Oppositional defiant disorder, 313.81	33
Depressive disorder, not otherwise specified, 311	9–38
Anxiety disorder, 300	25
Learning disorder, 315.2	12–30

Source: Adapted from Agency for Healthcare Policy and Research, U.S. Department of Health & Human Services.

Box 34-4 DSM-IV Diagnostic Criteria for ADHD

A. Either Criterion 1 or 2.
  1. Six or more of the following symptoms of inattention have persisted for at least 6 months to a degree that is maladaptive and inconsistent with developmental level:

Inattention
  a. Often fails to give close attention to details or makes careless mistakes in schoolwork, work, or other activities
  b. Often has difficulty sustaining attention in tasks or play activities
  c. Often does not seem to listen when spoken to directly
  d. Often does not follow through on instructions and fails to finish schoolwork, chores, or duties in workplace (not due to oppositional behavior or failure to understand instructions)
  e. Often has difficulty organizing tasks and activities
  f. Often avoids, dislikes, or is reluctant to engage in tasks requiring sustained mental effort (such as schoolwork or homework)
  g. Often loses things necessary for tasks or activities (e.g., toys, school assignments, pencils, books, or tools)
  h. Is often easily distracted by extraneous stimuli
  i. Is often forgetful in daily activities

  2. Six or more of the following symptoms of hyperactivity–impulsivity have persisted for at least 6 months to a degree that is maladaptive and inconsistent with developmental level:

Hyperactivity
  a. Often fidgets with hands/feet or squirms in seat
  b. Often leaves seat in classroom or in other situations in which remaining seated is expected
  c. Often runs about or climbs excessively in situations in which it is inappropriate (in adolescents or adults, may be limited to subjective feelings of restlessness)
  d. Often has difficulty playing or engaging in leisure activities quietly. Is often "on the go" or often acts as if "driven by a motor"
  e. Often talks excessively

Impulsivity
  a. Often blurts out answers before questions have been completed
  b. Often has difficulty waiting turn
  c. Often interrupts or intrudes on others (e.g., butts into conversations or games)

B. Some hyperactive–impulsive or inattentive symptoms that caused impairment were present before 7 years of age.
C. Some impairment from the symptoms is present in two or more settings (e.g., at school [or work] or at home).
D. There must be clear evidence of clinically significant impairment in social, academic, or occupational functioning.
E. Symptoms do not occur exclusively during course of pervasive developmental disorder, schizophrenia, or other psychotic disorder and are not better accounted for by another mental disorder (e.g., mood disorder, anxiety disorder, dissociative disorder, or personality disorder).

Code based on type:

314.01 attention-deficit/hyperactivity disorder, combined type: if both criteria A1 and A2 are met for past 6 months
314.00 attention-deficit/hyperactivity disorder, predominantly inattentive type: if criterion A1 is met but criterion A2 is not met for the past 6 months
314.01 attention-deficit/hyperactivity disorder, predominantly hyperactive, impulsive type: if criterion A2 is met but criterion A1 is not met for past 6 months
314.9 attention-deficit/hyperactivity disorder not otherwise specified: Child who presents with symptoms over the age of 7 and has predominantly inattentive type behaviors. Behavioral patterns include sluggishness, daydreaming, and hyperactivity.

Source: Reprinted with permission from the *Diagnostic and statistical manual of mental disorders,* text revision, 4th ed (DSM-IV). Copyright 2000, American Psychiatric Association.

3. Identifying at-risk child.
    a. Nurse practitioner plays integral role in identifying children at risk for ADHD by evaluating comprehensive medical history.
    b. Positive family history of one or more of hyperactivity disorder, conduct disorder, learning disorder, substance abuse, psychiatric disorder.
    c. Intrauterine exposure to smoking and drug/alcohol use, especially during first trimester.
    d. Parent, schoolteacher report that child displays impulsive and inattentive behaviors.
        •   School-age children tend to steal, tell lies, deliberately destroy property.
        •   Adolescents display behaviors associated with anger and mood lability: alcohol/substance abuse, smoking, sexually transmitted

infections, early pregnancy, low self-esteem, involvement in motor vehicle accidents.

4. Comprehensive medical history—include questions that elicit details concerning each of following parameters:
    a. Parental concerns.
        *   Onset and duration of symptoms.
        *   Parental approaches to displayed symptoms.
    b. Behavioral history.
        *   Hyperactivity as described by parents, caregivers, teachers.
        *   Behaviors that display impulsivity, inattentiveness to details.
        *   Ability to focus on interactive video games.
        *   Sleep patterns.
        *   General behavior at home and in school settings.
        *   Previous results of Denver Developmental Screening Tests and any formal psychological testing.
        *   School performance.
        *   Identification of any learning disabilities.
        *   Behaviors displayed while playing with other children.
        *   Parenting styles: what works, what does not work with the child.
    c. Significant past medical history.
        *   Prenatal, birth, neonatal history.
        *   Evaluation of growth charts.
        *   Evaluation of previous diagnostic testing including complete blood count (CBC) results, lead levels, visual and hearing test results.
        *   Seizures/seizure-like behaviors including staring episodes, tics, head trauma.
        *   Medication history (prescribed, OTC, illicit).
    d. Developmental history.
        *   Achievement of developmental milestones.
        *   Speech and language development.
        *   Gross motor and fine motor development.
        *   Coordination.
    e. Educational history.
        *   Type of educational program.
        *   Early intervention.
        *   Special education program.
        *   Participation in mainstream programs.
        *   One-on-one programs.
        *   Success/failure in each educational program.
        *   Mathematical ability.

    f. Behaviors at school.
- Reports from teachers, counselors.
- Relationships with children at home and school.
- Relationships with teacher, school nurse, counselor.

    g. Family history.
- Parents or siblings diagnosed with ADHD.
- Substance abuse.
- Mental illness.
- Learning disabilities.

    h. Psychosocial history.
- Family structure, function.
- Head of family.
- Parents' occupation, employment, level of education.
- Substance abuse by parents/child.
- Evaluate family–child interactions.
- Family stress level due to child's behavior.

    i. Manifestations consistent with comorbid conditions:
- Lack of motor control; clumsiness (developmental coordination disorder [dyspraxia]).
- •. Preschooler with speech, language delay (learning disability).
- Writes number in reverse order after age 7 (learning disability).
- Poor school performance: unable to learn to read, write, or do mathematics (learning disability).
- Insomnia.
- •. Enuresis, encopresis.
- Negative, hostile, defiant behaviors lasting at least 6 months (oppositional defiant disorder [ODD]).
- Violation of home/school rules (conduct disorder).
- Symptoms of depression.
- Inappropriate levels of anxiety.
- Low self-esteem.
- Autism spectrum disorders.
- Tic disorders.

G. Physical findings.
1. For diagnosis without comorbid conditions, physical examination is usually unremarkable.
2. Behavior during physical examination is often inappropriate for age: refuses to cooperate; refuses to respond to questions.
3. Dysmorphic features may be consistent with comorbid conditions.
4. Neurocutaneous lesions may be consistent with comorbid conditions.

H. Diagnostic tests.
  1. No specific diagnostic tests for definitive diagnosis.
  2. Diagnostics such as blood tests, brain scans, EEG, and psychological tests are not routinely necessary for children with AHDH without evidence of comorbid conditions.
  3. Laboratory tests that may assist in ruling out or verifying comorbid conditions.
      a. CBC with differential.
      b. Lead level (children 7 years and younger).
      c. Basic metabolic panel.
      d. Liver function panel.
      e. Thyroid studies including thyroid-stimulating hormone (TSH).
      f. ECG: to evaluate heart rate and QT interval (positive family history).
      g. EEG: recommended for all children who may be placed on medication therapy and have a past medical history of seizures and/or a family history of a seizure disorder.
  4. Diagnosis of ADHD.
      a. For definitive diagnosis, must use DSM-IV diagnostic criteria for ADHD (Box 34-4).
      b. AAP published evidenced-based guidelines for primary care diagnosis and clinical evaluation of children suspected of having ADHD. AAP guidelines require that a child meet the DSM-IV criteria.
      c. AAP guidelines require evidence directly obtained from the classroom teacher regarding the core symptoms of ADHD, the duration of symptoms, the degree of functional impairment, and coexisting conditions.
I. Differential diagnosis.
  1. Because diagnosis has several significant comorbid conditions, comprehensive history and physical examination essential to establish definitive diagnosis and formulate treatment plan.
  2. Differential diagnosis included in **Table 34-2.**
J. Treatment (**Box 34-5**).
  1. Both medication and behavior therapy.
  2. Evidence suggests that discontinuing treatment leads to reemergence of symptoms.
  3. Aimed at alleviating major symptoms child displays and improving child's ability to function within family unit, social and educational environments.
  4. In addition, if child also displays symptoms of one or more comorbid conditions, treatment is highly recommended to reduce or alleviate these symptoms.

Table 34-2 Differential Diagnosis of ADHD

Differential Diagnosis	Characteristic Symptoms or Presentation
Learning disability, 315.2	Language delay especially in preschool years
	Persistent reversal of numbers after 7 years of age
	Unsuccessful in achieving reading, writing, math skills
	Difficulty understanding concept of left and right
Sleep disorders, 780.5	Insomnia leading to attention deficit in school activities
	Sleeping during class
	Extended daytime naps at home or in school (preschool or kindergarten)
	Frequent episodes of night terrors or nightmares
Mild mental retardation, 317	Children who present with learning difficulties in elementary grades
Tourette syndrome, 307.23	Usually symptoms are evident after 7 years of age
	Reports by parents/caregivers that child has had 2+ motor tics and 1 vocal tic during 1-year interval
Oppositional defiant disorder, 313.81	Negativistic
	Hostile
	Defiant behaviors
	Uncontrolled temper
	Angry
	Refuses to comply with social rules at home, school
	Behaviors are associated with poor school performance
Conduct disorder, 312.9	Violates rights of others
	Violates societal norms
	Violates rules at home, school
	Participates in at-risk behaviors: smoking, substance abuse
	Often suspended from school

(continues)

Table 34-2 (Continued)

Differential Diagnosis	Characteristic Symptoms or Presentation
Anxiety disorder, 300	Feels threatened without apparent reason, cannot identify source of threat
	Feelings of uneasiness
	Apprehension
	History of breathlessness, palpitations, restlessness, chest tightness, trembling
Depression, 311	Low self-esteem, low self-image
	Reports feeling depressed
	Poor social relationships, does not participate in school activities
Bipolar disorder, 296.7	Mood lability, irritability
	Evidence of depression
Pervasive developmental disorders, 299.8; autism, Asperger's syndrome, 299.8; childhood disintegrative disorder, 299.1; Rett syndrome, 330.8	Language delay
	Abnormal social behaviors
	Ritualistic movements
	Impaired intellectual functioning

Box 34-5 Role of Nurse Practitioner in Managing Children with ADHD

1. Office assessment identifying parental concerns and child's behavior patterns.
2. Establish rapport with psychiatrist or psychologist to identify treatment plan.
3. Include parents, child, and school personnel in the treatment plan.
4. Monitor effects of stimulant medication to ensure desired treatment plan outcomes.
5. Follow up should include biannual physical examinations and appropriate laboratory studies including hemoglobin, because anemia is a side effect.
6. Emotional support measures for child and parents.

5. Mental health referrals for all children suspected of having comorbid psychiatric conditions.
6. Characteristics of treatment plan.
    a. Parent education.
        *   Provide education about ADHD and appropriate comorbid condition.
        *   Identify available resources and support groups for parents (**Table 34-3**).
    b. School-based strategies.
        *   Structured classroom setting.
        *   Consistent instruction and application of rules of conduct.

Table 34-3 Evidence-Based Treatment Guidelines for the School-Age Child

Recommendations	Description
Recommendation 1	Primary care clinicians should establish a strategy for diagnosing children with ADHD. ADHD is a chronic condition and requires a long-term management plan.
Recommendation 2	The treating nurse practitioner, parents, and the child, in collaboration with school personnel, should specify three to six target outcomes to guide management.
Recommendation 3	The clinician should recommend stimulant medication, as appropriate, to improve target outcomes in children with ADHD.
Recommendation 3A	For children on stimulants, if one stimulant does not work at the highest feasible dose, the clinician should recommend another.
Recommendation 4	When the selected management for a child with ADHD has not met target outcomes, clinicians should evaluate the original diagnosis, use of all appropriate treatments, adherence to the treatment plan, and presence of coexisting conditions.
Recommendation 5	The clinician should periodically provide a systematic follow-up visit for the child with ADHD. Initially, the patient should be followed every 2 to 4 weeks until a stable dose of medication is established. Once the child is stabilized, an office visit every 3 to 6 months is adequate. Monitoring should be directed to target outcomes and adverse effects by obtaining specific information from parents, teachers, and the child.

- Meets educational needs of child as identified through in-school testing.
  c. Behavior modification.
  - Strategies are consistent and followed at home and at school.
  - Inform child of rules of acceptable behavior.
  - Rewards for demonstrating positive behaviors (positive reinforcement).
  - Consequences for failure to meet the goals (punishment).
  - Repetitive application of the rewards and consequences shapes behavioral changes.
  d. Medication therapy.
  - Basic principles.
    i. Begin with lowest dosage and increase dosage every 5–7 days based on parent and teacher assessment of child's response (changes in behavior) to medication.
    ii. Once positive response to medication therapy is reported, increase dose at least one more time.
    iii. Medication administered every 12 hours has been shown to be most effective in controlling symptoms of ADHD.
  - Drugs of choice.
    i. May use immediate-release tablets: methylphenidate (Ritalin), dextroamphetamine levoamphetamine (Adderall), dextroamphetamine (Dexedrine), atomoxetime (Strattera)—a nonstimulant medication.
    ii. May use sustained-release tablets: methylphenidate (Ritalin SR; Concerta; Metadate ER; Metadate CD), dextroamphetamine levoamphetamine (Adderall XR), dextroamphetamine (Dexedrine Spansule).
  - Potential side effects:
    i. Decreased appetite, weight loss.
    ii. Insomnia.
    iii. Tachycardia.
    iv. Increased blood pressure.
    v. Nervousness.
    vi. Headache.
    vii. Dizziness.
    viii. Irritability.
    ix. Rebound moodiness.
    x. Leukopenia/anemia.
    xi. Skin rash.

       xii. Abnormal liver function tests.

       xiii. Exacerbations of tics and Tourette syndrome.

     • Management of side effects:

       i. Administer dose after meals to improve appetite; frequent high-calorie snacks.

       ii. Avoid caffeine intake.

       iii. Modify time of administration if sleep problems.

K. Follow up.

   1. Monitor height, weight, heart rate, blood pressure every 3 months in children younger than 12 years of age. School nurse can play integral role in monitoring these measurements in child every 3 months and report these findings to primary care provider.

   2. In children older than 12 years of age, monitor height, weight, heart rate, blood pressure every 6 months.

   3. Monitor CBC or hemoglobin every 6 months. Children are at increased risk for leukopenia/anemia while on psychostimulant drug therapy.

   4. Perform interval history, physical assessment every 6 months to evaluate child's response to treatment program.

   5. Consult with teacher and school psychologist prior to each 6-month healthcare evaluation for continuity of care.

   6. Follow up with psychiatric referrals, as appropriate.

L. Complications.

High blood pressure, 401.9	Tourette syndrome, 307.23
Increased heart rate, 785	Weight loss, 783.21
Tic disorder, not otherwise specified 307.2	

   1. Complications from medication therapy include weight loss, increased heart rate and blood pressure, growth suppression, exacerbations of tics and Tourette syndrome.

   2. Once medication is discontinued, symptoms related to complications of medication therapy resolve; however, evidence shows that ADHD symptoms return even with continuous behavior-modification therapy.

M. Education.

   1. Parent education is key to successful management.

      a. Parents should receive initial and updated education related to behavior modification strategies for successful treatment as child reaches each new developmental stage.

      b. Parents need to understand medication management.

      c. Know possible side effects of medication therapy.

    d. Support groups.

    e. Group and family therapy.

    f. Internet resources.

- American Academy of Child and Adolescent Psychiatry: www. aacap.org.
- American Academy of Pediatrics: www.aap.org.
- National Association of Pediatric Nurse Practitioners: www.nap-nap.org.
- Children and Adults with Attention Deficit/Hyperactivity Disorder (CHADD): www.chadd.org.
- National Resource Center on ADHD: www.help4ADHD.org.

III. AUTISTIC SPECTRUM DISORDER (ASD)

Asperger's syndrome, 299.8	Echolalia, 784.69
Autistic disorder, 299	Language disorder, 315.31
Autistic spectrum disorder, 299	Rett syndrome, 330.8
Childhood disintegrative disorder, 299.1	Social disorder, 313.22

A. ASD is a biologically based, neurobiological disorder that includes autistic spectrum disorder, Asperger's syndrome, childhood disintegrative disorder, pervasive developmental disorder, not otherwise specified, Rett syndrome (which will be removed in the DMS-V). Characterized by impairment in verbal and nonverbal communication, impaired cognitive abilities, and impaired social interactions.

B. Etiology.

    1. Genetic susceptibility: children with a diagnosis of tuberous sclerosis; fragile X; Rett syndrome (identified gene mutation).

    2. Genetic susceptibility and environmental factors: *no* single environmental factor identified, however, may be linked to prenatal exposure to thalidomides, valproic acid, and mesoprostol.

    3. There is *no* evidence that links the measles-mumps-rubella (MMR) vaccine or any immunizations to the autistic spectrum disorders.

C. Occurrence.

    1. Male-to-female ratio 3:1.

    2. In the United States: 1% of the population is affected.

    3. In the United States 1 child is affected for every 100 live births.

4. Recurrence rate in siblings of affected children is 2–8%.
5. Present in all racial, ethnic, and socioeconomic groups.
D. Clinical manifestations.
  1. Red flags.
    a. Significant impairment in social communication and interaction.
    b. Repetitive, restricted, and stereotyped patterns of behavior.
  2. Symptoms develop before 30 months of age.
    a. Lack of (or poorly developed) verbal and nonverbal communication skills.
     • Abnormal speech patterns; echolalia, nonsense rhyming.
     • Bruxism.
    b. Abnormal social play, solitary play, no friendships.
     • No eye contact.
     • No social smile.
     • Regression in language or social skills.
     • Repetitive body movements.
     • Ritualistic behaviors; need for sameness.
     • Preoccupation with an object.
     • Tantrums when ritual is disrupted.
     • Rocking behaviors.
    c. Impaired intellectual functioning.
     • Mental retardation (I.Q. < 70 in 40–62% of the children).
     • Occasionally child has particular talent (e.g., art, music).
E. Physical findings.
  1. Physical examination is most often normal.
  2. May have dysmorphic features.
    a. Long face and large eyes.
    b. Large head size not observed in infancy but observed in preschool years.
    c. May have microcephaly.
  3. Lack of communication skills and psychosocial skills in interactions in the home and during the office exam.
F. Diagnostic tests.
  1. No specific tests.
  2. Lead screening (children under 7 years old) and genetic testing may be indicated for identification of comorbid conditions.
  3. Refer to psychologist for cognitive and psychological testing.
  4. Refer to neurologist for full neurologic diagnostic workup including blood work, MRI with contrast, CT scan, EEG.

     5. Refer for early intervention services.

     6. Autistic measures (**Box 34-6**).

  G. Differential diagnosis.

Asperger's syndrome, 299.8	Mental retardation, 319
Childhood disintegrative disorder, 299.1	Obsessive-compulsive disorder, 300.3
Conduct disorder, 312.9	Pervasive disorder, 299.8
Fragile X syndrome, 759.83	Rett syndrome, 330.8
Hearing disorder, 389.9	Schizophrenia, 299.9
Lead poisoning, 984.9	Tourette syndrome, 307.23

     1. Obsessive-compulsive disorder, Tourette syndrome.

     2. Conduct disorder, mental retardation, hearing disorder.

     3. Schizophrenia of childhood.

     4. Lead poisoning.

     5. Fragile X syndrome.

     6. Additional pervasive disorders.

     7. Asperger's syndrome.

       a. Impairment is primarily in social interactions, which includes repetitive and obsessive behaviors.

       b. Children usually do not have language impairments characteristic of autism.

       c. Rare disorder characterized by normal development until 2–4 years old, at which time there is severe mental and social deterioration.

     8. Childhood disintegrative disorder.

     9. Rett syndrome.

       a. Development normal until 1 year of age, at which time language and motor development regress.

       b. Microcephaly is usually evident by 1 year of age.

  H. Treatment.

     1. No single best evidence-based treatment.

       a. Treatment is individualized to the child.

         • Management of challenging behaviors.

Box 34-6 Autistic Measures

Autistic Diagnostic Observation Schedule (ADOS)
Childhood Autism Rating Scale (CARS)

- Sleep problems.
- Social skills training.
  b. Medication.
    - For aggressive behaviors and irritability for children and teens with autism: resperidone and aripiprazole.
    - Stimulants for comorbid symptoms of ADHD.
    - Other comorbid conditions treated as appropriate by psychiatric specialists.
  c. Implement all early intervention services in home and school: speech therapy, occupational and physical therapy, behavior modification strategies.
2. Diagnosis.
   a. Denver Developmental II screening test: valuable tool used to assist in early recognition.
   b. Screening Tool for Autism in Toddlers and Young Children.
   c. Autism Spectrum Screening Questionnaire for 6–17 years old.
   d. Refer to developmental neurologist and Early Intervention services (under age 5) as soon as symptoms are suspected.
3. Comorbidity.
   a. ADHD.
   b. Intellectual disabilities.
   c. Mood disorders.
   d. Depression.
   e. Anxiety.
   f. Obsessive–compulsive behaviors.
   g. Phobias.
I. Follow up.
   1. Recognize early signs and symptoms of autism, Asperger's syndrome, childhood disintegrative disorder, Rett syndrome, and make appropriate referrals.
   2. Support for parents, other primary caregivers is essential. Families may benefit from connecting with the Autism Society (www.autism-society.org).
   3. Encourage parents to find respite care for child.
J. Complications.

Autism, 299

1. Autism is a chronic disease with no cure.

K. Education.
 1. Families need education about the disorder, what treatments have been proven to be successful; multidisciplinary interventions.
 2. Families need to be careful when investigating treatment programs and determine proven benefits from these programs. Families must consider own safety and that of their child.
 3. Internet resources.
  a. Autism Society: www.autism-society.org.
  b. Centers for Disease Control and Prevention: www.cdc.gov.
  c. American Academy of Pediatrics: www.aap.org.

IV. BREATH HOLDING

Apnea, 786.03	Cyanosis, 782.5
Bradycardia, 427.89	Cyanotic spells, 782.5
Breath holding spells, 786.9	Loss of consciousness, 780.09
Breath holding, 312.81	Pallid spells, 782.61
Cerebral anoxia, 348.1	Tonic seizure activity, 345.1
Clonic jerks, 333.2	

A. Characterized by episodes in which infant/young child holds breath, which leads to cerebral anoxia resulting in limp body and extremities, unresponsiveness. Two types: cyanotic spells and pallid spells.
B. Etiology.
 1. Unknown.
C. Occurrence.
 1. Usually begins after 6 months old.
 2. Highest incidence is at 2 years old.
 3. Usually resolves by 5 years old.
 4. Usually occurs in response to an upsetting, unexpected, or traumatic event.
 5. May occur with genetic conditions such as Rett syndrome.
 6. Associated with iron-deficiency anemia.
D. Clinical manifestations.
 1. Cyanotic spells.
  a. Brief shrill cry followed by forced expiration and apnea.
  b. Onset of cyanosis.
  c. Loss of consciousness.
  d. Generalized clonic jerks.
  e. Bradycardia.

2. Pallid spells.
   a. Usually follows fall in which child strikes head, causing pain.
   b. Cessation of normal breathing pattern; prolonged apneic episode.
   c. Loses consciousness.
   d. Pallor.
   e. Tonic seizure activity (occasional).
E. Physical findings.
   1. Normal physical exam findings.
F. Diagnostic tests.
   1. EEG. Referral to neurologist is recommended.
G. Differential diagnosis.

Seizure disorder, 780.39

1. Seizure disorder.
H. Treatment.
   1. No treatment necessary.
   2. Parental support and reassurance.
   3. Avoid situations that provoke the breath-holding episodes.
   4. Treat iron-deficiency anemia if present.
I. Follow up.
   1. Call within a few days to assess how family is dealing and answer questions.
   2. Parents' level of comfort with breath-holding spells determines further follow up.
J. Complications.
   1. Head injury if child falls during episode.
K. Education.
   1. Discussion of management plan that parents can follow consistently. Parents must feel comfortable with plan.
   2. Provide safe environment for child during and at conclusion of episode.
   3. Avoid reinforcement of these behaviors.
   4. Most children outgrow breath-holding episodes by 4 to 8 years old.

V. NIGHTMARES AND NIGHT TERRORS

Dilated pupil, 379.43	Nightmares, 307.47
Hyperventilation, 300.11	Tachycardia, 785
Night terrors, 307.46	

A. Etiology.
   1. Actual cause unknown.
   2. Dysfunctional family relationships should be suspected.
B. Occurrence.
   1. Occurs in 1–3% of children, mostly in boys between 5 and 7 years old.
C. Clinical manifestations.
   1. Night terrors: sudden, unexpected screams during sleep; usually occurs within 2 hours of the time the child goes to sleep.
   2. Nightmares: frightening dreams that awake the child and make the child afraid to return to sleep; usually occurs during the last third of the sleep cycle during REM sleep.
   3. Appears frightened; pupils dilated.
   4. Tachycardia, hyperventilation.
   5. Thrashing of extremities.
   6. Inconsolable, not aware of parents' presence.
   7. Panic.
   8. Sleepwalking.
   9. Returns to sleep.
   10. No recall of night terror in morning.
D. Physical findings.
   A. None.
E. Diagnostic tests.
   A. None necessary.
F. Differential diagnosis.

Anxiety, 300	Emotional disorder, V40.9
Depression, 311	Seizure, 780.39

   1. Rule out emotional disorder; anxiety; depression.
   2. Seizures.
G. Treatment.
   1. Child should be encouraged to lie down and be helped back to sleep (e.g., talking quietly, rubbing back).
   2. Turn on light or use a nightlight in the bedroom.
   3. Encourage family to wake child before episode for 1–2 weeks to attempt to break cycle.
   4. Protect child from injury.
   5. Prepare babysitter for possible episode.
   6. Leave bedroom door open.
   7. Provide comfort, reassurance to child.

      8.   Counseling may be necessary for children who have severe nighttime fears.

H. Follow up.

      1.   Refer to psychologist or psychiatrist if night terrors or nightmares persist.

      2.   Complete family evaluation may be necessary.

I. Complications.

Night terrors, 307.46

---

      1.   Injury.

      2.   Continued nighttime fears.

J. Education.

      1.   Often night terrors are self-limiting.

      2.   Family support may be necessary to reduce parental anxiety.

VI. SCHOOL REFUSAL

A. School-refusal behavior refers to any refusal to attend school or difficulty attending classes for an entire day by a child.

B. Occurrence.

      1.   5–28% of youths.

      2.   Prevalence: fairly equivalent among gender, racial, and economic status.

C. Triggers for school refusal.

      1.   Dysfunctional family patterns.

      2.   Impending school changes.

      3.   Illness.

      4.   Traumatic experiences.

D. Clinical manifestations.

      1.   Range of behaviors.

      2.   Depression.

      3.   Social anxiety.

      4.   Fears.

      5.   Fatigue.

      6.   Somatic complaints.

      7.   Noncompliance.

      8.   Aggression.

      9.   Clinging.

    10.   Temper tantrums.

    11.   Run away from home.

   E. Physical findings.

     1. No physical exam findings.

     2. Mental health assessment may reveal comorbid mental health problems.

   F. Diagnostic tests and assessment tools.

     1. Consider drug and alcohol screening based on presenting history.

     2. Consider pregnancy testing and screening for sexually transmitted disease if history of runaway.

     3. Anxiety Disorders Interview Schedule for DSM-IV (Parent and Child versions).

     4. The School Refusal Assessment Scale-Revised (SRAS-R).

   G. Treatment.

     1. Determine who will conduct the interventions: refer to school psychologist, social worker.

     2. Cognitive behavioral therapy.

     3. Relaxation therapy.

     4. Problem solving skills instruction.

     5. Parent interventions.

     6. Morning and evening routines.

   H. Education.

     1. Instructions for parents on effective parenting skills.

   I. Follow up.

     1. Monitor progress weekly and then monthly until problem resolves.

BIBLIOGRAPHY

Agency for Health Care Policy and Research. *Diagnosis of attention deficit/hyperactivity disorder* [Technical Review No. 3]. Rockville, MD: U.S. Department of Health and Human Services; 1999.

American Psychiatric Association. *Diagnostic and statistical manual of mental disorders, IV-TR* Washington, DC: Author; 2000.

Burns CE, Dunn AM, Brady MA, Starr NB, & Blosser CG. *Pediatric primary care.* 4th ed. St. Louis, MO: Saunders; 2009.

Conners CK. ADHD therapy: Optimizing functional outcomes. *Contemporary Pediatrics.* 2003;20(Suppl):4–6.

Dube SR, & Orpinas P. Understanding excessive school absenteeism as school refusal behavior. *Children and Schools.* 2009;31:87–95.

Forbes F. Improving recognition and management of ADHD. *Practitioner.* 2010;254(1728):34–38.

Kearnery CA, & Bates M. Addressing school refusal behavior: Suggestions for frontline professionals. *Children and Schools.* 2005;27:207–216.

Liu YH, & Leslie LK. Diagnosing ADHD: Putting AAP guidelines to the test—and into practice. *Contemporary Pediatrics.* 2003;20:51–73.

Melnyk BM, & Moldenhauer Z., eds. The KySS (keep your children/yourself safe and secure): Guide to child and adolescent mental health screening, early intervention and health promotion. National Association of Pediatric Nurse Practitioners and NAPNAP Foundation; 2006.

Salmeron PA. Childhood and adolescent attention-deficit hyperactivity disorder: Diagnosis, clinical practice guidelines, and social implications. *Journal of the American Academy of Nurse Practitioners*. 2009;21: 488–497.

Stein MT, & Perrin JM. Diagnosis and treatment of ADHD in school-age children in primary care settings: A synopsis of the AAP practice guidelines. *Pediatrics in Review*. 2003;24:92–98.

Wolraich ML. ADHD therapy: Optimizing functional outcomes. *Contemporary Pediatrics*, 2003;20(Suppl): 7–10.

CHAPTER 35

Mental Health Disorders

Kim Walton and Susan J. Kersey

I. ANXIETY DISORDERS

A. Presentation of anxiety disorder; includes both physical and emotional characteristics.

B. Etiology.
   1. Biochemical changes in brain.
      a. Possible genetic vulnerability.
      b. Post-traumatic stress disorder (PTSD) present in children who survive severe or terrifying physical or emotional event. Also occurs when witnessing an event that the child perceives as threatening; this includes domestic violence.
      c. Separation anxiety, note relative frequency in children of mothers with panic disorder.

C. Occurrence.
   1. Most common mental illness group occurring in children and adolescents.

2. Estimated prevalence of any anxiety disorder among children and adolescents is 13% in 6-month period.
D. Clinical manifestations.
1. Generalized anxiety disorder (also known as overanxious disorder in children).
   a. Characterized by at least 6 months of persistent, excessive anxiety/worry over everyday events; difficult to control the worry.
   b. Anxiety and worry are associated with at least one of following:
      • Restlessness.
      • Being easily fatigued.
      • Difficulty concentrating.
      • Irritability.
      • Muscle tension.
      • Sleep disturbance.
   c. Symptoms must cause significant distress or impairment in functioning.
2. Obsessive compulsive disorder (OCD).
   a. Obsessions: recurring thoughts or images that are disturbing, intrusive, cannot be controlled through rational reasoning.
      • Common obsessions:
        i. Contamination.
        ii. Fear of harm to self/family member.
        iii. Worry about acting on aggressive impulses.
        iv. Concern about order and symmetry.
      • Thoughts or images are not simply excessive worries about real-life problems.
      • Attempts to ignore or suppress such thoughts or images with some other thought/action.
   b. Compulsions: repetitive behaviors that one feels obliged to complete. Performance of compulsive behavior, at least temporarily, decreases anxiety, thereby reinforcing behavior.
      • Common compulsions:
        i. Handwashing.
        ii. Cleaning rituals.
        iii. Requesting reassurance.
        iv. Ordering and arranging.
        v. Complex touching habits.
        vi. Checking, counting, and repetition of routine activities.
      • Behaviors are aimed at preventing or reducing distress.

   c. Obsessions or compulsions must be time consuming (take > 1 hour a day), cause marked distress, interfere with daily activities.

   d. Often seen with comorbidities.

   e. Strong familial component.

   f. Immune response to streptococcal infections.

 3. PTSD.

   a. Must have exposure to traumatic event with *both* of following:

    • Actual or threatened death/serious injury or threat to physical integrity of self/others.

    • Response involving intense fear, helplessness, horror. May be expressed as disorganized/agitated behavior in children.

   b. Traumatic event is persistently reexperienced in one or more of following ways:

    • Recurrent, intrusive, distressing thoughts of event. In young children, may include repetitive play.

    • Recurrent distressing dreams. In children, may be frightening dreams without recognizable content.

    • Acting or feeling as if trauma were reoccurring. In young children, may include trauma-specific reenactment, often through play.

    • Intense psychologic distress on exposure to internal/external cues reminiscent of traumatic event.

    • Physiologic reactivity on exposure to internal/external cues reminiscent of traumatic event.

   c. Persistent *avoidance* of stimuli, numbing of general responsiveness with 3 or more of following:

    • Efforts to avoid thoughts, feelings, or talking about trauma.

    • Efforts to avoid activities, places, people that arouse memories.

    • Inability to recall important aspect of event.

    • Diminished interest/participation in activities.

    • Feelings of detachment/estrangement.

    • Restricted range of affect.

    • Sense of foreshortened future.

   d. Persistent symptoms of *arousal* with two or more of following:

    • Difficulty falling asleep/staying asleep.

    • Irritability or outbursts of anger.

    • Difficulty concentrating.

    • Hypervigilance.

    • Exaggerated startle response.

   e. Duration of symptoms for > 1 month.

      f. Disturbance causes significant distress or impairment in functioning.

      g. Diagnosis may be acute (symptoms < 3 months), chronic (symptoms ≥ 3 months), or delayed (onset of symptoms at least 6 months after stressor).

  4. Separation anxiety.

      a. Onset of excessive anxiety on separation from home/major attachment figure *beyond what is expected* for developmental level as evidenced by 3 or more of following:

- Recurrent excessive distress on separation from home or major attachment figure.
- Persistent/excessive worry about losing or harm coming to major attachment figure.
- Worry that untoward event will lead to separation (e.g., getting lost or kidnapped).
- Reluctance or refusal to go to school.
- Fearful or reluctant to be alone.
- Reluctance or refusal to go to sleep without being near attachment figure or to sleep away from home.
- Repeated nightmares with themes of separation.
- Repeated physical complaints when separation occurs or is anticipated.

      b. Symptoms must be present for at least 4 weeks and must begin before age 18.

      c. Symptoms must cause significant distress/impairment at home, school, with friends.

E. Physical findings.

  1. May present with symptoms of sleep disturbance, tiredness, school problems, restlessness, irritability, somatic complaints (sweating, nausea, diarrhea, shortness of breath, dizziness, headaches).

  2. For OCD, parents generally bring children in due to increase in temper tantrums, decline in school performance, food restriction, dermatitis. Children rarely request help; may be secretive about thoughts, behaviors.

F. Diagnostic tests.

  1. None. Requires interview with child and parent/caregiver.

  2. Consider collateral contact with school personnel, especially with separation anxiety.

  3. Assess recent life stressors (family move, death, divorce, new school setting, etc.).

G. Differential diagnosis.

Anxiety disorder, 300	Post-traumatic stress disorder (PTSD),
Attention deficit hyperactivity disorder	309.81
(ADHD), 314	Separation anxiety, 309.21
Obsessive-compulsive disorder (OCD),	Stress reaction, acute, 308.9
300.3	

   1. Attention deficit/hyperactivity disorder (ADHD).
   2. Differentiate among anxiety disorders such as PTSD, separation anxiety, generalized anxiety disorder, OCD.
   3. Consider acute stress reaction if exposed to traumatic event, symptoms present < 1 month.
H. Treatment.
   1. May require use of medications to reduce anxiety symptoms. Consider use of selective serotonin reuptake inhibitors (SSRIs). These may include:
      a. Fluoxetine (Prozac): starting dose of 5 mg/day; increase to 15–30 mg/day for children; 10–40 mg/day for teens.
      b. Fluvoxamine (Luvox): starting dose of 25 mg/day; increase to 50–200 mg/day for children; 150–300 mg/day for teens.
      c. Sertraline (Zoloft): starting dose of 25 mg/day; increase to 50–100 mg/day for children; 50–200 mg/day for teens.
   2. May also consider a tricyclic medication, such as clomipramine (Anafranil): starting dose of 10 mg/day; increase to 75–100 mg/day for children; 100–200 mg/day for teens.
   3. Cognitive behavioral therapy to help identify anxiety triggers, awareness of physiologic responses to anxiety. Develop plan for coping, evaluation of success of strategies.
   4. Family therapy to address ways family can support the child. Must allow 6–8 weeks before full benefit will be obtained. Follow black box warning regarding increase monitoring of SI.
I. Follow up.
   1. Follow-up appointment to monitor effectiveness of medications, address side effects of medications, compliance issues.
   2. Collaboration with family, mental health treatment provider, school personnel to assess success of treatment approaches and medications.
J. Complications.
   1. Poor school performance.

    2. Poor self-esteem, social skills, avoidance of peers.

    3. Potential for family stress and conflict.

    4. Development of comorbid diagnosis of substance abuse or major depression.

K. Education.

    1. Parent/caregiver and child need education about nature of anxiety, ways to identify, evaluate, change anxious thoughts.

    2. Child needs to learn to recognize physiologic symptoms of anxiety, use of positive "self-talk."

    3. Relaxation training may be beneficial.

II. EATING DISORDERS

Abdominal pain, 789	Hair loss, 704
Anorexia nervosa, 307.1	Hypotension, 458.9
Arrhythmias, 427.9	Hypothermia, 996.1
Brittle nails, 703.8	Insomnia, 780.52
Bulimia nervosa, 783.6	Lethargy, 780.79
Cold intolerance, 788.9	Leukopenia, 288
Constipation, 564	Metabolic acidosis, 276.2
Dehydration, 276.5	Metabolic alkalosis, 276.3
Dental caries, 525.09	Mild anemia, 285.9
Dental enamel erosion, 521.3	Nausea, 787.02
Dry skin, 701.1	Scars, 709.2
Eating disorders, 307.5	Sinus bradycardia, 427.89
Enlarged parotid glands, 240.9	Vomiting, 787.03
Expected weight gains, 783.41	Weakness, 780.79
Fatigue, 780.79	Weight loss, 783.21
Fluid and electrolyte imbalances, 276.9	

A. Serious, sometimes life threatening; tend to be chronic, usually arise in adolescence.

B. Etiology.

    1. Combination of genetic, neurochemical, psychodevelopmental, sociocultural factors.

       a. Increased risk among first-degree biological relatives of individuals with disorder. Often co-occurs with other mental health problems such as depression, anxiety, substance abuse, personality disorders.

C. Occurrence.
1. > 90% of all eating disorders occur in females.
2. Estimated 0.5% of adolescent females have anorexia nervosa; 1–5% meet criteria for bulimia nervosa.
3. Rarely begins before puberty, most common in ages 14–18 years.
4. Onset may be associated with stressful life event.

D. Clinical manifestations.
1. Anorexia nervosa.
    a. Most severe consequence with mortality rate from starvation, suicide, electrolyte imbalance.
    b. Characterized by refusal to maintain minimally normal body weight for age and height (< 85% of expected weight).
    c. Intense fear of gaining weight or becoming fat.
    d. Significant disturbance in perception of shape or size of body; sees self as overweight even when dangerously thin.
    e. In postmenarchal females, presence of amenorrhea.
2. Bulimia nervosa.
    a. Repeated episodes of binge eating characterized by:
      • Eating in discrete period of time (e.g., within 2 hours), amount of food larger than most people would eat during same period of time and under similar circumstances.
      • Sense of lack of control over eating during episode.
    c. Recurrent inappropriate compensatory behaviors to prevent weight gain such as self-induced vomiting, misuse of laxatives, diuretics, enemas, other medications, fasting, excessive exercise.
    d. Occurrence of *both* of above behaviors, on average at least twice a week for 3 months. Individuals place excessive emphasis on body shape, weight in self-evaluation.

E. Physical findings.
1. Anorexia nervosa.
    a. Reported by family members, individual presents with weight loss or failure to make expected weight gains.
    b. Leukopenia, mild anemia are common.
    c. May present with signs/symptoms of dehydration, sinus bradycardia, arrhythmias.
    d. May present with constipation, abdominal pain, cold intolerance, lethargy, hypotension, hypothermia, dry skin, dental enamel erosion.

2. Bulimia nervosa.
   a. Typically presents within normal weight range to slightly overweight.
   b. May present with complaints of abdominal pain, nausea, hair loss, brittle nails, fatigue, insomnia, or weakness.
   c. Fluid and electrolyte imbalances: metabolic alkalosis from vomiting or metabolic acidosis from laxative abuse.
   d. Loss of dental enamel, increased frequency of dental caries.
   e. Enlarged parotid glands.
   f. Possible calluses/scars on dorsal surface of hand from repeated self-induced vomiting.

F. Diagnostic tests.
   1. Ask all preteens, adolescents screening questions about eating patterns, satisfaction with body appearance.
   2. Monitor height, weight, body mass index (BMI) on all visits.
   3. Laboratory studies: complete blood count (CBC), electrolyte measurement, liver function tests, urinalysis, thyroid-stimulating hormone (TSH) test.
   4. Electrocardiogram.

G. Differential diagnosis.

AIDS, 042	Major depression, 311
Anxiety disorder, 300	Substance abuse, 995.5
Brain tumors, 348.8	Weight gain, 783.1
GI disease, 569.9	Weight loss, 783.21

   1. Rule out other possible medical causes for significant weight loss/failure to gain weight (GI disease, brain tumors, malignancies, AIDS, etc.), although these do not present with distorted body image.
   2. Comorbid diagnosis of substance abuse, major depression, anxiety disorder.

H. Treatment.
   1. Anorexia nervosa.
      a. Requires comprehensive treatment plan including medical care, monitoring, psychotherapy, nutritional counseling, medication (when appropriate). Involves three phases:
         • Restoring weight loss due to severe dieting, purging.
         • Treating psychologic disturbances such as distorted body image, low self-esteem, interpersonal conflicts.
         • Achieving long-term remission, rehabilitation.

       b. Treatment with medication, such as SSRIs; consider *only* after weight gain established.

       c. Acute inpatient hospitalization may be required to restore weight, address fluid and electrolyte imbalance or cardiac disturbances. May require nutrition via nasogastric tube/IV therapy.

       d. Intensive treatment may be needed in specialized day treatment program or intensive outpatient program.

       e. Refer for cognitive behavioral therapy and family therapy.

  2. Bulimia nervosa.

       a. Requires comprehensive treatment plan including medical care, monitoring, psychotherapy, nutritional counseling, medication (when appropriate).

       b. Primary goal: reduce/eliminate binge eating, purging behavior.
- Establish pattern of regular, nonbinging eating.
- Improve attitudes related to eating disorder.
- Encourage healthy, not excessive exercise.
- Resolution of co-occurring disorders such as depression, anxiety.

       c. Treatment approaches may include individual, group/family therapy.

       d. Cognitive behavioral therapy: useful to address cognitive distortions related to body image and to develop adaptive coping skills.

       e. Antidepressant medications, especially SSRIs, have been found to be effective.

I. Follow up.

  1. May need weekly visits to monitor weight, lab work.

  2. To achieve long-term remission and rehabilitation, treatment must include ongoing behavioral therapy, continued assessment of weight and physical health status.

  3. Ongoing assessment of anxiety/depressive symptoms.

  4. Collaboration between family and mental health provider to assess effectiveness of treatment approaches.

  5. Pharmacologic support has found conflicting evidence as benefit.

J. Complications.

Anorexia nervosa, 307.1	Fluid and electrolyte imbalances, 276.9
Bulimia nervosa, 783.6	Gastric rupture, 537.89
Cardiac arrhythmias, 427.9	Loss of dental enamel, 521.3
Cardiac complications, 429.9	Potential for development of depression, 311
Dehydration, 276.5	Potential for suicide, 300.9

Dental caries, 525.09	Renal failure, 584.9
Depression, 300.4	Starvation, 994.2
Esophagitis, 530.1	Ulceration of esophagus, 530.2
Family stress and conflict, 308.9	Vomiting, 787.03

1. Anorexia nervosa.
   a. Starvation, fluid and electrolyte imbalances, dehydration.
   b. Cardiac complications.
   c. Renal failure.
   d. Potential for suicide.
   e. Development of anxiety/depression.
   f. Potential for family stress and conflict.
2. Bulimia nervosa.
   a. Dental caries, loss of dental enamel.
   b. Potential for development of depression, substance abuse.
   c. Gastric rupture from acute gastric dilatation secondary to vomiting.
   d. Esophagitis and ulceration of esophagus.
   e. Potential for cardiac arrhythmias.
K. Education.
   1. Educate family on potential complications of disorder, as well as how to best support adolescent in treatment.
   2. Adolescent and family may benefit from nutritional counseling.

III. MOOD DISORDERS

Appetite changes, 783	Mania, 296.9
Attention deficit/hyperactivity disorder (ADHD), 314.01	Mood disorders, 296.9
	Oppositional behavior, 313.81
Bipolar disorder, 296.7	Self-harm, 300.9
Depression, 311	Sleep, 307.4
Fatigue, 780.79	Stomachache, 789
Headache, 784	

A. Etiology.
   1. Close family member with depression or bipolar disorder may be single largest contributor to likelihood of disorder in child.

B. Occurrence.
  1. For depression, prevalence is 2% in children, 6% in adolescents, with life-time prevalence in adolescents estimated to be 20%.
  2. 1% of adolescents 14–18 years of age meet criteria for bipolar disorder. Recent reports indicate a 40-fold increase in the diagnosis of bipolar disorder in children and teens.
C. Clinical manifestations.
  1. Major depression.
     a. Characterized by five or more of the following symptoms present daily for at least 2 weeks:
        • Persistent sadness or irritable mood.
        • Loss of interest in activities once enjoyed.
        • Significant change in appetite or body weight.
        • Difficulty sleeping or oversleeping.
        • Psychomotor agitation or slowing.
        • Loss of energy.
        • Feelings of worthlessness or inappropriate guilt.
        • Difficulty concentrating.
        • Recurrent thoughts of death or suicide.
     b. Other signs associated with depression include:
        • Frequent, vague, nonspecific physical complaints such as stomach-aches, headaches, muscle aches, tiredness.
        • Frequent absences from school or poor school performance.
        • Talk of or efforts to run away from home.
        • Outbursts of shouting, complaining, unexplained irritability or crying.
        • Being bored or lack of interest in playing with friends.
        • Alcohol or substance abuse.
        • Social isolation, poor communication, difficulty with relationships.
        • Fear of death.
        • Extreme sensitivity to rejection/failure.
        • Increased irritability, anger, hostility.
        • Reckless behavior.
  2. Bipolar disorder.
     a. Bipolar I: experiences alternating episodes of intense mania and depression.
     b. Bipolar II: experiences episodes of hypomania (markedly elevated or irritable mood with increased physical and mental energy) between recurrent periods of depression.

    c. Bipolar not specified (NOS): being used more to describe bipolar spectrum symptoms. Next edition of *Diagnostics and Statistical Manual of Mental Disorders* to include Temper Dysregulation Disorder that will better capture developmental aspect of symptoms.

    d. *Manic symptoms* include:
- Severe or rapid changes in mood: extremely irritable or overly silly, elated mood.
- Overly inflated self-esteem, grandiosity.
- Exaggerated beliefs about personal talents/abilities.
- Increased energy, decreased need for sleep; able to go with very little/no sleep for days without tiring.
- Talks too much, too fast, changes subjects too quickly.
- Distractibility, hyperactivity: attention shifts from one thing to another quickly.
- Increased sexual thoughts, feelings, behaviors, or use of explicit sexual language.
- Increased goal-directed activity or physical agitation.
- Excessive involvement in risky, daredevil behaviors/activities.

    e. *Depressive symptoms* include:
- Pervasive/overwhelming sadness, crying spells.
- Sleeping too much or inability to sleep.
- Agitation, irritability.
- Withdrawal from activities formerly enjoyed.
- Drop in grades, inability to concentrate.
- Thoughts of death and suicide.
- Low energy.
- Significant loss of appetite.

    f. May also present: explosive/destructive rages, separation anxiety, defiance of authority, bedwetting, night terrors, strong and frequent cravings, impaired judgment, impulsivity.

    g. Presents with depressive symptoms and also exhibits ADHD–like symptoms that are very severe: Refer to mental health professional for further evaluation, particularly if family history of bipolar disorder.

D. Physical findings.
1. Specifically ask about thoughts of suicide or self-harm: suicide is third leading cause of death among 10–24-year olds.
2. Major depression may present with multiple, vague somatic complaints (e.g., headache, stomachache, fatigue, sleep, appetite changes).
3. Bipolar disorder may present with symptoms of ADHD, depression, mania, oppositional behavior.

E. Diagnostic tests.
1. Several screening tools useful for children/adolescents, including Children's Depression Inventory for ages 7–17 and Beck Depression Inventory for adolescents. Positive screens indicate need for comprehensive diagnostic evaluation by mental health professional.
2. Requires intensive interview with child/adolescent and family as well as detailed family history.
F. Differential diagnosis.

Adjustment disorder, 309.9	Intermittent explosive disorder, 312.34
Attention-deficit/hyperactivity disorder (ADHD), 314.01	Oppositional defiant disorder, 313.81

1. Adjustment disorder.
2. ADHD.
3. Intermittent explosive disorder.
4. Oppositional defiant disorder.
G. Treatment.
1. Major depression.
   a. Antidepressant medication may be indicated.
   • Consider SSRI medications:
      i. Fluoxetine (Prozac): starting dose of 5 mg/day; increase to 15–40 mg/day for children, 10–60 mg/day for teens.
      ii. Fluvoxamine (Luvox): starting dose of 25 mg/day; increase to 50–200 mg/day for children, 100–300 mg/day for teens.
      iii. Sertraline (Zoloft): starting dose of 25 mg/day; increase to 50–150 mg/day for children, 50–200 mg/day for teens.
   • Following remission of symptoms, continue medications *with* therapy for at least several months given high rate of relapse, recurrence of depression. Gradually discontinue medications over 6 weeks or longer.
   b. Short-term psychotherapy such as cognitive behavioral therapy (CBT).
   • CBT based on premise that young people with depression have distorted view of themselves, world, future. CBT focuses on changing distortions through time-limited therapy.
   • Continued therapy for several months after remission of symptoms may help consolidate skills learned, cope with after effects of depression, address environmental stressors, understand how young person's thoughts and behaviors could contribute to relapse.

2. Bipolar disorder.
   a. Use of mood-stabilizing medications such as lithium (Eskalith, Lithobid, lithium carbonate), valproic acid (Depakote), carbamazepine (Tegretol), lamotrigrine (Lamictal), tiagabine (Gabitril).
      • Start lithium at 25 mg/kg/day, gradually increase until serum level reaches therapeutic range of 0.9–1.1 mEq/L.
      • Valproic acid (Depakote): start at 15 mg/kg/day, gradually increase until serum level reaches therapeutic range of 80–120 mg/mL.
      • Carbamazepine (Tegretol): starting dose of 100 mg/day with increase to 300–800 mg/day in children, 800–1000 mg/day in teens; monitor for serum level to reach therapeutic range of 8–12 mcg/mL.
   b. Consider polypharmacy with addition of antipsychotic medications, calcium channel blockers, antianxiety agents.
   c. Do not use antidepressant medication alone; may lead to mania or rapid cycling.
   d. Psychostimulant medications frequently used to treat ADHD may worsen manic symptoms.
   e. CBT, interpersonal therapy, multifamily support groups essential part of overall treatment plan.
H. Follow up.
   1. Monitor effectiveness of medications; address side effects, compliance issues.
   2. Monitor closely for suicidal thoughts and/or behaviors. *Note*: FDA Black Box warning on use of SSRI antidepressants in children and teens.
   3. Monitor blood levels to assess appropriate medication dosing.
   4. Collaborate with family, mental health treatment provider, school personnel to assess success of treatment approaches.
I. Complications.

Conduct disorder, 312.9	Risk for suicide, 300.9
Poor psychosocial functioning, V71.02	Substance abuse, 995.5

   1. Increased risk for suicidal behavior: attempts may rise, particularly among adolescent males, if depression accompanied by conduct disorder or substance abuse.
   2. Increased risk for poor psychosocial functioning.
   3. School truancy or poor academic performance.
   4. Substance abuse.

J. Education.
    1. Monitor effectiveness of medications.
    2. Educate families on signs/symptoms of both depression and mania and signs/symptoms of suicidal ideation.

BIBLIOGRAPHY

American Psychiatric Association. *Diagnostic and statistical manual of mental disorders.* 4th ed. Washington, DC: Author; 2000.
National Institute of Mental Health. *Brief notes on the mental health of children and adolescents.* Bethesda, MD: Author; 2002.
National Institute of Mental Health. NIH Publication No. 00-4744. Bethesda, MD: Author; 2002.
National Institute of Mental Health. NIH Publication No. 00-4778. Bethesda, MD: Author; 2002.
National Institute of Mental Health. NIH Publication No. 01-4901. Bethesda, MD: Author; 2002.
Scahill L. Child and adolescent psychiatric nursing. In NL Keltner, CE Bostrom, & T McGuinness, eds. *Psychiatric nursing.* 6th ed. pp. 459–468. St. Louis: Mosby; 2011.

Recommended Immunization Schedule

Recommended Immunization Schedule for Persons Aged 0 Through 6 Years—United States • 2011
For those who fall behind or start late, see the catch-up schedule

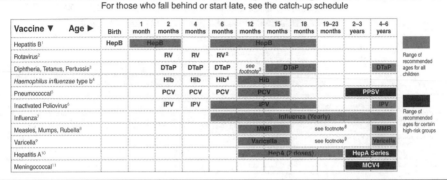

Vaccine ▼ Age ►	Birth	1 month	2 months	4 months	6 months	12 months	15 months	18 months	19–23 months	2–3 years	4–6 years	
Hepatitis B[1]	HepB	HepB				HepB						
Rotavirus[2]			RV	RV	RV[2]							Range of recommended ages for all children
Diphtheria, Tetanus, Pertussis[3]			DTaP	DTaP	DTaP	see footnote[3]	DTaP				DTaP	
Haemophilus influenzae type b[4]			Hib	Hib	Hib[4]	Hib						
Pneumococcal[5]			PCV	PCV	PCV	PCV				PPSV		
Inactivated Poliovirus[6]			IPV	IPV		IPV					IPV	
Influenza[7]						Influenza (Yearly)						Range of recommended ages for certain high-risk groups
Measles, Mumps, Rubella[8]						MMR		see footnote[8]			MMR	
Varicella[9]						Varicella		see footnote[9]			Varicella	
Hepatitis A[10]						HepA (2 doses)				HepA Series		
Meningococcal[11]											MCV4	

This schedule includes recommendations in effect as of December 21, 2010. Any dose not administered at the recommended age should be administered at a subsequent visit, when indicated and feasible. The use of a combination vaccine generally is preferred over separate injections of its equivalent component vaccines. Considerations should include provider assessment, patient preference, and the potential for adverse events. Providers should consult the relevant Advisory Committee on Immunization Practices statement for detailed recommendations: http://www.cdc.gov/vaccines/pubs/acip-list.htm. Clinically significant adverse events that follow immunization should be reported to the Vaccine Adverse Event Reporting System (VAERS) at http://www.vaers.hhs.gov or by telephone, 800-822-7967. Use of trade names and commercial sources is for identification only and does not imply endorsement by the U.S. Department of Health and Human Services.

1. **Hepatitis B vaccine (HepB).** (Minimum age: birth)
   At birth:
   - Administer monovalent HepB to all newborns before hospital discharge.
   - If mother is hepatitis B surface antigen (HBsAg)-positive, administer HepB and 0.5 mL of hepatitis B immune globulin (HBIG) within 12 hours of birth.
   - If mother's HBsAg status is unknown, administer HepB within 12 hours of birth. Determine mother's HBsAg status as soon as possible and, if HBsAg-positive, administer HBIG (no later than age 1 week).
   Doses following the birth dose:
   - The second dose should be administered at age 1 or 2 months. Monovalent HepB should be used for doses administered before age 6 weeks.
   - Infants born to HBsAg-positive mothers should be tested for HBsAg and antibody to HBsAg 1 to 2 months after completion of at least 3 doses of the HepB series, at age 9 through 18 months (generally at the next well-child visit).
   - Administration of 4 doses of HepB to infants is permissible when a combination vaccine containing HepB is administered after the birth dose.
   - Infants who did not receive a birth dose should receive 3 doses of HepB on a schedule of 0, 1, and 6 months.
   - The final (3rd or 4th) dose in the HepB series should be administered no earlier than age 24 weeks.
2. **Rotavirus vaccine (RV).** (Minimum age: 6 weeks)
   - Administer the first dose at age 6 through 14 weeks (maximum age: 14 weeks 6 days). Vaccination should not be initiated for infants aged 15 weeks 0 days or older.
   - The maximum age for the final dose in the series is 8 months 0 days
   - If Rotarix is administered at ages 2 and 4 months, a dose at 6 months is not indicated.
3. **Diphtheria and tetanus toxoids and acellular pertussis vaccine (DTaP).** (Minimum age: 6 weeks)
   - The fourth dose may be administered as early as age 12 months, provided at least 6 months have elapsed since the third dose.
4. **Haemophilus influenzae type b conjugate vaccine (Hib).** (Minimum age: 6 weeks)
   - If PRP-OMP (PedvaxHIB or Comvax [HepB-Hib]) is administered at ages 2 and 4 months, a dose at age 6 months is not indicated.
   - Hiberix should not be used for doses at ages 2, 4, or 6 months for the primary series but can be used as the final dose in children aged 12 months through 4 years.
5. **Pneumococcal vaccine.** (Minimum age: 6 weeks for pneumococcal conjugate vaccine [PCV]; 2 years for pneumococcal polysaccharide vaccine [PPSV])
   - PCV is recommended for all children aged younger than 5 years. Administer 1 dose of PCV to all healthy children aged 24 through 59 months who are not completely vaccinated for their age.
   - A PCV series begun with 7-valent PCV (PCV7) should be completed with 13-valent PCV (PCV13).
   - A single supplemental dose of PCV13 is recommended for all children aged 14 through 59 months who have received an age-appropriate series of PCV7.
   - A single supplemental dose of PCV13 is recommended for all children aged 60 through 71 months with underlying medical conditions who have received an age-appropriate series of PCV7.

   - The supplemental dose of PCV13 should be administered at least 8 weeks after the previous dose of PCV7. See MMWR 2010:59(No. RR-11).
   - Administer PPSV at least 8 weeks after last dose of PCV to children aged 2 years or older with certain underlying medical conditions, including a cochlear implant.
6. **Inactivated poliovirus vaccine (IPV).** (Minimum age: 6 weeks)
   - If 4 or more doses are administered prior to age 4 years an additional dose should be administered at age 4 through 6 years.
   - The final dose in the series should be administered on or after the fourth birthday and at least 6 months following the previous dose.
7. **Influenza vaccine (seasonal).** (Minimum age: 6 months for trivalent inactivated influenza vaccine [TIV]; 2 years for live, attenuated influenza vaccine [LAIV])
   - For healthy children aged 2 years and older (i.e., those who do not have underlying medical conditions that predispose them to influenza complications), either LAIV or TIV may be used, except LAIV should not be given to children aged 2 through 4 years who have had wheezing in the past 12 months.
   - Administer 2 doses (separated by at least 4 weeks) to children aged 6 months through 8 years who are receiving seasonal influenza vaccine for the first time or who were vaccinated for the first time during the previous influenza season but only received 1 dose.
   - Children aged 6 months through 8 years who received no doses of monovalent 2009 H1N1 vaccine should receive 2 doses of 2010–2011 seasonal influenza vaccine. See MMWR 2010;59(No. RR-8):33–34.
8. **Measles, mumps, and rubella vaccine (MMR).** (Minimum age: 12 months)
   - The second dose may be administered before age 4 years, provided at least 4 weeks have elapsed since the first dose.
9. **Varicella vaccine.** (Minimum age: 12 months)
   - The second dose may be administered before age 4 years, provided at least 3 months have elapsed since the first dose.
   - For children aged 12 months through 12 years the recommended minimum interval between doses is 3 months. However, if the second dose was administered at least 4 weeks after the first dose, it can be accepted as valid.
10. **Hepatitis A vaccine (HepA).** (Minimum age: 12 months)
   - Administer 2 doses at least 6 months apart.
   - HepA is recommended for children aged older than 23 months who live in areas where vaccination programs target older children, who are at increased risk for infection, or for whom immunity against hepatitis A is desired.
11. **Meningococcal conjugate vaccine, quadrivalent (MCV4).** (Minimum age: 2 years)
   - Administer 2 doses of MCV4 at least 8 weeks apart to children aged 2 through 10 years with persistent complement component deficiency and anatomic or functional asplenia, and 1 dose every 5 years thereafter.
   - Persons with human immunodeficiency virus (HIV) infection who are vaccinated with MCV4 should receive 2 doses at least 8 weeks apart.
   - Administer 1 dose of MCV4 to children aged 2 through 10 years who travel to countries with highly endemic or epidemic disease and during outbreaks caused by a vaccine serogroup.
   - Administer MCV4 to children at continued risk for meningococcal disease who were previously vaccinated with MCV4 or meningococcal polysaccharide vaccine after 3 years if the first dose was administered at age 2 through 6 years.

The Recommended Immunization Schedules for Persons Aged 0 Through 18 Years are approved by the Advisory Committee on Immunization Practices (http://www.cdc.gov/vaccines/recs/acip), the American Academy of Pediatrics (http://www.aap.org), and the American Academy of Family Physicians (http://www.aafp.org).
Department of Health and Human Services • Centers for Disease Control and Prevention

Recommended Immunization Schedule for Persons Aged 7 Through 18 Years—United States • 2011

For those who fall behind or start late, see the schedule below and the catch-up schedule

Vaccine ▼ Age ▶	7–10 years	11–12 years	13–18 years	
Tetanus, Diphtheria, Pertussis[1]		Tdap	Tdap	■ Range of recommended ages for all children
Human Papillomavirus[2]	see footnote [2]	HPV (3 doses)(females)	HPV Series	
Meningococcal[3]	MCV4	MCV4	MCV4	
Influenza[4]	Influenza (Yearly)			□ Range of recommended ages for catch-up immunization
Pneumococcal[5]	Pneumococcal			
Hepatitis A[6]	HepA Series			
Hepatitis B[7]	Hep B Series			
Inactivated Poliovirus[8]	IPV Series			□ Range of recommended ages for certain high-risk groups
Measles, Mumps, Rubella[9]	MMR Series			
Varicella[10]	Varicella Series			

This schedule includes recommendations in effect as of December 21, 2010. Any dose not administered at the recommended age should be administered at a subsequent visit, when indicated and feasible. The use of a combination vaccine generally is preferred over separate injections of its equivalent component vaccines. Considerations should include provider assessment, patient preference, and the potential for adverse events. Providers should consult the relevant Advisory Committee on Immunization Practices statement for detailed recommendations: **http://www.cdc.gov/vaccines/pubs/acip-list.htm**. Clinically significant adverse events that follow immunization should be reported to the Vaccine Adverse Event Reporting System (VAERS) at **http://www.vaers.hhs.gov** or by telephone, **800-822-7967.**

1. **Tetanus and diphtheria toxoids and acellular pertussis vaccine (Tdap).** (Minimum age: 10 years for Boostrix and 11 years for Adacel)
   * Persons aged 11 through 18 years who have not received Tdap should receive a dose followed by Td booster doses every 10 years thereafter.
   * Persons aged 7 through 10 years who are not fully immunized against pertussis (including those never vaccinated or with unknown pertussis vaccination status) should receive a single dose of Tdap. Refer to the catch-up schedule if additional doses of tetanus and diphtheria toxoid–containing vaccine are needed.
   * Tdap can be administered regardless of the interval since the last tetanus and diphtheria toxoid–containing vaccine.
2. **Human papillomavirus vaccine (HPV).** (Minimum age: 9 years)
   * Quadrivalent HPV vaccine (HPV4) or bivalent HPV vaccine (HPV2) is recommended for the prevention of cervical precancers and cancers in females.
   * HPV4 is recommended for prevention of cervical precancers, cancers, and genital warts in females.
   * HPV4 may be administered in a 3-dose series to males aged 9 through 18 years to reduce their likelihood of genital warts.
   * Administer the second dose 1 to 2 months after the first dose and the third dose 6 months after the first dose (at least 24 weeks after the first dose).
3. **Meningococcal conjugate vaccine, quadrivalent (MCV4).** (Minimum age: 2 years)
   * Administer MCV4 at age 11 through 12 years with a booster dose at age 16 years.
   * Administer 1 dose at age 13 through 18 years if not previously vaccinated.
   * Persons who received their first dose at age 13 through 15 years should receive a booster dose at age 16 through 18 years.
   * Administer 1 dose to previously unvaccinated college freshmen living in a dormitory.
   * Administer 2 doses at least 8 weeks apart to children aged 2 through 10 years with persistent complement component deficiency and anatomic or functional asplenia, and those every 5 years thereafter.
   * Persons with HIV infection who are vaccinated with MCV4 should receive 2 doses at least 8 weeks apart.
   * Administer 1 dose of MCV4 to children aged 2 through 10 years who travel to countries with highly endemic or epidemic disease and during outbreaks caused by a vaccine serogroup.
   * Administer MCV4 to children at continued risk for meningococcal disease who were previously vaccinated with MCV4 or meningococcal polysaccharide vaccine after 3 years (if first dose administered at age 2 through 6 years) or after 5 years (if first dose administered at age 7 years or older).
4. **Influenza vaccine (seasonal).**
   * For healthy nonpregnant persons aged 7 through 18 years (i.e., those who do not have underlying medical conditions that predispose them to influenza complications), either LAIV or TIV may be used.
   * Administer 2 doses (separated by at least 4 weeks) to children aged 6 months through 8 years who are receiving seasonal influenza vaccine for the first

time or who were vaccinated for the first time during the previous influenza season but only received 1 dose.
   * Children 6 months through 8 years of age who received no doses of monovalent 2009 H1N1 vaccine should receive 2 doses of 2010-2011 seasonal influenza vaccine. See *MMWR* 2010;59(No. RR-8):33–34.
5. **Pneumococcal vaccines.**
   * A single dose of 13-valent pneumococcal conjugate vaccine (PCV13) may be administered to children aged 6 through 18 years who have functional or anatomic asplenia, HIV infection or other immunocompromising condition, cochlear implant or CSF leak. See *MMWR* 2010;59(No. RR-11).
   * The dose of PCV13 should be administered at least 8 weeks after the previous dose of PCV7.
   * Administer pneumococcal polysaccharide vaccine at least 8 weeks after the last dose of PCV to children aged 2 years or older with certain underlying medical conditions, including a cochlear implant. A single revaccination should be administered after 5 years to children with functional or anatomic asplenia or an immunocompromising condition.
6. **Hepatitis A vaccine (HepA).**
   * Administer 2 doses at least 6 months apart.
   * HepA is recommended for children aged older than 23 months who live in areas where vaccination programs target older children, or who are at increased risk for infection, or for whom immunity against hepatitis A is desired.
7. **Hepatitis B vaccine (HepB).**
   * Administer the 3-dose series to those not previously vaccinated. For those with incomplete vaccination, follow the catch-up schedule.
   * A 2-dose series (separated by at least 4 months) of adult formulation Recombivax HB is licensed for children aged 11 through 15 years.
8. **Inactivated poliovirus vaccine (IPV).**
   * The final dose in the series should be administered on or after the fourth birthday and at least 6 months following the previous dose.
   * If both OPV and IPV were administered as part of a series, a total of 4 doses should be administered, regardless of the child's current age.
9. **Measles, mumps, and rubella vaccine (MMR).**
   * The minimum interval between the 2 doses of MMR is 4 weeks.
10. **Varicella vaccine.**
   * For persons aged 7 through 18 years without evidence of immunity (see *MMWR* 2007;56[No. RR-4]), administer 2 doses if not previously vaccinated or the second dose if only 1 dose has been administered.
   * For persons aged 7 through 12 years, the recommended minimum interval between doses is 3 months. However, if the second dose was administered at least 4 weeks after the first dose, it can be accepted as valid.
   * For persons aged 13 years and older, the minimum interval between doses is 4 weeks.

The Recommended Immunization Schedules for Persons Aged 0 Through 18 Years are approved by the Advisory Committee on Immunization Practices (**http://www.cdc.gov/vaccines/recs/acip**), the American Academy of Pediatrics (**http://www.aap.org**), and the American Academy of Family Physicians (**http://www.aafp.org**).
Department of Health and Human Services • Centers for Disease Control and Prevention

Catch-up Immunization Schedule for Persons Aged 4 Months Through 18 Years Who Start Late or Who Are More Than 1 Month Behind—United States • 2011

The table below provides catch-up schedules and minimum intervals between doses for children whose vaccinations have been delayed. A vaccine series does not need to be restarted, regardless of the time that has elapsed between doses. Use the section appropriate for the child's age

Vaccine	Minimum Age for Dose 1	Minimum Interval Between Doses			
		Dose 1 to Dose 2	Dose 2 to Dose 3	Dose 3 to Dose 4	Dose 4 to Dose 5
PERSONS AGED 4 MONTHS THROUGH 6 YEARS					
Hepatitis B[1]	Birth	4 weeks	8 weeks (and at least 16 weeks after first dose)		
Rotavirus[2]	6 wks	4 weeks	4 weeks[2]		
Diphtheria, Tetanus, Pertussis[3]	6 wks	4 weeks	4 weeks	6 months	6 months[3]
Haemophilus influenzae type b[4]	6 wks	4 weeks if first dose administered at younger than age 12 months / 8 weeks (as final dose) if first dose administered at age 12–14 months / No further doses needed if first dose administered at age 15 months or older	4 weeks[4] if current age is younger than 12 months / 8 weeks (as final dose)[4] if current age is 12 months or older and first dose administered at younger than age 12 months and second dose administered at younger than 15 months / No further doses needed if previous dose administered at age 15 months or older	8 weeks (as final dose) This dose only necessary for children aged 12 months through 59 months who received 3 doses before age 12 months	
Pneumococcal[5]	6 wks	4 weeks if first dose administered at younger than age 12 months / 8 weeks (as final dose for healthy children) if first dose administered at age 12 months or older or current age 24 through 59 months / No further doses needed for healthy children if first dose administered at age 24 months or older	4 weeks if current age is younger than 12 months / 8 weeks (as final dose for healthy children) if current age is 12 months or older / No further doses needed for healthy children if previous dose administered at age 24 months or older	8 weeks (as final dose) This dose only necessary for children aged 12 months through 59 months who received 3 doses before age 12 months or for children at high risk who received 3 doses at any age	
Inactivated Poliovirus[6]	6 wks	4 weeks	4 weeks	6 months[6]	
Measles, Mumps, Rubella[7]	12 mos	4 weeks			
Varicella[8]	12 mos	3 months			
Hepatitis A[9]	12 mos	6 months			
PERSONS AGED 7 THROUGH 18 YEARS					
Tetanus, Diphtheria / Tetanus, Diphtheria, Pertussis[10]	7 yrs[10]	4 weeks	4 weeks if first dose administered at younger than age 12 months / 6 months if first dose administered at 12 months or older	6 months if first dose administered at younger than age 12 months	
Human Papillomavirus[11]	9 yrs	Routine dosing intervals are recommended (females)[11]			
Hepatitis A[9]	12 mos	6 months			
Hepatitis B[1]	Birth	4 weeks	8 weeks (and at least 16 weeks after first dose)		
Inactivated Poliovirus[6]	6 wks	4 weeks	4 weeks[6]	6 months[6]	
Measles, Mumps, Rubella[7]	12 mos	4 weeks			
Varicella[8]	12 mos	3 months if person is younger than age 13 years / 4 weeks if person is aged 13 years or older			

1. **Hepatitis B vaccine (HepB).**
   - Administer the 3-dose series to those not previously vaccinated.
   - The minimum age for the third dose of HepB is 24 weeks.
   - A 2-dose series (separated by at least 4 months) of adult formulation Recombivax HB is licensed for children aged 11 through 15 years.
2. **Rotavirus vaccine (RV).**
   - The maximum age for the first dose in the series is 14 weeks 6 days. Vaccination should not be initiated for infants aged 15 weeks 0 days or older.
   - The maximum age for the final dose in the series is 8 months 0 days.
   - If Rotarix was administered for the first and second doses, a third dose is not indicated.
3. **Diphtheria and tetanus toxoids and acellular pertussis vaccine (DTaP).**
   - The fifth dose is not necessary if the fourth dose was administered at age 4 years or older.
4. **Haemophilus influenzae type b conjugate vaccine (Hib).**
   - 1 dose of Hib vaccine should be considered for unvaccinated persons aged 5 years or older who have sickle cell disease, leukemia, or HIV infection, or who have had a splenectomy.
   - If the first 2 doses were PRP-OMP (PedvaxHIB or Comvax), and administered at age 11 months or younger, the third (and final) dose should be administered at age 12 through 15 months and at least 8 weeks after the second dose.
   - If the first dose was administered at age 7 through 11 months, administer the second dose at least 4 weeks later and a final dose at age 12 through 15 months.
5. **Pneumococcal vaccine.**
   - Administer 1 dose of 13-valent pneumococcal conjugate vaccine (PCV13) to all healthy children aged 24 through 59 months with any incomplete PCV schedule (PCV7 or PCV13).
   - For children aged 24 through 71 months with underlying medical conditions, administer 1 dose of PCV13 if 3 doses of PCV were received previously or administer 2 doses of PCV13 at least 8 weeks apart if fewer than 3 doses of PCV were received previously.
   - A single dose of PCV13 is recommended for certain children with underlying medical conditions through 18 years of age. See age-specific schedules for details.
   - Administer pneumococcal polysaccharide vaccine (PPSV) to children aged 2 years or older with certain underlying medical conditions, including a cochlear implant, at least 8 weeks after the last dose of PCV. A single revaccination should be administered after 5 years to children with functional or anatomic asplenia or an immunocompromising condition. See *MMWR* 2010;59(No. RR-11).

6. **Inactivated poliovirus vaccine (IPV).**
   - The final dose in the series should be administered on or after the fourth birthday and at least 6 months following the previous dose.
   - A fourth dose is not necessary if the third dose was administered at age 4 years or older and at least 6 months following the previous dose.
   - In the first 6 months of life, minimum age and minimum intervals are only recommended if the person is at risk for imminent exposure to circulating poliovirus (i.e., travel to a polio-endemic region or during an outbreak).
7. **Measles, mumps, and rubella vaccine (MMR).**
   - Administer the second dose routinely at age 4 through 6 years. The minimum interval between the 2 doses of MMR is 4 weeks.
8. **Varicella vaccine.**
   - Administer the second dose routinely at age 4 through 6 years.
   - If the second dose was administered at least 4 weeks after the first dose, it can be accepted as valid.
9. **Hepatitis A vaccine (HepA).**
   - HepA is recommended for children aged older than age 23 months who live in areas where vaccination programs target older children, or who are at increased risk for infection, or for whom immunity against hepatitis A is desired.
10. **Tetanus and diphtheria toxoids (Td) and tetanus and diphtheria toxoids and acellular pertussis vaccine (Tdap).**
    - Doses of DTaP are counted as part of the Td/Tdap series.
    - Tdap should be substituted for a single dose of Td in the catch-up series for children aged 7 through 10 years or as a booster for children aged 11 through 18 years; use Td for other doses.
11. **Human papillomavirus vaccine (HPV).**
    - Administer the series to females at age 13 through 18 years if not previously vaccinated or have not completed the vaccine series.
    - Quadrivalent HPV vaccine (HPV4) may be administered in a 3-dose series to males aged 9 through 18 years to reduce their likelihood of genital warts.
    - Use recommended routine dosing intervals for series catch-up (i.e., the second and third doses should be administered at 1 to 2 and 6 months after the first dose). The minimum interval between the first and second doses is 4 weeks. The minimum interval between the second and third doses is 12 weeks, and the third dose should be administered at least 24 weeks after the first dose.

Information about reporting reactions after immunization is available online at http://www.vaers.hhs.gov or by telephone, 800-822-7967. Suspected cases of vaccine-preventable diseases should be reported to the state or local health department. Additional information, including precautions and contraindications for immunization, is available from the National Center for Immunization and Respiratory Diseases at http://www.cdc.gov/vaccines or telephone, **800-CDC-INFO** (800-232-4636).
Department of Health and Human Services • Centers for Disease Control and Prevention

Recommended Dietary Flouride Supplement Schedule

FLUORIDE SUPPLEMENT DOSAGE SCHEDULE—2010

Approved by the American Dental Association Council on Scientific Affairs

Age	Fluoride Ion Level in Drinking Water (ppm)*		
	< 0.3	0.3-0.6	> 0.6
Birth–6 months	None	None	None
6 months–3 years	0.25 mg/day**	None	None
3–6 years	0.50 mg/day	0.25 mg/day	None
6–16 years	1.0 mg/day	0.50 mg/day	None

*1.0 part per million (ppm) = 1 milligram per liter (mg/l)

** 2.2 mg sodium fluoride contains 1 mg fluoride ion

Children's Growth Charts

Birth to 36 months: Boys
Length-for-age and Weight-for-age percentiles

NAME _____

RECORD # _____

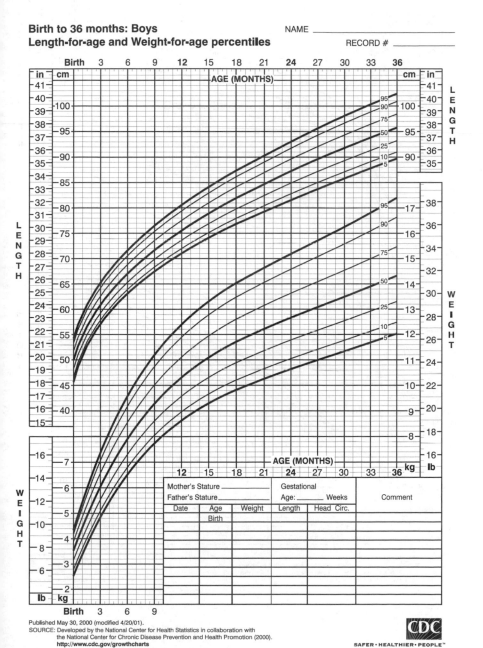

Published May 30, 2000 (modified 4/20/01).
SOURCE: Developed by the National Center for Health Statistics in collaboration with
the National Center for Chronic Disease Prevention and Health Promotion (2000).
http://www.cdc.gov/growthcharts

CDC
SAFER·HEALTHIER·PEOPLE™

Birth to 36 months: Boys
Head circumference-for-age and
Weight-for-length percentiles

NAME _____

RECORD # _____

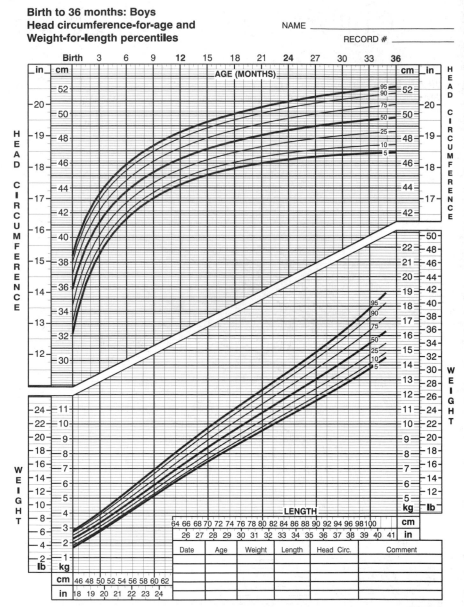

Published May 30, 2000 (modified 10/16/00).
SOURCE: Developed by the National Center for Health Statistics in collaboration with
the National Center for Chronic Disease Prevention and Health Promotion (2000).
http://www.cdc.gov/growthcharts

SAFER · HEALTHIER · PEOPLE™

Birth to 36 months: Girls
Length-for-age and Weight-for-age percentiles

NAME _____

RECORD # _____

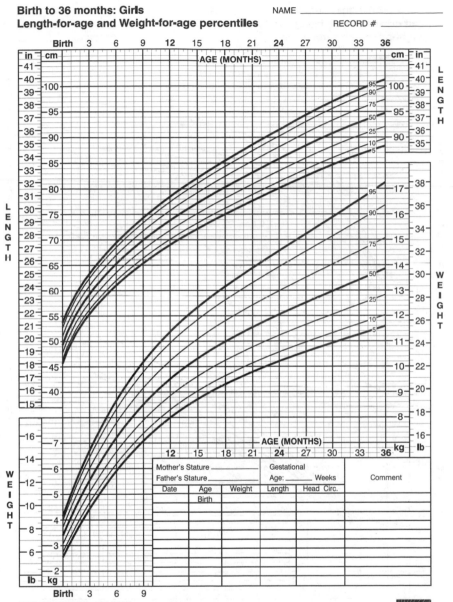

Published May 30, 2000 (modified 4/20/01).
SOURCE: Developed by the National Center for Health Statistics in collaboration with
the National Center for Chronic Disease Prevention and Health Promotion (2000).
http://www.cdc.gov/growthcharts

SAFER·HEALTHIER·PEOPLE™

Birth to 36 months: Girls
Head circumference-for-age and
Weight-for-length percentiles

NAME _____

RECORD # _____

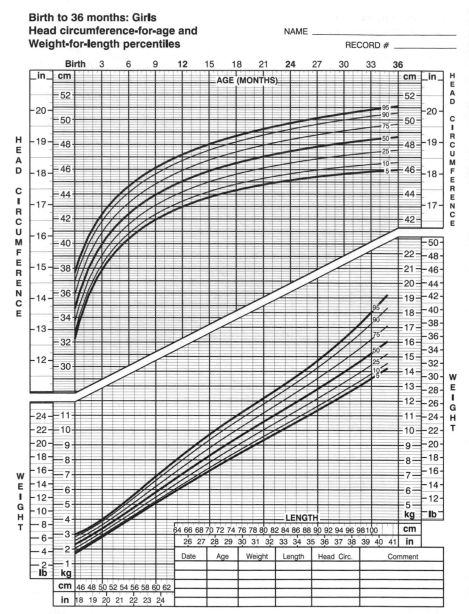

Published May 30, 2000 (modified 10/16/00).
SOURCE: Developed by the National Center for Health Statistics in collaboration with
the National Center for Chronic Disease Prevention and Health Promotion (2000).
http://www.cdc.gov/growthcharts

SAFER · HEALTHIER · PEOPLE™

2 to 20 years: Boys
Stature-for-age and Weight-for-age percentiles

NAME _____

RECORD # _____

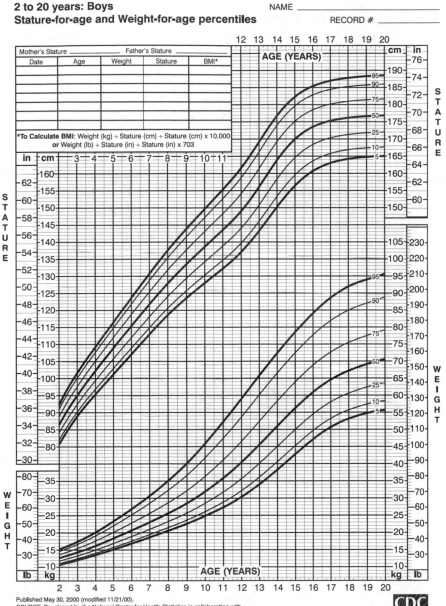

Published May 30, 2000 (modified 11/21/00).
SOURCE: Developed by the National Center for Health Statistics in collaboration with
the National Center for Chronic Disease Prevention and Health Promotion (2000).
http://www.cdc.gov/growthcharts

2 to 20 years: Boys
Body mass index-for-age percentiles

NAME _____

RECORD # _____

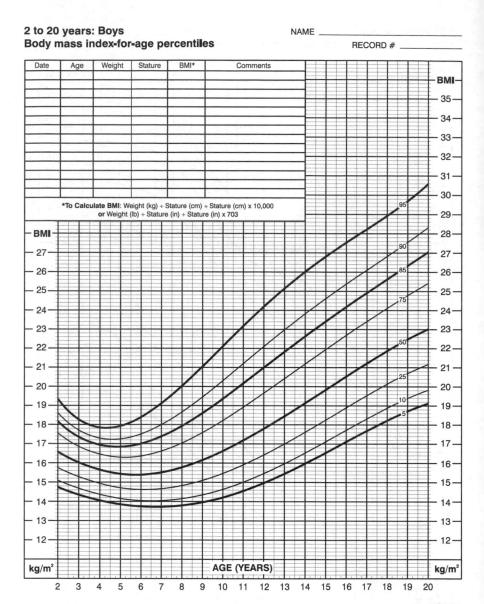

Date	Age	Weight	Stature	BMI*	Comments

*To Calculate BMI: Weight (kg) ÷ Stature (cm) ÷ Stature (cm) x 10,000
or Weight (lb) ÷ Stature (in) ÷ Stature (in) x 703

AGE (YEARS)

Published May 30, 2000 (modified 10/16/00).
SOURCE: Developed by the National Center for Health Statistics in collaboration with
the National Center for Chronic Disease Prevention and Health Promotion (2000).
http://www.cdc.gov/growthcharts

SAFER·HEALTHIER·PEOPLE™

2 to 20 years: Girls
Stature-for-age and Weight-for-age percentiles

NAME _____

RECORD # _____

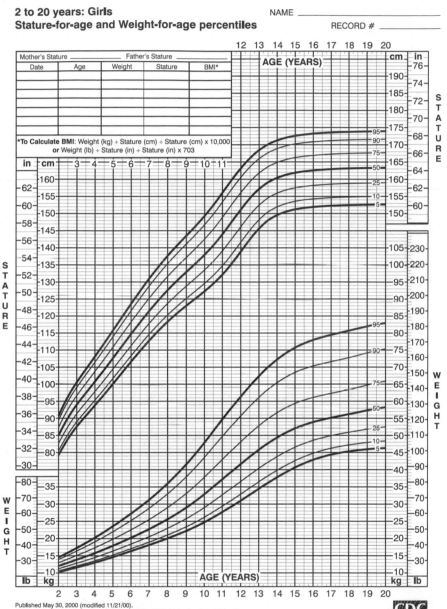

Published May 30, 2000 (modified 11/21/00).
SOURCE: Developed by the National Center for Health Statistics in collaboration with
the National Center for Chronic Disease Prevention and Health Promotion (2000).
http://www.cdc.gov/growthcharts

SAFER · HEALTHIER · PEOPLE™

BMI Table

Category	Normal						Overweight					Obese										Extreme Obesity														
BMI	19	20	21	22	23	24	25	26	27	28	29	30	31	32	33	34	35	36	37	38	39	40	41	42	43	44	45	46	47	48	49	50	51	52	53	54
Height (inches)												Body Weight (pounds)																								
58	91	96	100	105	110	115	119	124	129	134	138	143	148	153	158	162	167	172	177	181	186	191	196	201	205	210	215	220	224	229	234	239	244	248	253	258
59	94	99	104	109	114	119	124	128	133	138	143	148	153	158	163	168	173	178	183	188	193	198	203	208	212	217	222	227	232	237	242	247	252	257	262	267
60	97	102	107	112	118	123	128	133	138	143	148	153	158	163	168	174	179	184	189	194	199	204	209	215	220	225	230	235	240	245	250	255	261	266	271	276
61	100	106	111	116	122	127	132	137	143	148	153	158	164	169	174	180	185	190	195	201	206	211	217	222	227	232	238	243	248	254	259	264	269	275	280	285
62	104	109	115	120	126	131	136	142	147	153	158	164	169	175	180	186	191	196	202	207	213	218	224	229	235	240	246	251	256	262	267	273	278	284	289	295
63	107	113	118	124	130	135	141	146	152	158	163	169	175	180	186	191	197	203	208	214	220	225	231	237	242	248	254	259	265	270	278	282	287	293	299	304
64	110	116	122	128	134	140	145	151	157	163	169	174	180	186	192	197	204	209	215	221	227	232	238	244	250	256	262	267	273	279	285	291	296	302	308	314
65	114	120	126	132	138	144	150	156	162	168	174	180	186	192	198	204	210	216	222	228	234	240	246	252	258	264	270	276	282	288	294	300	306	312	318	324
66	118	124	130	136	142	148	155	161	167	173	179	186	192	198	204	210	216	223	229	235	241	247	253	260	266	272	278	284	291	297	303	309	315	322	328	334
67	121	127	134	140	146	153	159	166	172	178	185	191	198	204	211	217	223	230	236	242	249	255	261	268	274	280	287	293	299	306	312	319	325	331	338	344
68	125	131	138	144	151	158	164	171	177	184	190	197	203	210	216	223	230	236	243	249	256	262	269	276	282	289	295	302	308	315	322	328	335	341	348	354
69	128	135	142	149	155	162	169	176	182	189	196	203	209	216	223	230	236	243	250	257	263	270	277	284	291	297	304	311	318	324	331	338	345	351	358	365
70	132	139	146	153	160	167	174	181	188	195	202	209	216	222	229	236	243	250	257	264	271	278	285	292	299	306	313	320	327	334	341	348	355	362	369	376
71	136	143	150	157	165	172	179	186	193	200	208	215	222	229	236	243	250	257	265	272	279	286	293	301	308	315	322	329	338	343	351	358	365	372	379	386
72	140	147	154	162	169	177	184	191	199	206	213	221	228	235	242	250	258	265	272	279	287	294	302	309	316	324	331	338	346	353	361	368	375	383	390	397
73	144	151	159	166	174	182	189	197	204	212	219	227	235	242	250	257	265	272	280	288	295	302	310	318	325	333	340	348	355	363	371	378	386	393	401	408
74	148	155	163	171	179	186	194	202	210	218	225	233	241	249	256	264	272	280	287	295	303	311	319	326	334	342	350	358	365	373	381	389	396	404	412	420
75	152	160	168	176	184	192	200	208	216	224	232	240	248	256	264	272	279	287	295	303	311	319	327	335	343	351	359	367	375	383	391	399	407	415	423	431
76	156	164	172	180	189	197	205	213	221	230	238	246	254	263	271	279	287	295	304	312	320	328	336	344	353	361	369	377	385	394	402	410	418	426	435	443

Source: Reprinted from National Heart, Lung, and Blood Institute. (2008). Body mass index table. Retrived May 10, 2008, from http://www.nhlbi.nih.gov/ guidelines/obesity/bmi_tbl.pdf.

MyPlate

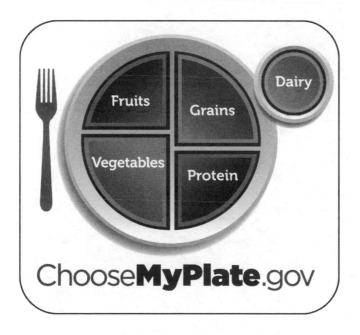

Predicted Peak Flow Measurements

MaineHealth

AH! Asthma Health

Predicted Peak Flow Measurements
(based on Personal Best® peak flow meter)

Normal Children and Adolescents

Height (in)	(cm)	Males & Females
43	109	147
44	112	160
45	114	173
46	117	187
47	119	200
48	122	214
49	124	227
50	127	240
51	130	254
52	132	267
53	135	280
54	137	293
55	140	307
56	142	320
57	145	334
58	147	347
59	150	360
60	152	373
61	155	387
62	157	400
63	160	413
64	163	427
65	165	440
66	168	454

Normal Adult Males

Age (Yrs)	(in) 60 (cm)152	65 165	70 178	75 191	80 203
20	554	575	594	611	626
25	580	603	622	640	656
30	594	617	637	655	672
35	599	622	643	661	677
40	597	620	641	659	675
45	591	613	633	651	668
50	580	602	622	640	656
55	566	588	608	625	640
60	551	572	591	607	622
65	533	554	572	588	603
70	515	535	552	568	582
75	496	515	532	547	560

Normal Adult Females

Age (Yrs)	(in) 55 (cm)140	60 152	65 165	70 178	75 191
20	444	460	474	486	497
25	455	471	485	497	509
30	458	475	489	502	513
35	458	474	488	501	512
40	453	469	483	496	507
45	446	462	476	488	499
50	437	453	466	478	489
55	427	442	455	467	477
60	415	430	443	454	464
65	403	417	430	441	451
70	390	404	416	427	436
75	377	391	402	413	422

Asthma Management Plan

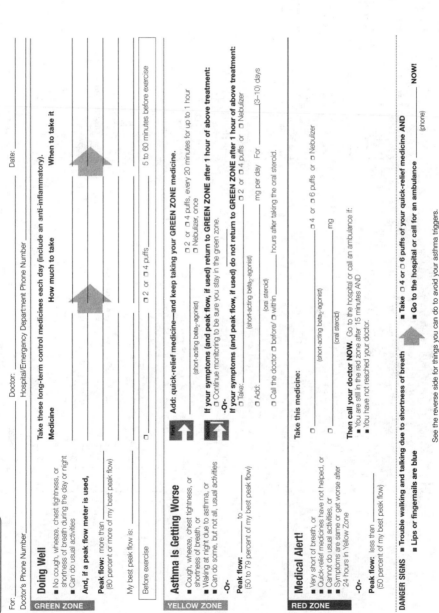

Asthma Action Plan

For: _____ Doctor: _____ Date: _____

Doctor's Phone Number: _____ Hospital/Emergency Department Phone Number: _____

GREEN ZONE — Doing Well

- No cough, wheeze, chest tightness, or shortness of breath during the day or night
- Can do usual activities

And, if a peak flow meter is used,

Peak flow: more than _____ (80 percent or more of my best peak flow)

My best peak flow is: _____

Take these long-term control medicines each day (include an anti-inflammatory).

Medicine	How much to take	When to take it
Before exercise	☐ 2 or ☐ 4 puffs	5 to 60 minutes before exercise

YELLOW ZONE — Asthma Is Getting Worse

- Cough, wheeze, chest tightness, or shortness of breath, or
- Waking at night due to asthma, or
- Can do some, but not all, usual activities

-Or-

Peak flow: _____ to _____ (50 to 79 percent of my best peak flow)

FIRST Add: quick-relief medicine—and keep taking your GREEN ZONE medicine.

_____ (short-acting beta₂-agonist) ☐ 2 or ☐ 4 puffs, every 20 minutes for up to 1 hour ☐ Nebulizer, once

SECOND If your symptoms (and peak flow, if used) return to GREEN ZONE after 1 hour of above treatment:

☐ Continue monitoring to be sure you stay in the green zone.

-Or-

If your symptoms (and peak flow, if used) do not return to GREEN ZONE after 1 hour of above treatment:

☐ Take: _____ (short-acting beta₂-agonist) ☐ 2 or ☐ 4 puffs or ☐ Nebulizer

☐ Add: _____ (oral steroid) _____ mg per day For _____ (3–10) days

☐ Call the doctor ☐ before/ ☐ within _____ hours after taking the oral steroid.

RED ZONE — Medical Alert!

- Very short of breath, or
- Quick-relief medicines have not helped, or
- Cannot do usual activities, or
- Symptoms are same or get worse after 24 hours in Yellow Zone

-Or-

Peak flow: less than _____ (50 percent of my best peak flow)

Take this medicine:

☐ _____ (short-acting beta₂-agonist) ☐ 4 or ☐ 6 puffs or ☐ Nebulizer

☐ _____ (oral steroid) _____ mg

Then call your doctor NOW. Go to the hospital or call an ambulance if:

- You are still in the red zone after 15 minutes AND
- You have not reached your doctor.

DANGER SIGNS
- Trouble walking and talking due to shortness of breath
- Lips or fingernails are blue

→ Take ☐ 4 or ☐ 6 puffs of your quick-relief medicine AND

→ Go to the hospital or call for an ambulance _____ (phone) NOW!

See the reverse side for things you can do to avoid your asthma triggers.

How To Control Things That Make Your Asthma Worse

This guide suggests things you can do to avoid your asthma triggers. Put a check next to the triggers that you know make your asthma worse and ask your doctor to help you find out if you have other triggers as well. Then decide with your doctor what steps you will take.

Allergens

☐ Animal Dander

Some people are allergic to the flakes of skin or dried saliva from animals with fur or feathers.

The best thing to do:

- Keep furred or feathered pets out of your home.

If you can't keep the pet outdoors, then:

- Keep the pet out of your bedroom and other sleeping areas at all times, and keep the door closed.
- Remove carpets and furniture covered with cloth from your home. If that is not possible, keep the pet away from fabric-covered furniture and carpets.

☐ Dust Mites

Many people with asthma are allergic to dust mites. Dust mites are tiny bugs that are found in every home—in mattresses, pillows, carpets, upholstered furniture, bedcovers, clothes, stuffed toys, and fabric or other fabric-covered items.

Things that can help:

- Encase your mattress in a special dust-proof cover.
- Encase your pillow in a special dust-proof cover or wash the pillow each week in hot water. Water must be hotter than 130° F to kill the mites. Cold or warm water used with detergent and bleach can also be effective.
- Wash the sheets and blankets on your bed each week in hot water.
- Reduce indoor humidity to below 60 percent (ideally between 30—50 percent). Dehumidifiers or central air conditioners can do this.
- Try not to sleep or lie on cloth-covered cushions.
- Remove carpets from your bedroom and those laid on concrete, if you can.
- Keep stuffed toys out of the bed or wash the toys weekly in hot water or cooler water with detergent and bleach.

☐ Cockroaches

Many people with asthma are allergic to the dried droppings and remains of cockroaches.

The best thing to do:

- Keep food and garbage in closed containers. Never leave food out.
- Use poison baits, powders, gels, or paste (for example, boric acid). You can also use traps.
- If a spray is used to kill roaches, stay out of the room until the odor goes away.

☐ Indoor Mold

- Fix leaky faucets, pipes, or other sources of water that have mold around them.
- Clean moldy surfaces with a cleaner that has bleach in it.

☐ Pollen and Outdoor Mold

What to do during your allergy season (when pollen or mold spore counts are high):

- Try to keep your windows closed.
- Stay indoors with windows closed from late morning to afternoon, if you can. Pollen and some mold spore counts are highest at that time.
- Ask your doctor whether you need to take or increase anti-inflammatory medicine before your allergy season starts.

Irritants

☐ Tobacco Smoke

- If you smoke, ask your doctor for ways to help you quit. Ask family members to quit smoking, too.
- Do not allow smoking in your home or car.

☐ Smoke, Strong Odors, and Sprays

- If possible, do not use a wood-burning stove, kerosene heater, or fireplace.
- Try to stay away from strong odors and sprays, such as perfume, talcum powder, hair spray, and paints.

Other things that bring on asthma symptoms in some people include:

☐ Vacuum Cleaning

- Try to get someone else to vacuum for you once or twice a week, if you can. Stay out of rooms while they are being vacuumed and for a short while afterward.
- If you vacuum, use a dust mask (from a hardware store), a double-layered or microfilter vacuum cleaner bag, or a vacuum cleaner with a HEPA filter.

☐ Other Things That Can Make Asthma Worse

- Sulfites in foods and beverages: Do not drink beer or wine or eat dried fruit, processed potatoes, or shrimp if they cause asthma symptoms.
- Cold air: Cover your nose and mouth with a scarf on cold or windy days.
- Other medicines: Tell your doctor about all the medicines you take. Include cold medicines, aspirin, vitamins and other supplements, and nonselective beta-blockers (including those in eye drops).

For More Information, go to: www.nhlbi.nih.gov

NIH Publication No. 07-5251
April 2007

U.S. Department of Health and Human Services
National Institutes of Health

National Heart
Lung and Blood Institute

Pediatric Dosage Schedules

IBUPROFEN SUSPENSION (ADVIL, MOTRIN) every 6 hours					
		Fever 102.5°F (39.2°C) or below 5 mg/kg		Fever 102.5°F (39.2°C) or below 10mg/kg	
Age	Weight (lb)	mg	tsp	mg	tsp
6–11 mo	13–17	25	1/4	50	1/2
12–23 mo	18–23	50	1/2	100	1
2–3 yr	24–35	75	3/4	150	1 1/2
4–5 yr	36–47	100	1	200	2
6–8 yr	48–59	125	1 1/4	250	2 1/2
9–10 yr	60–71	150	1 1/2	300	3
11–12 yr	72–95	200	2	400	4

ACETAMINOPHEN (TYLENOL) every 4–6 hours			
Weight (lb)	**Age**	**Dose**	**Dose**
		Tylenol Oral Suspension (160 mg/5 mL)	Tylenol Extra Strength (500 mg Tablet)
6–11	0–3 mos	1.25 mL	–
12–17	4–11 mos	2.5 mL	–
18–23	12–23 mos	3.75 mL	–
24–35	24–36 mos	5 mL	–
36–47	4–5 years	7.5 mL	–
48–59	6–8 years	10 mL	–
60–71	9–10 years	12.5 mL	–
72–95	11 years	15 mL	1 tablet
96 and over	12 years	–	1 tablet

Pediatric Medications

ACYCLOVIR—ANTIVIRAL

Brand Name

Zovirax, Avirax

Uses

Antiviral, used to treat initial and recurrent episodes of mucocutaneous herpes simplex virus (HSV-1 and HSV-2) infections in immunocompromised patients; varicella (chickenpox) infections in immunocompromised patients; acute herpes zoster infection in immunocompetent patients; herpes simplex encephalitis.

Availability

Suspension: 200 mg/5 mL. Tablets: 400 mg, 800 mg. Capsules: 200 mg. Injection: 500 mg/vial, 1 g/vial. Cream, Ointment.

Indications/Routes/Dosage

Varicella infection in immunocompromised patients: Children age 12 years or older: 800 mg PO q4h (5 times/day while awake) for 5 days. Children age 2 years or older and weighing < 40 kg: 20 mg/kg (max: 800 mg/dose) PO qid for 5 days.

Acute herpes zoster: Children age 12 years or older: 800 mg PO q4h (5 times/day) for 7–10 days.

Genital herpes (initial episode): Adults: 200 mg q4h (5 times/day) for 10 days.

Genital herpes (recurrent episode): Adults: 200 mg q4h (5 times/day) for 5 days.

Usual topical dosage: Adults: 3–6 times/day for 7 days.

Labial herpes: Apply cream to affected area 4–6 times/day for 10 days; apply ointment q3h 6 times/day for 7 days—use glove or applicator stick to apply.

Adverse Reactions

Malaise, headache, encephalopathic changes, nausea, vomiting, diarrhea hematuria, acute renal failure, thrombocytopenia, leukopenia, rash, itching, urticaria, inflammation or phlebitis at injection site.

Implications

- May increase blood urea nitrogen (BUN) and creatinine levels. May decrease white blood count (WBC) and increase or decrease platelet count.
- Use cautiously in patients with neurologic problems, renal disease, or dehydration. Monitor renal function.
- Drink adequate fluids, do not touch lesions with fingers to prevent spreading infection to new site, use finger cot or rubber glove to apply topical ointment.
- Avoid sexual intercourse while lesions present to prevent spread to partner.

ALBUTEROL—BRONCHODILATOR

Brand Name

Ventolin, Proventil

Uses

Relaxes bronchial, uterine, and vascular smooth muscle, to prevent or treat bronchospasm.

Availability

Aerosol inhaler: 90 mcg/metered spray, 100 mcg/metered spray. Albuterol sulfate: Capsules for inhalation: 200 mcg. Solution for inhalation: 0.083% mg/mL, 0.5% mg/mL, 0.63 mg/mL, 1.25 mg/3 mL. Syrup: 2 mg/5 mL. Tablets: 2 mg, 4 mg. Tablets, extended-release: 4 mg, 8 mg.

Indications/Routes/Dosage

Prevention/treatment of bronchospasm in patients with reversible obstructive airway disease: Aerosol inhalation: Children 4 years old or older: 1 or 2 inhalations q4–6h. Capsules for inhalation: Children 4 years old or older: 200 mcg inhaled q4–6h. Solution for inhalation: Children 12 years old or older: 2.5 mg tid or qid by nebulizer. Children

2–12 years old: initially, 0.1–0.15 mg/kg by nebulizer, with subsequent dosing titrated to response, not to exceed 2.5 mg tid or qid by nebulization.

Syrup or oral tablets: Children 2–6 years: initially, 0.1 mg/kg PO tid. Starting dose should not exceed 2 mg (1 tsp) tid. Do not exceed 4 mg tid. Children 6–14 years: 2 mg PO tid or qid. Do not exceed 24 mg daily. Adults, children 14 years old or older: 2–4 mg PO tid or qid. Do not exceed 8 mg qid.

Extended-release tablets: Children 6–12 years old: 4 mg PO q12h. Adults, children older than 12 years: 4–8 mg PO q12h.

To prevent exercise-induced bronchospasm: 2 aerosol inhalations 15–30 min before exercise.

Adverse Reactions

Nervousness, dizziness, headache, weakness, insomnia, nasal congestion, hoarseness, tachycardia, hypertension, nausea, vomiting, heartburn, increased appetite, hypokalemia, muscle cramps, bronchospasm, cough, increased sputum.

Implications

- Use caution in patients with diabetes mellitus, hypertension, or hyperthyroidism.
- Teach family how to use inhaler properly.
- Increase fluid intake.
- Do not take more than 2 inhalations at any one time to prevent paradoxical bronchoconstriction.
- Rinse mouth after inhalation.

AMOXICILLIN—ANTIBIOTIC

Brand Name

Amoxil (generic also available)

Uses

Treat otitis media, upper and lower respiratory tract, soft tissue, skin, GI, GU, and gonorrhea infections. Used to treat: Gram-positive cocci: *Staphylococcus aureus, Streptococcus pyogenes, Streptococcus faecalis, Streptococcus pneumoniae.* Gram-negative cocci: *Neisseria gonorrhoeae, Neisseria meningitides.* Gram-positive bacillus: *Corynebacterium diphtheriae, Listeria monocytogenes.* Gram-negative bacillus: *Haemophilus influenzae,*

Escherichia coli, Proteus mirabilis, Salmonella; also used in bacterial endocarditis prophylaxis.

Availability

Suspension: 125/5 mL, 200/5 mL, 250/5 mL, 400/5 mL. Tablets: 500 mg, 875 mg. Pediatric drops: 50 mg/mL. Tablets, chewable: 125 mg, 200 mg, 250 mg, 400 mg. Capsules: 250 mg, 500 mg.

Indications/Routes/Dosage

Ear, nose, throat, GU, skin/structure infections: Children < 20 kg: 20–40 mg/kg/day divided q8–12h. Children, adults > 20 kg: 250–500 mg q8h or 500–875 mg 2 times/day.

Lower respiratory tract infections: Children < 20 kg: 40 mg/kg/day divided q8–12h. Children, adults > 20 kg: 500 mg q8h or 875 mg tablets 2 times/day.

Acute uncomplicated gonorrhea, epididymitis-orchitis: Adults: 3 g once with 1 g probenecid PO follow with tetracycline or erythromycin.

Acute otitis media: Children: 80–90 mg/kg/day divided bid for those at high risk.

Adverse Reactions

Mild diarrhea, rash, oral/vaginal candidiasis; superinfection, colitis, allergic reaction–anaphylaxis.

Implications

- Take all of medication.
- Report rash or severe diarrhea.
- Discard suspension after 14 days.

AMOXICILLIN-CLAVULANATE—POTASSIUM ANTIBIOTIC

Brand Name

Augmentin

Uses

Treat lower respiratory infection, otitis media, sinusitis, skin infections, urinary tract infections caused by susceptible strains of Gram-positive and Gram-negative organisms.

Availability

Oral suspension: 125 mg/5 mL, 200 mg/5 mL, 250 mg/5 mL, 400 mg/5mL. Tablets: 250 mg, 500 mg, 875 mg. Tablets, chewable: 125 mg, 200 mg, 250 mg, 400 mg.

Indications/Routes/Dosage

Recurrent or persistent otitis media caused by *Streptococcus pneumoniae, Haemophilus influenzae,* or *Moraxella catarrhalis:* Augmentin ES-600. Children older than 3 months: 90 mg/kg/day, based on amoxicillin component, PO q12h for 10 days.

Lower respiratory infections, otitis media, sinusitis, skin infections, urinary tract infections caused by susceptible strains of Gram-positive and Gram-negative organisms: Adults, children weighing > 40 kg: 250 mg (based on amoxicillin component) PO q8h or 500 mg q12h. May use 500 mg PO q8h OR 875 mg PO q12h for more severe infections. Children weighing < 40 kg: 20 to 45 mg/kg, based on amoxicillin component and severity of infection, PO daily in divided doses q8–12h.

Children 3 months of age or older: 30 mg/kg/day PO in divided doses q12h.

Adverse Reactions

Nausea, vomiting, diarrhea, agitation, confusion, dizziness, insomnia, enterocolitis, pseudomembranous colitis, abdominal pain, vaginitis, anemia, thrombocytopenia, hypersensitivity reactions.

Implications

- May decrease effectiveness of hormonal contraceptives.
- *Note:* oral suspensions have varying clavulanic acid content.
- Continue antibiotic for full length of treatment, take with meals.

AZITHROMYCIN—MACROLIDE ANTIBIOTIC

Brand Name

Zithromax

Uses

Treat community-acquired pneumonia, otitis media, pharyngitis, tonsillitis, dental prophylaxis in patients allergic to penicillin, uncomplicated gonococcal infections, chlamydial infections.

Availability

Powder for oral suspension: 100 mg/5 mL, 200 mg/5 mL, 1000 mg/packet. Tablets: 250 mg, 500 mg, 600 mg. Injection: 500 mg.

Indications/Routes/Dosage

Otitis media: Children older than 6 months: 10 mg/kg PO daily for 3 days OR 10 mg/kg PO on day 1 then 5 mg/kg once daily on days 2–5.

Pharyngitis, tonsillitis: Children older than 2 years: 12 mg/kg (max 500 mg) PO daily for 5 days.

Dental prophylaxis: Adults: 500 mg PO 1 hour before procedure. Children: 15 mg/kg PO 1 h before procedure.

Chlamydial infections: Adults, adolescents older than 16 years: 1 g PO as a single dose.

Adverse Reactions

Dizziness, headache, fatigue, palpitations, chest pain, nausea, vomiting, diarrhea, abdominal pain, cholestatic jaundice, pseudomembranous colitis, candidiasis, vaginitis, rash, photosensitivity, angioedema.

Implications

- Use cautiously with liver impairment.
- Give oral suspension 1 hour before or 2 hours after meals.
- Do not give with antacids.

BENZOCAINE—TOPICAL OTIC ANALGESIC

Brand Name

Auralgan Otic Solution

Uses

Topical analgesic to reduce pain associated with acute otitis media.

Availability

10-mL bottle.

Indications/Routes/Dosage

Instill drops until ear canal is full, put wick into ear canal. May repeat every 1–2 hours as needed.

Adverse Reactions

Irritation of ear canal.

Implications

- Do not let dropper touch ear canal, do not rinse ear dropper after use, keep out of the reach of children.
- Have child lay on side and tilt the affected ear upward, pull ear lobe up and instill medication, have child lay on side for 5 minutes then insert wick.
- Do not use on perforated eardrum.

BUDESONIDE—INHALATION CORTICOSTEROID ANTI-INFLAMMATORY

Brand Name

Entocort EC, Pulmicort, Rhinocort

Uses

Manage symptoms of seasonal or perennial allergic rhinitis.

Availability

Nasal inhaler: 32 mcg/metered spray (Rhinocort AQ). Nasal spray: 50 mcg/dose (Pulmicort). Powder for inhalation: 200 mcg/inhalation (Pulmicort Turbuhaler). Suspension for oral inhalation: 0.25 mg/2 mL, 0.5 mg/2 mL (Pulmicort Respules).

Indications/Routes/Dosage

Intranasal: Children older than 6 years, adults: Rhinocort: 2 sprays each nostril 2 times/day or 4 sprays to each nostril in morning. Rhinocort Aqua: 1 spray to each nostril once daily. Children younger than 12 years: 4 sprays/day. Children older than 12 years: 8 sprays/day.

Nebulization: Children 1–8 years: 0.25–1 mg/day titrated to lowest effective dosage.
Inhalation: Children older than 6 years, adults: initially 200–400 mcg 2 times/day to max 400 mcg 2 times/day.

Rhinitis: Nasal inhalation: Children older than 6 years: initial, 2 sprays/nostril twice daily. Adult: initial 2 sprays/nostril bid or 4 sprays/nostril in the morning. Max 4 sprays/nostril per day. Nasal spray: Children older than 6 years: initial, 1 spray/nostril once a day. Max dose 4 sprays/nostril/day. Children younger than 12 years: 2 sprays/nostril once a day. Not recommended for children younger than 6 years. Children older than 12 years: 4 sprays/nostril, once a day. Nasal spray: initial, 1 spray/nostril once daily, max 4 sprays/nostril once a day.

Adverse Reactions

Mild nasopharyngeal irritation, burning stinging, headache, throat irritation, epistaxis, Cushing's syndrome, cataract, adrenal suppression, glaucoma.

Implications

- Use caution in patients with cataracts, diabetes mellitus, exposure to viral infections, glaucoma, liver cirrhosis, peptic ulcer.
- Do not consume grapefruit juice during oral treatment.
- Reduce dose for hepatic insufficiency.
- May take 3–7 days for full effect.

CEFDINIR—THIRD-GENERATION CEPHALOSPORIN ANTIBIOTIC

Brand Name

Omnicef

Uses

Treat susceptible infections due to *Streptococcus pyogenes, S. pneumoniae, Haemophilus influenzae, H. parainfluenzae, Moraxella catarrhalis*, acute maxillary sinusitis, chronic bronchitis, community-acquired pneumonia, otitis media, pharyngitis/tonsillitis, skin infections.

Availability

Suspension: 125 mg/5 mL; 250 mg/5mL; Capsule: 300 mg.

Indications/Routes/Dosage

Children older than 6 mos: 7 mg/kg PO q12h for 10 days or 14 mg/kg PO once a day for 10 days, max 600 mg/day.

Children: < 20 kg: 2.5 mL (0.5tsp) q12h or 5 mL (1 tsp) q24h. 20–40 lbs: 5 mL (1 tsp) q12h or 10 mL (2 tsp) q24h. 41–60 lbs: 7.5 mL (1.5 tsp) q12h or 15 mL (3 tsp) q24h. 61–80 lbs: 10 mL (2 tsp) q12h or 20 mL (4 tsp) q24h. 81–85 lbs: 12 mL (2.5 tsp) q12h or 24 mL (5 tsp) q24h.

Adults: 300 mg PO q12h or 600 mg PO once a day for 10 days.

Adverse Reactions

Diarrhea, nausea, oral and vaginal candidiasis, headache.

Implications

- May take with or without food.
- Take antacids 2 hours before or after taking medication.
- Take for full length of treatment.
- Suspension can be stored at room temperature, discard after 10 days.
- Adjust dose in renal impairment.

CEFPROZIL—SECOND-GENERATION CEPHALOSPORIN ANTIBIOTIC

Brand Name

Cefzil

Uses

Treat susceptible infections due to *Streptococcus pneumoniae, S. pyogenes, Staphylococcus aureus, Haemophilus influenzae, Moraxella catarrhalis*, acute or chronic bronchitis, secondary bacterial infection, acute sinusitis, otitis media, pharyngitis/tonsillitis, skin infections.

Availability

Oral suspension: 125 mg/5 mL, 250 mg/5 mL. Tablets: 250 mg, 500 mg.

Indications/Routes/Dosage

Acute sinusitis: Children 6 months–12 years: 7.5–15 mg/kg PO q12h for 10 days. Adults: 500 mg PO q12h for 10 days.

  Otitis media: Children 6 mos–12 years: 15 mg/kg PO q12h for 10 days (max 1 g/day).

  Bronchitis: Adult: 500 mg PO q12h for 10 days.

  Pharyngitis/tonsillitis: Children 2–12 years: 7.5 mg/kg PO q12h for 10 days. Adults: 500 mg PO q24h for 10 days.

  Skin infections: Children 2–12 years: 20 mg/kg PO q24h for 10 days. Adults: 250 mg–500 mg PO q12–24h for 10 days.

Adverse Reactions

Diarrhea, nausea, vomiting; diaper rash, oral and vaginal candidiasis, dizziness, elevation of liver enzymes, severe hypersensitivity reactions.

Implications

- Refrigerate suspension, discard after 14 days.
- May take with or without food.
- Adjust dose for renal impairment.

CEFTRIAXONE—THIRD-GENERATION CEPHALOSPORIN ANTIBIOTIC

Brand Name

Rocephin

Uses

Treat susceptible infections due to Gram-negative bacilli: *Haemophilus influenzae, Escherichia coli, Proteus mirabilis, Klebsiella, Enterobacter, Salmonella, Shigella,*

Neisseria, Serratia; Gram-positive organisms: *Streptococcus pneumoniae, S. pyogenes, Staphylococcus aureus;* serious lower respiratory tract, urinary tract, gonorrhea, meningitis, septicemia, bone, joint infections.

Availability

Powder for injection: 500 mg, 1 g, 2 g, 10 g.

Indications/Routes/Dosage

Children: 50–75 mg/kg/day divided q12h; adult 1–2 g daily. Max 2 g q12h.
   Uncomplicated gonorrhea: adults: 250 mg IM as a single dose.
   Meningitis: Children, adult: 100 mg/kg/day IM divided q12h. Max 4 g/day.

Adverse Reactions

Nausea, vomiting, diarrhea, anorexia, hypersensitivity, nephrotoxicity.

Implications

● Assess sensitivity to penicillin and other cephalosporins (10% cross over).
● Watch for adverse reactions.

CEFUROXIME SODIUM, CEFUROXIME AXETIL—SECOND-GENERATION CEPHALOSPORIN ANTIBIOTICS

Brand Name

Kefurox, Zinacef, Cefuroxime Axetil, Ceftin

Uses

Treat susceptible infections due to Group B streptococci, pneumococci, staphylococci, *Haemophilus influenzae, Escherichia coli, Enterobacter, Klebsiella*, bone and joint infection, gonorrhea, lower respiratory tract infections, meningitis, preoperative prophylaxis, septicemia, urinary tract infections.

Availability

Suspension: 125 mg/5 mL, 250 mg/5 mL. Tablet: 250 mg, 500 mg. Infusion: 1.5 g/50 mL, 750 mg/50 mL. Injection: 1.5 g, 7.5 g, 750 mg.

Indications/Routes/Dosage

Pharyngitis/tonsillitis: Tablets: 125 mg PO bid for 10 days. Children 3 mos–12 years: 30 mg/kg/day PO in 2 divided doses for 10 days. Max 500 mg/day.

Impetigo, otitis media, sinusitis: Children 3 mos–12 years: 30 mg/kg/day PO in 2 divided doses for 10 days. Max 1 g/day. Tablets: 250 mg PO bid for 10 days.

Susceptible infections: Neonates: 20–100 mg/kg/day IV in divided doses q12h. Children older than 3 months: 50–100 mg/kg/day IV/IM divided q6–8h.

Bone and joint infections: Children older than 3 mos: 150 mg/kg/day IV/IM divided q8h.

Meningitis: Children 3 months old or older: 200–240 mg/kg/day IV/IM divided q6–8h. Max 9 g/day.

Bronchitis: Adults: 250 or 500 mg PO bid for 10 days.

Gonorrhea: Adults: 1 g PO as a single dose; 1.5 g IM as a single dose with 1.5 g probenecid PO.

Gonococcal infections: Adults: 750 mg IV/IM q8h.

Pharyngitis/tonsillitis/sinusitis: Adults: 250 mg PO bid for 10 days.

Skin infections: Adults: 250–500 mg PO bid for 10 days.

Urinary tract infections: Adults: 125mg or 250 mg PO bid for 7–10 days.

Adverse Reactions

Local reactions at IV/IM site; diarrhea, abdominal cramping, nausea; oral and vaginal candidiasis.

Implications

- Adjust dose for renal impairment.
- Take antibiotic for full length of treatment.

CEPHALEXIN HYDROCHLORIDE—FIRST-GENERATION CEPHALOSPORIN ANTIBIOTIC

Brand Name

Keftab, Keflex, Biocef

Uses

Treat infections of respiratory tract, GI tract, skin, soft tissue, bone, joints, and otitis media caused by *Escherichia coli* and other coliform bacteria, Group A beta-hemolytic streptococci, *Klebsiella* species, *Proteus mirabilis, Streptococcus pneumoniae,* and staphylococci.

Availability

Cephalexin hydrochloride: Tablets: 500 mg. Cephalexin monohydrate: Oral suspension: 125 mg/5 mL, 250 mg/5 mL. Tablets: 250 mg, 500 mg, 1 g. Capsules: 250 mg, 500 mg.

Indications/Routes/Dosage

Children: 25–50 mg/kg/day PO in 2 to 4 equally divided doses. Adults: 250 mg–1 g PO q6h or 500 mg q12h. Max 4 g daily. Dose can be doubled in severe infections.

Adverse Reactions

Dizziness, headache, confusion, fatigue, hallucinations, nausea, vomiting, diarrhea, pseudomembranous colitis, oral candidiasis, vaginitis, genital pruritus, interstitial nephritis, neutropenia, anemia, thrombocytopenia, arthritis, joint pain, rash, urticaria, hypersensitivity reactions.

Implications

- Take with food or milk.
- There is a possibility of cross-sensitivity with penicillin and other beta-lactam antibiotics.
- Adjust dose for renal impairment.
- Avoid using with aminoglycosides, increases risk of nephrotoxicity.

CETIRIZINE—ANTIHISTAMINE

Brand Name

Zyrtec

Uses

Rhinitis, allergic symptoms.

Availability

Syrup: 5 mg/5 mL. Tablets: 5 mg, 10 mg.

Indications/Routes/Dosage

Child 2–6 years: 2.5 mg daily may increase to 5 mg daily or 2.5 mg bid.
Child older than 6 years, adult: 5–10 mg daily.
Zyrtec D (5 mg with 120 mg pseudoephedrine) once bid.

Adverse Reactions

Thickening of bronchial secretions, dry mouth, headache, drowsiness.

Implications

- Avoid driving if drowsiness occurs; use sunscreen when in sunlight.
- Notify provider of difficulty voiding.

CIPROFLOXACIN HYDROCHLORIDE— FLUOROQUINOLONE ANTI-INFECTIVE

Brand Name

Cipro

Uses

Treat conjunctival keratitis, keratoconjunctivitis, corneal ulcers, blepharitis, dacryocystitis, blepharoconjunctivitis.

Availability

Ophthalmic: 0.03%; Otic (Ciprodex).

Indications/Routes/Dosage

Conjunctivitis: 1–2 drops q2h for 2 days, then q4h next 5 days.
Corneal ulcer: 2 drops q15min for 6h, then 2 drops q30min remainder first day; 2 drops q1h second day; then q4h days 3–14.
Otic: older than 6 months, 4 drops in ear bid for 7 days.

Adverse Reactions

Ophthalmic: Sensitization may contraindicate later systemic use of ciprofloxacin.

Implications

- Tilt patient's head back, put drops in conjunctival sac.
- Do not use ophthalmic solution as injection.

CLARITHROMYCIN—MACROLIDE ANTIBIOTIC

Brand Name

Biaxin, Biaxin XL

Uses

Treat bronchitis, otitis media, acute maxillary sinusitis, pharyngitis, tonsillitis, pneumonia, skin infections.

Availability

Suspension: 125/5 mL, 250/5 mL. Tablets: 250 mg, 500 mg. Tablets, extended-release: 500 mg.

Indications/Routes/Dosages

Acute otitis media: Children: 15 mg/kg/day in 2 divided doses for 10 days.

Respiratory/skin infections: Children: 15 mg/kg/day in 2 divided doses for 10 days. Usual adult dose: 250–500 mg q12h for 7–14 days. Extended release: Two 500-mg tablets daily for 7–14 days.

Adverse Reactions

Antibiotic-associated colitis (severe abdominal pain, fever, watery diarrhea), superinfection, hepatotoxicity, thrombocytopenia.

Implications

- Monitor bowel activity and stool consistency.
- For minor GI effects take with food.
- Doses should be evenly spaced.
- Take with 8 oz water.

CLINDAMYCIN—ANTIBIOTIC

Brand Name

Cleocin

Uses

Treat infections from staphylococci, streptococci, Rickettsia, *Pneumocystis carinii* pneumonia.

Availability

Oral solution: 75 mg/mL. Capsules: 75 mg, 150 mg, 300 mg.

Indications/Routes/Dosage

Children younger than 1 month: 15–20 mg/kg/day divided q6–8h. Children older than 1 month 8–25 mg/kg/day divided q6–8h. Adult: 150–450 mg q6h. Max 1.8 g/day.

Adverse Reactions

Nausea, vomiting, diarrhea, pseudomembranous colitis (severe diarrhea), urinary frequency, vaginitis.

Implications

- Take with full glass of water.
- Give with food to reduce GI symptoms.
- Antiperistaltic drugs may worsen diarrhea.
- Do not break, crush, or chew capsules.
- Call provider for diarrhea.

CLOMIPRAMINE HYDROCHLORIDE—TRICYCLIC ANTIDEPRESSANT

Brand Name

Anafranil

Uses

Treat obsessive-compulsive disorder manifested as repetitive tasks producing marked distress; off label: mental depression, panic disorder, neurogenic pain, bulimia.

Availability

Capsules: 25 mg, 50 mg, 75 mg.

Indications/Routes/Dosage

Children: starting dose of 10 mg/day; increase to 75–100 mg/day. Teens: starting dose of 10 mg/day increase to 100–200 mg/day.

Adverse Reactions

Dry mouth, dizziness, sleepiness, tremors, decreased libido, headache, aggressiveness, high doses may produce cardiovascular effects (severe postural hypotension, dizziness, tachycardia, palpitations, arrhythmias, seizures). Abrupt withdrawal from prolonged therapy may produce headache, malaise, nausea, vomiting.

Implications

- Contraindicated within 14 days of MAO inhibitor ingestion.
- Caution with history of seizures, hyperthyroidism, cardiac/hepatic/renal disease, diabetes mellitus.
- May cause dry mouth, blurred vision, constipation, drowsiness.
- Ability to tolerate postural hypotension, sedative, and anticholinergic effects occurs during early therapy.
- Maximum therapeutic effect occurs in 2–4 weeks.
- Do not abruptly stop medication.
- Avoid tasks that require alertness, motor skills until drug response is established.
- Wear sunscreen to prevent photosensitivity.

CROTAMITON—SCABICIDE, ANTIPRURITIC

Brand Name

Eurax

Uses

Treat parasitic infestation (scabies), pruritus.

Availability

Topical cream: 10%. Topical lotion: 10%.

Indications/Routes/Dosage

For itching, apply locally, massaging affected area until medication absorbed.

Adverse Reactions

Dermatitis, skin irritation.

Implications

- Patient should wash entire body with soap and water.
- Avoid application to face, eyes, mouth, or mucous membranes; avoid applying to inflamed skin or raw, oozing skin surfaces.
- Remove any crusting and apply a thin layer of cream over entire body from the chin down.
- Apply second coat. Wash medication off 48 hours after second coat applied.
- Repeat treatment in 7–10 days if new lesions develop.

DIPHENHYDRAMINE HYDROCHLORIDE— ANTIHISTAMINE, ANTIPRURITIC, ANTITUSSIVE

Brand Name

Benadryl, Nytol, Allerdryl

Uses

Treat allergy symptoms, rhinitis, motion sickness, urticaria.

Availability

Elixir: 125 mg/5 mL. Syrup: 12.5 mg/5 mL. Tablets: 25 mg, 50 mg. Tablets, chewable: 25 mg. Capsules: 25 mg, 50 mg.

Indications/Routes/Dosage

Children younger than 2 years: 2 mg/kg q4–6h.

Children 2–6 years: 6.25 mg q4–6h. Max 37.5 mg/day. 6–12 years: 12.5–25 mg q4–6h. Max 150 mg/day. Children older than 12 years, adults: 25–50 mg q4–6h. Max 300 mg/day.

Moderate to severe allergic reaction: Children: 5 mg/kg/day divided q6–8h. Max 300 mg/day. Adults: 25–50 mg q4h. Max 400 mg/day.

Adverse Reactions

Dizziness, drowsiness, dry nose, throat.

Implications

● Avoid tasks that require alertness, motor skills until response to drug is established, avoid alcohol.

ERYTHROMYCIN—ANTIBIOTIC

Brand Name

Erythromycin, EES

Uses

Treat upper and lower respiratory infections such as pneumonia, bronchitis, pharyngitis, otitis media, pertussis, Legionnaires' disease, prophylaxis for rheumatic fever, oral surgery, intestinal and skin infections, gonorrheal pelvic inflammatory infection (if penicillin is contraindicated), Lyme disease (younger than 9 years).

Availability

Tablets: 250 mg, 333 mg, 500 mg. Tablets, delayed-release: 333 mg. Capsules, delayed-release: 250 mg.

Estolate: Oral suspension: 125 mg/5 mL, 250 mg/5 mL. Tablets: 500 mg. Capsules: 250 mg.

Ethylsuccinate: Oral suspension: 200 mg/5 mL, 400 mg/5 mL. Tablets: 400 mg. Tablets, chewable: 200 mg.

Stearate: Tablets: 250 mg, 500 mg.

Indications/Routes/Dosage

Base and ethylsuccinate: Children: 30–50 mg/kg/day divided q6–8h up to 60–100 mg/kg/day for severe infections for 10 days, not to exceed 2 g/day. Adults: delayed-release: 333 mg q8h increase up to 4 g/day.

Ethylsuccinate: Adults: 400–800 mg q6–12h.

Estolate: 30–50 mg/kg/day divided q6–12h. Do not exceed 2 g/day. Adults: 250–500 mg q6–12h.

Stearate: 30–50 mg/kg/day divided q6h. Do not exceed 2 g/day. Adults: 250–500 mg q6–12h.

Pertussis: 40–50 mg/kg/day divided q6h for 14 days.

Prophylaxis for rheumatic fever: 250 mg bid if penicillin allergy.

Chlamydia trachomatis: 50 mg/kg/day divided q6h for 10–14 days.

Adverse Reactions

Nausea, vomiting, abdominal pain, diarrhea, rash, anaphylaxis.

Implications

- Avoid milk and acidic beverages 1 hour before or after a dose.
- Take with food or snack to decrease GI upset.
- Do not break or chew tablets or capsules.
- Suspension is stable for 14 days at room temperature.

FERROUS SULFATE—IRON PREPARATION

Brand Name

Feosol, Fer-In-Sol

Uses

Treat iron-deficiency anemia.

Availability

Feosol: Tablets: 200 mg (65 mg elemental iron). Fer-In-Sol: Drops: 75 mg/0.6 mL (15 mg elemental iron/0.6 mL).

Indications/Routes/Dosage

Mild to moderate iron deficiency: 3 mg elemental iron/kg/day in 1–2 divided doses.
  Severe iron deficiency: 4–6 mg elemental iron/kg/day in 3 divided doses.

Adverse Reactions

Nausea, diarrhea, black stools, constipation, black urine, teeth staining.

Implications

- Interactions: antacids, tetracycline will reduce absorption. Vitamin C enhances absorption.
- Give between meals with orange juice; do not give with milk. Give with a straw or brush teeth after giving.
- May cause abdominal discomfort, keep out of the reach of small children.

FEXOFENADINE HYDROCHLORIDE—ANTIHISTAMINE

Brand Name

Allegra

Uses

Treat seasonal allergic rhinitis.

Availability

Tablets: 30 mg, 60 mg, 180 mg. Capsules: 60 mg. Capsules, extended-release: 180 mg.

Indications/Routes/Dosage

Children older than 12 years: 60 mg bid or 180 mg once daily.
  Children 6–11 years: 30 mg bid.

Adverse Reactions

Dry mouth, nose, headache, fatigue, nausea, vomiting.

Implications

- Avoid tasks that require alertness, motor skills until response to drug is known.
- Avoid alcohol, coffee, or tea; may decrease drowsiness.

FLUOXETINE—SELECTIVE SEROTONIN REUPTAKE INHIBITOR (SSRI), ANTIDEPRESSANT

Brand Name

Prozac, Sarafem (Prozac weekly)

Uses

Treat major depression, obsessive-compulsive disorder (OCD), bulimia nervosa, premenstrual dysphoric disorder (PMDD).

Availability

Oral solution: 20 mg/5 mL. Tablets: 10 mg, 20 mg. Capsules: 10 mg, 20 mg, 40 mg.

Indications/Routes/Dosage

Anxiety disorders: starting dose of 5 mg/day, increase to 15–30 mg/day for children and 10–40 mg/day for teens.

Major depression: starting dose of 5 mg/day increase to 15–40 mg per day for children, 10–60 mg/day for teens.

Adverse Reactions

Headache, nervousness, insomnia, drowsiness, anxiety, tremor, dizziness, sedation, poor concentration, abnormal dreams, decreased libido, dry mouth, diarrhea, weight loss.

Implications

- Take with food and milk for GI symptoms.
- Can crush tablet if patient unable to swallow.
- Take at night to decrease oversedation.
- Therapeutic effect may take 1–4 weeks.

- Use sunscreen to prevent photosensitivity.
- Avoid alcohol and other CNS depressants.
- Notify prescriber if pregnant, plan to become pregnant, or are breastfeeding.
- Change position slowly due to orthostatic hypotension.
- Educate parents about FDA concerns of suicide risk in patients on SSRI antidepressants, monitor suicidal risk closely during course of treatment especially in the first 30 days of treatment.

FLUVOXAMINE—SELECTIVE SEROTONIN REUPTAKE INHIBITOR, ANTIDEPRESSANT, ANTIANXIETY

Brand Name

Luvox

Uses

Treat obsessive-compulsive disorder (OCD), major depression, anxiety disorders.

Availability

Tablets: 25 mg, 50 mg, 100 mg.

Indications/Routes/Dosage

Starting dose of 25 mg/day, increase to 50–200 mg/day for children and 150–300 mg/day for teens.

Adverse Reactions

Headache, drowsiness, dizziness, convulsions, nausea, vomiting, anorexia, constipation, diarrhea, decreased libido, increased effect with St. John's wort. Fatal reactions: MAO inhibitor interactions increase action of propranolol, diazepam, lithium, warfarin, carbamazepine, theophylline.

Implications

- Give with food, milk for GI distress.
- Therapeutic effects may take 2–3 weeks. Use caution when driving.

- Do not use with other CNS depressants, e.g., alcohol, barbiturates, benzodiazepines, St. John's wort.
- Educate parents about FDA concerns of suicide risk in patients on SSRI antidepressants; monitor suicidal risk closely during course of treatment especially in the first 30 days of treatment.

FOLIC ACID—NUTRITION SUPPLEMENT

Brand Name

Folate, Folvite

Uses

Treat anemia due to folate deficiency, nutritional supplement to prevent neural tube defects.

Availability

Tablets: 0.4 mg, 0.8 mg, 1.0 mg.

Indications/Routes/Dosage

Recommended daily intake for children: 6 months–3 years: 50 mcg (15 mcg/kg/day). 4–6 years: 75 mcg. 7–10 years: 100 mcg. 11–14 years: 150 mcg. Older than15 years: 200 mcg.

Dosage: Infants: 15 mcg/kg/daily. Children: 1 mg/day initial dosage. Maintenance dose, 1–10 years: 0.1–0.4 mg/day. Children older than 11 years, adults: 1 mg/day initial dose; maintenance dose 0.5 mg/day.

Adverse Reactions

Flushing, irritability, difficulty sleeping, malaise, rash, itching, GI upset, hypersensitivity reactions.

Implications

- Take everyday.
- Call provider if adverse reactions.

LACTULOSE—HYPEROSMOTIC LAXATIVE

Brand Name

Constilac, Constulose, Enulose

Uses

Treat constipation.

Availability

Syrup: 10 mg/15 mL. Packets: 10 g, 20 g.

Indications/Routes/Dosage

Children: 7.5 mL/day after breakfast. Adults: 15–30 mL/day up to 60 mL/day.

Adverse Reactions

Cramping, flatulence, increased thirst, abdominal discomfort, diarrhea indicates an overdose.

Implications

- Drink water, juice, milk with each dose.
- Evacuation occurs in 24–48 hours of initial dose.
- Patients should also be on a high-fiber diet and exercise to promote defecation.

LEVALBUTEROL—BRONCHODILATOR

Brand Name

Xopenex

Uses

Prevention of bronchospasm due to reversible obstructive airway disease.

Availability

Solution for nebulization: 0.63 mg OR 1.25 mg in 3-mL vials (no dilution necessary).

Indications/Routes/Dosage

Children older than12 years: 0.63–1.25 mg q6–8h (tid), with max of 1.25 mg tid.

Adverse Reactions

Tremors, nervousness, headache, throat dryness/irritation, palpitations, chest pain, extrasystole.

Implications

- Monitor rate, depth, rhythm, and type of respiration.
- Increase fluid intake.
- Rinse mouth with water after inhalation.
- Avoid caffeine.

LITHIUM CARBONATE—ANTIMANIC, ANTIDEPRESSANT

Brand Name

Eskalith, Dura-Lith

Uses

Prophylaxis, treatment of acute mania, manic phase of bipolar disorder.

Availability

Syrup: 300 mg/5 mL. Tablets: 300 mg. Tablets, slow-release: 300 mg, 450 mg. Capsules: 150 mg, 300 mg, 600 mg.

Indications/Routes/Dosage

Start at 25 mg/kg/day, gradually increase until serum level reaches therapeutic range of 0.9–1.1 mEq/L.

Adverse Reactions

Headache, drowsiness, dizziness, anorexia, nausea, vomiting, diarrhea, hypotension, dry mouth. May increase effects of antithyroid medication, iodinate glycerol, potassium iodide. Nonsteroidal anti-inflammatory drugs (NSAIDs) and diuretics may increase concentration, toxicity. May decrease absorption of phenothiazines.

Implications

- Give with meals, milk.
- Limit alcohol, caffeine.
- May cause dry mouth.
- Do not crush, chew, or break extended-release or film-coated tablets.
- Assess serum lithium levels q3–4 days during initial phase of therapy, q1–2 months thereafter and weekly if no improvement.
- Monitor for signs of lithium toxicity vomiting, diarrhea, drowsiness, incoordination, hand tremor, muscle twitching, mental confusion, ataxia.

LORATADINE—ANTIHISTAMINE

Brand Name

Claritin

Uses

Treat seasonal rhinitis.

Availability

Syrup: 5 mg/5 mL. Tablet: 10 mg.

Indications/Routes/Dosage

Children 2–12 years: 5 mg daily. Children older than12 years, adult: 10 mg daily.

Adverse Reactions

Sedation is more common with larger doses, headache.

Implications

- Use sunscreen (photosensitive).
- Avoid driving if drowsiness occurs.
- Additive CNS effects with alcohol and antidepressants.

MEBENDAZOLE—ANTHELMINTIC

Brand Name

Vermox

Uses

Treatment of *Enterobius vermicularis* (pinworms), *Ascaris lumbricoides* (roundworm), *Trichuris trichiura* (whipworm), and *Ancylostoma duodenale* (common hookworm).

Availability

Tablets, chewable: 100 mg.

Indications/Routes/Dosage

Enterobiasis: Children, adults: 100 mg PO as a single dose. *Other infestations:* Children, adults: 100 mg 2 bid for 3 days.

Adverse Reactions

GI transient abdominal pain. Carbamazepine and phenytoin can increase metabolism of mebendazole.

Implications

- Tablets may be chewed, swallowed, or crushed and mixed with food.
- Do not administer to children younger than 2 years or pregnant and lactating women.
- If patient is not cured in 3 weeks following treatment, retreatment is necessary.
- All family members should be treated at the same time.
- Discuss hygiene, transmission, and reinfection.

MONTELUKAST—ANTIASTHMATIC

Brand Name

Singulair

Uses

Prophylaxis and chronic treatment of asthma.

Availability

Tablets: 10 mg. Tablets, chewable: 4 mg, 5 mg. Oral granules: 4 mg.

Indications/Routes/Dosages

Children 1–5 years: one 4-mg tablet taken in the evening. 6–14 years: one 5-mg chewable tablet taken in the evening. Children older than 14, adults: 10 mg daily taken in the evening.

Adverse Effects

Headache, abdominal pain, fever, restlessness, irritability.

Implications

- Do not use to reverse bronchospasm as in an acute asthma attack.
- Increase fluid intake.
- Continue other asthma medications while taking this one.
- Chewable table contains phenylalanine.
- Patients sensitive to aspirin should avoid aspirin and NSAIDs while on this medication.

NITROFURANTOIN—ANTIBIOTIC

Brand Name

Furadantin, Macrobid, Macrodantin

Uses

Treat urinary tract infections caused by *Escherichia coli, Klebsiella, Pseudomonas, Proteus vulgaris, Staphylococcus aureus, Salmonella, Shigella.*

Availability

Suspension: 25 mg/5 mL. Tablets: 50 mg, 100 mg. Capsules: 25 mg, 50 mg, 100 mg.

Indications/Routes/Dosage

Active infections: Children 1 month old to 3 years: 5–7 mg/kg/day divided qid; 1–3 mg/kg/day for long-term treatment. Children older than 12 years, adult: 50–100 mg qid PO or 50–100 mg at bedtime for long-term treatment.

Chronic suppression: Children: 1 mg/kg/day every night. Adults: 50–100 mg every night.

Adverse Reactions

Dizziness, headache, nausea, vomiting, abdominal pain, diarrhea.

Implications

- Do not use in infants younger than 1 month old.
- Take with food or milk.
- Avoid alcohol.
- Drowsiness may occur; do not drive or operate machinery until response to drug is established.
- Do not crush tabs or open capsules.
- May turn urine rust-yellow to brown.

OFLOXACIN—FLUOROQUINOLONE ANTIINFECTIVE

Brand Name

Floxin Optic, Floxin Otic Drops, Ocuflox

Uses

Ophthalmic: Treat bacterial conjunctivitis, corneal ulcers. Otic: Treat otitis externa, acute/chronic otitis media.

Availability

Ophthalmic solution: 3 mg/mL. Otic solution: 0.3%.

Indications/Routes/Dosage

Bacterial conjunctivitis: 1–2 drops q2–4h for 2 days then 4 times/day for 5 days.

Corneal ulcers: Ophthalmic: 1–2 drops q30min while awake for 2 days, then q60min while awake for 5–7 days, then 4 times/day. Otic: twice daily.

Adverse Reactions

Allergic reaction.

Implications

Ophthalmic:
- Tilt patient's head back, place solution in conjunctival sac.
- Do not use ophthalmic solution for injection.

Otic:
- Eardrops should be at room temperature.
- Instruct patient to lie down with head turned so affected ear is upright.
- Pull the auricle down and posterior in children, pull up and posterior in older adolescents and adults.
- Instill toward canal wall.

OMEPRAZOLE — GASTRIC ACID PUMP INHIBITOR

Brand Name

Prilosec

Uses

Short-term treatment (4–8 weeks) and maintenance of erosive esophagitis, gastro-esophageal reflux disease (GERD), poorly responsive to other treatments. Unlabeled treatment of *Helicobacter pylori*–associated duodenal ulcer.

Availability

Tablets: 10 mg, 20 mg, 40 mg.

Indications/Routes/Dosage

Children older than 2 years: 20 mg/day, < 20 kg 10 mg/day.

Adverse Reactions

May increase concentration of oral anticonvulsants diazepam; phenytoin may increase serum glutamic oxaloacetic transaminase (SGOT), serum glutamic pyruvic transaminase (SGPT), alanine aminotransferase (ALT).

Implications

- Report headache to provider.
- Take before meals.
- Swallow capsule whole; do not crush or chew.

PAROXETINE HYDROCHLORIDE—SELECTIVE SEROTONIN REUPTAKE INHIBITOR, ANTIDEPRESSANT, ANTIPANIC, ANTIANXIETY

Brand Name

Paxil, Paxil CR

Uses

Treat major depressive disorder, obsessive-compulsive disorder (OCD), panic and generalized anxiety disorders.

Availability

Oral suspension: 10 mg/kg. Tablets: 10 mg, 20 mg, 30 mg, 40 mg. Tablets, controlled-release (CR): 12.5 mg, 25 mg, 37.5 mg.

Indications/Routes/Dosage

Children, adolescents: initial dose 5–10 mg, titrate up to 20 mg and monitor for side effects. Paxil CR: Children, adolescents: initial dose 12 mg titrate up to 25 mg.

Adverse Reactions

Nausea, headache, nervousness, insomnia, sedation, agitation, fatigue, dry mouth, constipation, diarrhea, decreased libido/sexual dysfunction.

Implications

- Dose changes should occur at 1-week intervals for both drugs.
- Do not use with MAO inhibitor.
- Use with cimetidine may increase concentrations.
- Use with phenytoin may decrease concentrations.
- Use with risperidone may increase paroxetine concentration enough to cause extrapyramidal symptoms.
- May cause dry mouth; avoid alcohol.
- Therapeutic effect may occur in 1–4 weeks.
- Do not abruptly discontinue medication.
- Avoid tasks that require alertness or motor skills until response to drug is established.
- Give with food or milk if GI symptoms.
- Educate parents about FDA concerns of suicide risk in patients on SSRI antidepressants, monitor suicidal risk closely during course of treatment especially in the first 30 days of treatment.

PENICILLIN V POTASSIUM—ANTIBIOTIC

Brand Name

Pen VK, V-cillin-K

Uses

Treatment of mild to moderate infections of respiratory tract, skin/skin structures, otitis media, prophylaxis for rheumatic fever, dental procedures.

Availability

Oral solution: 125 mg/5 mL, 250 mg/5 mL. Tablets: 125 mg, 250 mg, 500 mg.

Indications/Routes/Dosage

Children younger than 12 years: 25–50 mg/kg/day divided q6–8h. Max 3 g/day.
Children older than 12 years, adults: 125–500 mg q6–8h.

Rheumatic fever prophylaxis: Children, adults: 250 mg 2–3 times/day.

Adverse Reactions

Hypersensitivity reaction, colitis, fever, rash, pruritus.

Implications

- Question history of drug allergies.
- Continue antibiotic for full treatment.
- Notify provider of rash, sensitivity reaction.

PREDNISOLONE—ANTI-INFLAMMATORY

Brand Name

Pediapred, Prelone, Orapred

Uses

Treat reactive airway disease and asthma flare.

Availability

Syrup: 5 mg/5 mL, 15 mg/5 mL. Tablets: 5 mg.

Indications/Routes/Dosage

1–2 mg/kg/day in divided doses bid usually for 5 days, although longer may be required.

Adverse Reactions

Insomnia, heartburn, nervousness, abdominal distention, mood swings, increased sweating, and delayed healing. Long term: hypocalcemia, hypokalemia, muscle wasting especially the arms and legs, osteoporosis, spontaneous fractures, amenorrhea, cataracts, glaucoma, peptic ulcer disease.

Implications

- Notify healthcare provider of fever, sore throat, muscle aches, swelling, weight gain.
- Avoid alcohol, caffeine.
- Avoid exposure to chickenpox or measles.

RANTIDINE—ANTIULCER AGENT, GASTRIC ACID SECRETION INHIBITOR

Brand Name

Zantac

Uses

To prevent and treat gastric and duodenal ulcers.

Availability

Syrup 15 mg/5 mL; Tablets 75 mg, 150 mg, 300 mg; effervescent capsules 150 mg, 300 mg.

Indications/Routes/Dosage

GERD and ulcers: Children 1 month–16 years. 2–4 mg/kg bid; effervescent tabs 2.5–5 mg/kg bid; adults and adolescents 150 mg bid.

SERTRALINE—SEROTONIN SELECTIVE REUPTAKE INHIBITOR, ANTIDEPRESSANT, ANTIPANIC AGENT

Brand Name

Zoloft

Uses

Treat major depression, obsessive-compulsive disorder (OCD), post-traumatic stress disorder, panic disorder, PMDD.

Availability

Oral liquid: 20 mg/mL. Tablets: 25 mg, 50 mg, 100 mg.

Indications/Routes/Dosage

Anxiety: Children: starting dose of 25 mg/day increase to 50–100 mg/day; 50–200 mg/day for teens.

Major depression: Children: starting dose of 25 mg/day increase to 50–150 mg/day; 50–200 mg/day for teens.

Adverse Reactions

Headache, nausea, diarrhea, insomnia, drowsiness, fatigue, rash, dry mouth, anxiety, sexual dysfunction.

Implications

- Do not give within 14 days of MAO inhibitor.
- Therapeutic effect may take 2–3 weeks.
- Avoid tasks that require alertness, motor skills until response to drug is established.
- Take with food or milk, avoid alcohol.
- Weigh weekly: appetite may decrease.
- Notify provider if intending to become pregnant, are pregnant, or are breastfeeding.
- Do not use with St. John's wort, Sam-e.
- Avoid CNS depressants.
- Do not stop quickly, need to taper.
- Educate parents about FDA concerns of suicide risk in patients on SSRI antidepressants, monitor suicidal risk closely during course of treatment especially in the first 30 days of treatment.

SULFAMETHOXAZOLE/TRIMETHOPRIM—ANTI-INFECTIVE

Brand Name

Bactrim, Septra

Uses

Treat acute/complicated and recurrent urinary tract infections, *Shigella*, enteritis, otitis media, traveler's diarrhea, enteritis, *Pneumocystis carinii* pneumonia.

Availability

Oral suspension: 40 mg trimethoprim/200 mg, 400 mg sulfamethoxazole/5 mL. Tablets: 80 mg trimethoprim/400 mg sulfamethoxazole; 160 mg/800 mg.

Indications/Routes/Dosage

Urinary tract infection caused by *Escherichia coli, Klebsiella, Proteus mirabilis, Enterobacter*, enteritis, acute otitis media: Children older than 2 months: 7.5–8 mg/kg/day divided q12h for 10 days. Adults: 160 mg q12h for 7–14 days.

Weight: lbs, kg	Suspension	Tablets
22, 10	1 tsp (5 mL)	½
44, 20	2 tsp (10 mL)	1
66, 30	3 tsp (15 mL)	1½
88, 40	4 tsp (20 mL)	2 tablets or 1 DS tablet

Travelers' diarrhea, bronchitis: Adults: 1 double-strength tablet q12h for 5 days.

Adverse Reactions

Anorexia, nausea, vomiting urticaria, diarrhea, abdominal pain, rash, fever, sore throat, cough, shortness of breath.

Implications

- Take each dose with one glass water and increase fluid intake.
- Take for full treatment time as prescribed.
- Do not use in children younger than 2 months.
- Do not use in patients sensitive to sulfa drugs.

Note: all patients weighing > 100 pounds should be dosed according to adult dosage guidelines.

Abbreviations

AAP—American Academy of Pediatrics

ABG—arterial blood gas

ABO—blood types

ABR—auditory brainstem response

AC—air conduction

ACE—angiotensin converting enzyme

AD—atopic dermatitis

ADD—attention deficit disorder

ADH—antidiuretic hormone

ADHD—attention deficit hyperactivity disorder

ADL—activity of daily living

AFP—alpha fetal protein

ANA—antinuclear antibody

AOM—acute otitis media

AOME—acute otitis media with effusion

ASO—antistreptolysin enzyme

AVN—avascular necrosis

BAER—brainstem auditory-evoked response

BC—bone conduction

bid—twice daily

BM—bowel movement

BMI—body mass index

BP—blood pressure

BPM—beats per minute

BUN—blood urea nitrogen

CBC—complete blood count

CBT—cognitive behavioral therapy

CDC—Centers for Disease Control and Prevention

CF—cystic fibrosis

CHF—congestive heart failure

cm—centimeter

CMV—cytomegalovirus

CNS—central nervous system

CP—cerebral palsy

C/S—culture/sensitivity

CSF—cerebrospinal fluid

CT—computed tomography (X-ray exam)

CVA—costal-vertebral angle

CXR—chest X-ray

DDAVP—synthetic vasopressin (posterior pituitary hormone)

DDH—developmental dysplasia of the hip

DRSP—drug-resistant *Streptococcus pneumoniae*
DTaP—diphtheria-tetanus-acellular pertussis (vaccine)
DTP—diphtheria-tetanus-pertussis (vaccine)

EBV—Epstein-Barr virus
EC—emergency contraception
ECG—electrocardiogram (aka EKG)
ED—emergency department
EDC—estimated date of confinement
EEG—electroencephalogram
EENT—eye, ear, nose, throat
ENS—enteral nutritional support
ENT—ear, nose, throat
EOAE—evoked otoacoustic emissions
ESR—erythrocyte sedimentation rate
ETD—eustachian tube dysfunction
ETOH—alcohol

FEV—forced expiratory volume

g—gram
GABHS—Group A beta-hemolytic streptococcus
GD—gestational diabetes
GER—gastroesophageal reflux
GI—gastrointestinal
GU—genitourinary

h—hour
H. flu—*Haemophilus influenzae* b (bacteria)

HAB—hepatitis A virus
HBsAg—hepatitis B surface antigen
HBV—hepatitis B virus
HCG—human chorionic gonadotropin
Hct—hematocrit
HCV—hepatitis C virus
HDL—high-density lipoprotein
HEENT—head, eyes, ear, nose, throat
Hep—hepatitis
Hep B—hepatitis B vaccine
Hgb—hemoglobin
Hib—*Haemophilus influenzae* b (vaccine)
HIV—human immunodeficiency virus
HPV—human papillomavirus
HR—heart rate
HS—at bedtime
HSV—herpes simplex virus

IBD—inflammatory bowel disease
IBS—irritable bowel syndrome
ICP—intracranial pressure
Ig—immunoglobulin
IgC—immunoglobulin C
IgE—immunoglobulin E
IgM—immunoglobulin M
IM—intramuscular
I&O—intake and output
IPV—inactivated poliovirus vaccine
IV—intravenous

JRA—juvenile rheumatoid arthritis

kcal—kilocalorie

kg—kilogram

KOH—potassium chloride

KUB—kidneys, ureters bladder (X-ray examination)

lbs—pounds

LDLs—low-density lipoproteins

LES—lower esophageal sphincter

LFT(s)—liver function test(s)

LMP—last menstrual period

LOC—level of consciousness

LP—lumbar puncture

LRI—lower respiratory infection

LTB—laryngotracheobronchitis

LTBP—laryngotracheobroncho-pneumonia

MAO(I)—monoamine oxidase (inhibitor)

MCV—mean corpuscular volume

mg—milligram

min—minute

mL—milliliter

mm—millimeter

MMR—measles-mumps-rubella (vaccine)

MMWR—*Morbidity and Mortality Weekly Report* (www.cdc.gov)

mo(s)—month(s)

MRI—magnetic resonance imaging (X-ray examination)

NCHS—National Center for Health Statistics

NPO—nothing by mouth

NSAID—nonsteroidal antiinflammatory drug

N/V—nausea and vomiting

OD—right eye

OFC—occipital frontal circumference

OM—otitis media

O&P—ova and parasites

OS—left eye

OTC—over the counter

OU—both eyes

Pap—Papanicolaou

PCOS—polycystic ovary syndrome

PCV—Prevnar or pneumococcal vaccine

PID—pelvic inflammatory disease

PIH—pregnancy-induced hypertension

PMNs—polymorphonucleotides

PnC—pneumococcal conjugate

PO—by mouth

Postop—postoperative

PPD—purified protein derivative

PPI—proton pump inhibitors

Preop—preoperative

PRN—as required

PS—pyloric stenosis

PT—prothrombin time

PTT—partial thromboplastin time

PUD—peptic ulcer disease

q—every

qd—every day

qh—every hour

q2h—every 2 hours

q3h—every 3hours

q4h—every 4 hours

q6h—every 6 hours

q12h—every 12 hours

qid—four times daily

RAP—recurrent abdominal pain syndrome

RBC—red blood cell

Rh—blood group on surface of erythrocytes

R/O—rule out

ROM—range of motion

RSV—respiratory syncytial virus

SBE—subacute bacterial endocarditis

SD—standard deviation

SGOT—serum glutamic-oxaloacetic transaminase

SGPT—serum glutamic-pyruvic transaminase

SIADH—syndrome of inappropriate antidiuretic hormone

SIDS—sudden infant death syndrome

SMR—sexual maturity rating

SSRI—selective serotonin reuptake inhibitor

STI—sexually transmitted infection (aka STD – sexual transmitted disease)

TB—tuberculosis

TBSA—total body surface area

Tbsp—tablespoon

Td—tetanus toxoid

TD—tetanus and diphtheria vaccine

Temp—temperature

TIBC—total iron-binding capacity

tid—three times daily

TM—tympanic membrane

TMJ—temporomandibular joint dysfunction

TMP-SMX—trimethoprim-sulfamethoxazole

TSH—thyroid-simulating hormone

tsp—teaspoon

UA—urinalysis

UCG—urine chorionic gonadotropin (pregnancy test)

URI—upper respiratory infection

UTI—urinary tract infection

VBAC—vaginal birth after cesarean

VCUG—voiding cystourethrogram

WBC—white blood count

wk(s)—week(s)

WNL—within normal limits

wt—weight

yr(s)—year(s)

> — greater than

< — less than

≥ — greater than or equal to

≤ — less than or equal to

Index

Note: Italicized page locators indicate figures; tables are noted with *t*.

PMNs. *See* Polymorphonucleotides
Pneumococcal vaccine (PCV)
    acute otitis media and, 220
    seven-to-ten-year visit, 132
    six-year visit, 121
Pneumonia, 265, 286–294
    bacterial, 289
    clinical manifestations, 289–290
    diagnosis of, 291–292
    education, 293–294
    etiology, 287–288
    follow up, 293
    influenza and, 270
    occurrence, 288–289
    physical findings, 290–291
    secondary, pertussis and, 278
    treatment, 292–293
    viral, 288–289
Podolox, for genital warts, 406
Podophyllin
    for molluscum contagiosum, 178
    for viral warts, 179*t*
    for warts, 178
Podophyllin resin 1-25%, for genital warts, 406
Poison control information, 88
Poisoning, toddler safety and, 103
Poisonous plants, removing, 95
Polycystic ovarian syndrome, 435–436, 540
    amenorrhea and, 398
    diagnosis, 435–436
    etiology, occurrence, clinical manifestation, and
        physical findings, 435
    treatment, follow up, and complications, 436
Polyethylene glycol/PEG 3350, for constipation,
    339
Polymerase chain reaction
    encephalitis and, 482
    meningitis and, 479
    pertussis and, 276
Polymorphonucleotides, croup and, 261
Portion sizes, for toddlers, 98
Positive reinforcement, toddlers and, 102
Post-traumatic stress disorder
    clinical manifestations, 571–572
    etiology, 569
Postural proteinuria, 393
Posturing, of newborn, abnormal findings, 28
Potassium hydroxide, for molluscum contagiosum,
    178
Potty chairs
    choosing, 99
    two-year visit, 111
Pottying routine, for toddlers, 99
PPD # 1, six-year visit, 121
PPI. *See* Proton pump inhibitor
PPSV. *See* Pneumococcal vaccine
Prader-Willi syndrome, 540

Praise
    three-year visit, 117
    toddlers and, 102
Preadolescence, rapid change, emotional turbulence
    during, 141
Precocious puberty, evaluating
    in boys, 130
    in girls, 129
Precordial catch, 308
Pregnancy
    acute vomiting and, in postmenarchal girls, 371
    amenorrhea and, 398
    eleven-to-thirteen-year visit, 146
    fifth disease and, 179
    fourteen-to-eighteen-year visit, 160
    history, 26
Pregnancy-induced hypertension, 26
Pregnancy termination, fourteen-to-eighteen-year visit,
    155
Premarin cream, for female genitalia disorders, 383
Premature infants
    cryptorchidism in, 373
    inguinal hernia and, 352
    metatarsus adductus and, 464
    physical assessment of, 27
Prenatal care, 26
Prenatal history, initial history, 4
Preschool-age children, elements of interval history, 11.
    See also Three–year visit (preschool)
Prescriptions, initial history, 5
Preseptal cellulitis (periorbital cellulitis), 201–203
Prevacid
    for GERD, 351
    for *H. pylori* infection, 364
Prevnar, acute otitis media and, 220
PRICE (protect, rest, ice, compression, elevation), for
    sprain, strain, overuse, 440
Prilosec, for GERD, 351
Primary amenorrhea, 397
Primary dysmenorrhea, 401
Primary peptic ulcer disease, etiology, 362
Processus vaginalis, hydrocele and, 375
Prolactin, lactation and, 35, *36*
Promethazine
    for migraine headaches, 496
    for treating headaches in children, 499
Propionibacterium acnes, 165, 167
Propranolol
    hyperthyoidism and, 417
    for migraine headaches, 495
    for treating headaches in children, 498
Propylthiouracil, hyperthyroidsm and, 417
Protective enclosures, around water sites, 84, 88, 94
Protein requirements, two-year visit, 109
Proteinuria, 392–395
    complications and education, 395
    diagnosis, treatment and follow up, 394

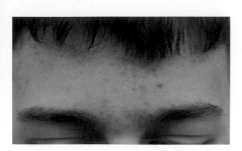

Figure 1 Acne vulgaris of the forehead. © F.C.G./Fotolia.com

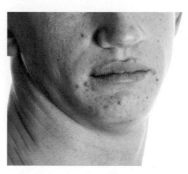

Figure 2 Acne vulgaris of the lower face. © Olga Sapegina/Fotolia.com

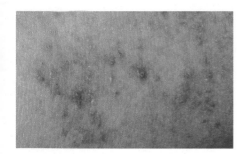

Figure 3 Atopic dermatitis. Minute excoriations with lichenification in the antecubital fossa seen. © iStockphoto/Thinkstock

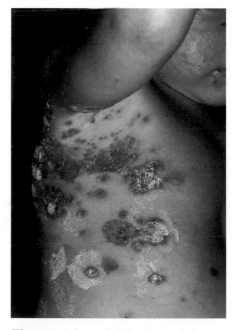

Figure 4 Impetiginized atopic dermatisis. © Dr. P. Marazzi/Photo Researchers, Inc.

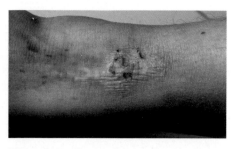

Figure 5 Flexural involvement of popliteal fossa in atopic dermatisis. © Jingling Water/Fotolia.com

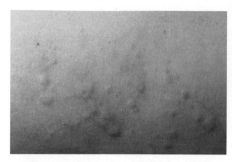

Figure 6 Urticaria. © Rob Byron/ ShutterStock, Inc.

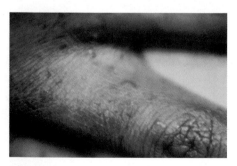

Figure 7 Scabies. Courtesy of CDC

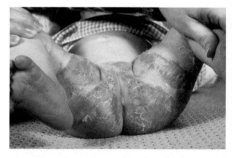

Figure 8 Irritant diaper dermatitis. © Biophoto Associates/Photo Researchers, Inc.

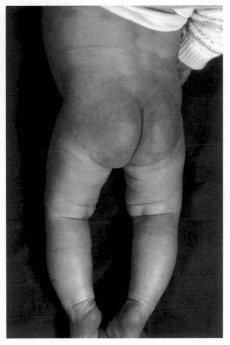

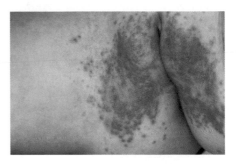

Figure 10 Candidiasis in the diaper area. A positive culture for Candida can be obtained from satellite pustules. © Dr. P. Marazzi/Photo Researchers, Inc.

Figure 9 Chafing type of diaper dermatitis. © Medical-on-Line/Alamy

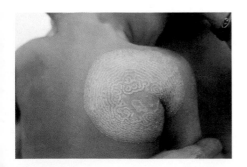

Figure 11 Inflammatory superficial fungal infection. Courtesy of K. Mae Lennon/CDC

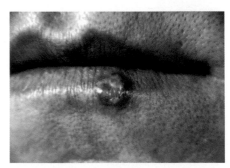

Figure 12 Recurrent herpes simplex. Courtesy of Dr. Hermann/CDC

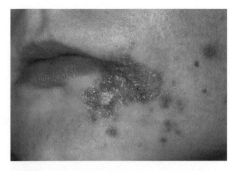

Figure 13 Impetigo. Spread of infection to top of nose from beneath the nose in an infant with impetigo. © Dr. P. Marazzi/Photo Researchers, Inc.

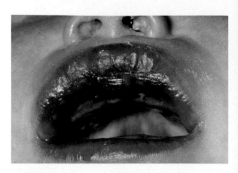

Figure 14 Infant with primary herpes gingivostomatitis. © Dr. P. Marazzi/Photo Researchers, Inc.

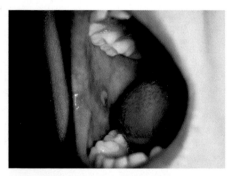

Figure 15 Erosion of the tongue in a child with hand-foot-and-mouth syndrome. © Dr. P. Marazzi/Photo Researchers, Inc.

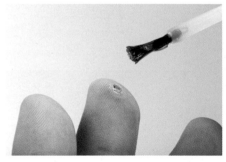

Figure 16 Common warts on child's finger. © leschnyhan/Fotolia.com

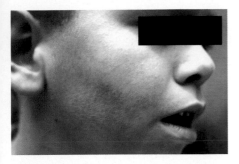

Figure 17 Slapped-cheek appearance of a child with parvovirus B19 infection (erythema infectiosum). Courtesy of CDC

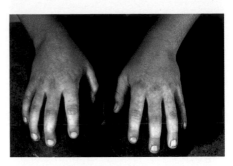

Figure 18 Lacy pink eruption over the palms in erythema infectiosum. Courtesy of CDC

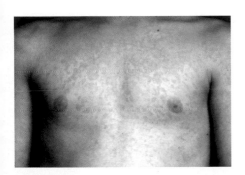

Figure 19 Lacy pink eruption of erythema infectiosum on chest and upper abdomen. Courtesy of Dr. Gary P. Williams, M. D.

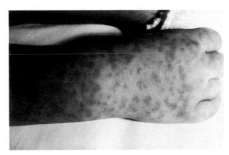

Figure 20 CDC-1962. RMSF, acral dusky oval purpuric lesions. Courtesy of CDC

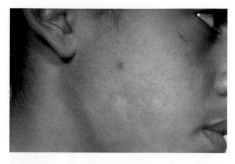

Figure 21 Pityriasis alba. In some atopic patients, subtle inflammation may result in poorly demarcated areas of hypopigmentation, known as pityriasis alba. Lesions are most prominent in darkly pigmented individuals. © Medical-on-Line/Alamy

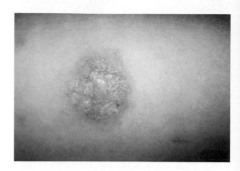

Figure 22 Pityriasis rosea. The large herald patch on the chest of this 10-year old girl shows central clearing, which mimics tinea corporis. Courtesy of Dr. Sellars/CDC

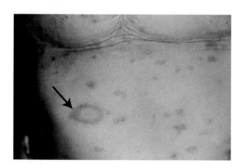

Figure 23 Pityriasis rosea. Numerous oval lesions on the chest of a Caucasian teenager. Courtesy of CDC

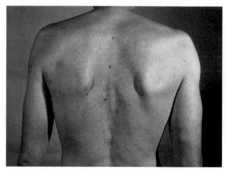

Figure 24 Tinea versicolor. The well-demarcated, scaly papules appear darker than surrounding skin on the back of a Caucasian adolescent. Courtesy of Dr. Lucille K. Georg/CDC

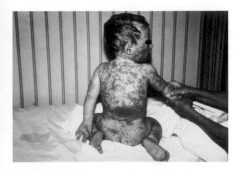

Figure 25 Roseaola/exanthema subitum. A generalized, pink, maculopapular rash suddenly appeared on this infant after 3 days of high fever. Courtesy of Arthur E. Kaye/CDC

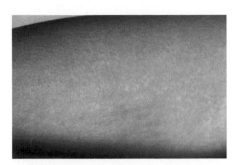

Figure 26 Scarlet fever. A generalized, bright red, sandpaper-like papular rash developed in a 7-year-old boy with a streptococcal pharyngitis. Courtesy of CDC

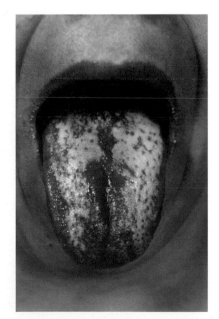

Figure 27 Scartlet fever. A white strawberry tongue precedes red-strawberry tongue. Courtesy of Jere J. Mammino, DO, FAOCD

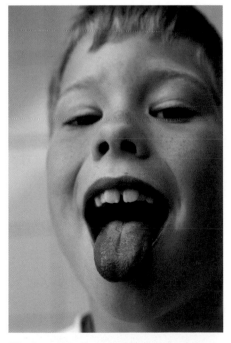

Figure 28 Scarlett fever. A red-strawberry tongue as the erythrotoxin-mediated enanthema evolves. © imagebroker/Alamy Images

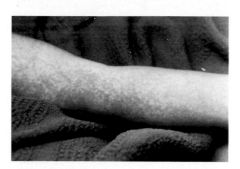

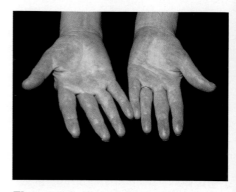

Figure 29 Kawasaki syndrome. A generalized, morbilliform, erythema multiforme-like rash is a characteristic clinical finding. Courtesy of CDC

Figure 30 Kawasaki syndrome. Palmar and plantar erythema with edema of the hands and feet is a characteristic clinical finding. © Ralph Hutchings/Visuals Unlimited, Inc.

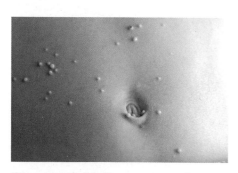

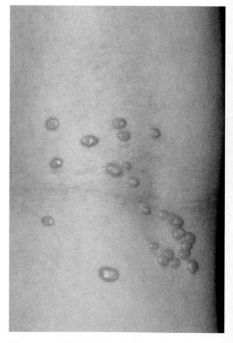

Figure 31 Mollesum contagiosum. Individual lesions are 2- to 5- mm, flesh colored, dome-shaped umbilicated paules. © Jarrod Erbe/ShutterStock, Inc.

Figure 32 Molluscum contagiosum spreads rapidly in eczematous skin. This patient has atopic dermatitis of the popliteal fossa. © Dr. P. Marazzi/Photo Researchers, Inc.